Y. Victoria Zhang • Uttam Garg
Editors

Practical Guide to Implementing Liquid Chromatography Mass Spectrometry in Clinical Laboratories

Springer

Editors
Y. Victoria Zhang
Pathology and Laboratory Medicine
University of Rochester Medical Center
Rochester, NY, USA

Uttam Garg
Pathology and Laboratory Medicine
Children's Mercy Hospital and University of Missouri-Kansas City School of Medicine
Kansas City, MO, USA

ISBN 978-3-032-03851-7 ISBN 978-3-032-03852-4 (eBook)
https://doi.org/10.1007/978-3-032-03852-4

This Springer imprint is published by the registered company Springer Nature Switzerland AG
The registered company address is: Gewerbestrasse 11, 6330 Cham, Switzerland

Preface

Mass spectrometry coupled with liquid chromatography has long been a cornerstone of research laboratories, but its migration into the clinical setting marks one of the most transformative shifts in modern laboratory medicine. The ability of liquid chromatography–tandem mass spectrometry (LC-MS/MS) to provide highly specific, sensitive, and multiplexed analyses has opened new frontiers in diagnostics—from therapeutic drug monitoring to endocrinology, toxicology, and beyond. Yet for many clinical laboratories, the transition from theoretical interest to practical implementation remains challenging.

This book was designed to bridge that gap.

Practical Guide to Implementing Liquid Chromatography Mass Spectrometry in Clinical Laboratories was developed to provide a clear and structured roadmap for laboratories looking to implement or expand LC-MS/MS technologies. Whether you are a medical technologist building your first assay, a pathologist overseeing validation, or a laboratory director shaping long-term strategy, this guide aims to offer relevant and practical insights at every step.

The chapters walk through foundational principles, instrumentation considerations, method development and validation, sample preparation, troubleshooting, quality assurance, regulatory expectations, and real-world clinical applications. A dedicated chapter at the end of the book includes multiple-choice questions based on each chapter, designed to reinforce key concepts and support teaching, training, and self-assessment.

The authors have drawn from their collective experience across academic medical centers, hospital systems, and reference laboratories. We hope the lessons, tools, and practical advice shared in these pages empower laboratory professionals to embrace mass spectrometry with confidence and purpose.

Above all, we hope this book serves not only as a technical manual but also as a catalyst to inspire laboratories to advance diagnostic science and improve patient care through thoughtful, rigorous implementation of liquid chromatography mass spectrometry in clinical laboratories.

Rochester, NY, USA — Y. Victoria Zhang
Kansas City, MO, USA — Uttam Garg

Contents

Introduction to Implementation of LC-MS/MS in Clinical Laboratory

1

Uttam Garg, Alan L. Rockwood, David Herold, and Y. Victoria Zhang

Brief History of Liquid Chromatography and Mass Spectrometry

Liquid chromatography (LC) and mass spectrometry (MS) have become indispensable analytical techniques across various scientific disciplines, including pharmaceutical development, proteomics, environmental analysis, and clinical diagnostics. The integration of LC and MS has revolutionized modern analytical workflows, enabling highly sensitive and specific detection of complex biological and chemical samples, particularly for clinical applications.

The origins of LC date back to 1903, when Mikhail Tswett introduced adsorption chromatography to separate plant pigments [1]. Over the following decades, key advancements—including partition chromatography, paper chromatography, and

U. Garg
Pathology and Laboratory Medicine, Children's Mercy Hospital and University of Missouri-Kansas City School of Medicine, Kansas City, MO, USA
e-mail: ugarg@cmh.edu

A. L. Rockwood
Emeritus Professor (Clinical) of Pathology, University of Utah School of Medicine, Salt Lake City, UT, USA
e-mail: alan@rockwood-scientific-consulting.com

D. Herold
Department of Pathology, University of California, San Diego, CA, USA

VA Healthcare System, San Diego, CA, USA
e-mail: dherold@ucsd.edu

Y. V. Zhang (✉)
Department of Pathology and Laboratory Medicine, University of Rochester Medical Center, Rochester, NY, USA
e-mail: Victoria_Zhang@URMC.Rochester.edu

Y. V. Zhang, U. Garg (eds.), *Practical Guide to Implementing Liquid Chromatography Mass Spectrometry in Clinical Laboratories*,
https://doi.org/10.1007/978-3-032-03852-4_1

gel permeation chromatography—laid the foundation for modern liquid-phase separations [2, 3]. A major breakthrough occurred in the 1960s, and Csaba Horváth and Seymour Lipsky developed high-performance liquid chromatography (HPLC) [4]. Subsequent innovations, including reverse-phase HPLC (RP-HPLC) in the 1970s, capillary LC in the 1980s, and ultra-high-performance liquid chromatography (UHPLC) in the 1990s, further enhanced the technique's capabilities [5–9].

In parallel, MS has undergone significant technological advancements since its inception by J. J. Thomson in 1912, when he first demonstrated the separation of charged particles based on their mass-to-charge ratio (m/z) [10, 11]. FW Aston improved the resolution of mass spectrometry for isotopic analysis and he was awarded the 1922 Nobel Prize in Chemistry [10, 12, 13]. The mid-twentieth century saw major breakthroughs that improved mass resolution and separation capabilities, including the development of time-of-flight (TOF) MS, quadrupole mass analyzers, and ion trapping techniques [14–19]. These innovations, particularly the triple quadrupole analyzer, became essential for clinical diagnostics.

The development of new ionization methods expanded MS applications in biological analysis. Soft ionization techniques introduced in the 1980s and 1990s were of particular significance. Electrospray ionization (ESI), developed by John Fenn, and matrix-assisted laser desorption/ionization (MALDI), developed by Koichi Tanaka, Franz Hillenkamp, and Michael Karas, enabled the analysis of large biomolecules, revolutionizing proteomics, metabolomics, and clinical diagnostics [20–25]. Fenn and Tanaka were awarded the 2002 Nobel Prize in Chemistry for their contributions. The continuous advancement of tandem mass spectrometry (MS/MS), ion trap technologies, and high-resolution MS analyzers has further solidified MS as a cornerstone of modern analytical science.

One of the earlier clinical applications of MS was newborn errors of metabolism screening from dried blood spots [26, 27]. By quantifying amino acids, organic acids, and acylcarnitines, the MS platform allowed for the diagnosis of inherited metabolic disorders of amino acids, organic acids, and fatty acid oxidation disorders such as phenylketonuria (PKU), maple syrup urine disease (MSUD), propionic acidemia, and medium-chain acyl-CoA dehydrogenase (MCAD) deficiency. Early detection of inherited metabolic disorders enabled prompt medical intervention, improving patient outcomes.

By the late twentieth century, LC was successfully coupled with MS, combining the separation power of chromatography with the high sensitivity and specificity of mass spectrometry [28, 29]. This integration has transformed forensic science, environmental analysis, and clinical diagnostics, enabling unprecedented analytical performance.

Applications of LC-MS/MS in Clinical Diagnostics

The adoption of LC-tandem mass spectrometry (LC-MS/MS) in clinical laboratories has significantly enhanced diagnostic capabilities by providing accurate, precise, and highly specific measurements of a wide range of analytes for clinical diagnostics, toxicology, and therapeutic drug monitoring purposes.

LC-MS/MS has revolutionized drug of abuse testing by offering high sensitivity and specificity confirmatory testing for detecting a broad range of illicit and prescription drugs that traditional immunoassays were not able to. Its high specificity has established LC-MS/MS as the gold standard for forensic and clinical toxicology testing. It is widely used for detecting opioids, cannabinoids, amphetamines, benzodiazepines, and other substances in various biological matrices such as urine, blood, oral fluid, and meconium [30–34].

Another major clinical application is therapeutic drug monitoring (TDM), where LC-MS/MS is used to measure drug concentrations in patient samples to ensure optimal drug dosing and prevent toxicity [35–37]. Some examples include immunosuppressant drugs, antiepileptics, and certain antibiotics.

In endocrinology, LC-MS/MS has become the preferred method for measuring steroid hormones again due to its high specificity to be able to distinguish structurally similar steroids [38–40]. Some examples include cortisol, testosterone, 17-hydroxyprogesterone, estradiol, and other steroid hormones and particularly in patient populations that have lower concentrations than the traditional immunoassay detection limit.

The evolution of LC-MS/MS has enabled both targeted and non-targeted analysis of complex body fluid samples. The technique continues to expand its role in clinical diagnostics, providing reliable solutions for a broad range of medical conditions.

Developing LC-MS/MS assays for clinical use requires extensive time and collaboration among scientists. We use the testosterone assay as an example to illustrate the evolution of analytical methods over time.

Historically, testosterone measurement relied on immunoassays, which were prone to interference, especially at low concentrations. Advancing alternative technologies became necessary to ensure accurate and precise testosterone measurements, minimizing interferences that could significantly impact validity testing in women and children.

In 1970, Siekmann et al. [41] reported a mass fragmentographic determination and quantification of testosterone without an internal standard. Chapman [42] later commented that it is advisable to use an internal standard that can be tracked in mass fragmentographic recordings. In 1974, Dehennin et al. [43] introduced a GC method using 4-methyl-19-nortestosterone as an internal standard, which completely separated from testosterone. Chapman [42] later noted that this approach might be disadvantageous since the ions from the two compounds are not detected simultaneously. That same year, Chapman and Bailey [42] reported a method for analyzing testosterone in male plasma spiked with a deuterium-labeled internal standard. While the method was precise and accurate at higher concentrations, it lacked reliability at lower concentrations due to the internal standard's impurity, limiting its usefulness for women and children.

In 1975, Björkhem et al. [44] developed a method using radioactive testosterone as an internal standard. The assay involved multiple steps, including ether extraction, thin-layer chromatography purification, further extraction with methanol, and derivatization. The amounts of unlabeled and labeled testosterone were analyzed at m/z 432 and 434, respectively. The method demonstrated a standard deviation of approximately 2.7% with a strong correlation ($r = 0.83$) to a radioimmunoassay. However, Björkhem noted that, as expected, the mass spectrometry method yielded significantly lower values than the radioimmunoassay, likely due to cross-reactivity with dihydrotestosterone and possibly other compounds. In 1979, Siekmann [45] reported a refined workflow utilizing ^{14}C-labeled testosterone as an internal standard. After several preparation steps, the assay used m/z 680 relative to m/z 682 to monitor the unlabeled and ^{14}C-labeled testosterone. The reported lower limit of detection was 10.4 nmol/L (300 ng/dL), with a precision of 1% based on two analyses.

In 1981, Finlay and Gaskell [46] presented a highly specific GC–MS method using [^{2}H] testosterone and unlabeled 17-epitestosterone as internal standards, along with multiple sample preparation and derivatization steps. Their findings indicated that routine immunoassays often overestimate testosterone concentrations, as demonstrated by consistently higher mean values compared to GC–MS results. Despite the strong correlation between the methods ($r = 0.997$), the discrepancy suggested potential immune-cross-reactivity issues. This work highlighted the sensitivity and specificity advantages of GC–MS as a reference method for evaluating the performance of routine steroid hormone assays. However, the method was not adopted for clinical laboratory use due to the high cost and complexity of the instrumentation. Additionally, it was limited to male subjects and required 10 mL of serum due to sensitivity constraints.

Subsequent methods improved sensitivity through deuterated labeling. Salerno et al. [47] reported a method with a limit of quantification (LOQ) of 1 ng/dL and an intra-assay precision of 7.4% (n = 5). Furuta et al. [48] and Legrand et al. [49] demonstrated good accuracy at higher concentrations, but broad-range quantification across clinically relevant levels remained a challenge.

In 1996, Fitzgerald and Herold [50] developed an electron capture negative chemical ionization GC-MS procedure involving liquid–liquid extraction of serum samples and the synthesis of a pentafluorobenzyloxime/silyl ether derivative of testosterone, which exhibited excellent chromatographic and electron-capturing properties. This assay successfully quantified serum testosterone in the clinically relevant range of 0.69–69.3 nmol/L (20–2000 ng/dL).

This publication sparked discussions and debates regarding the cost-effectiveness of mass spectrometry compared to the accuracy of radioimmunoassay [51–55]. These questions were resolved when commercially available immunoassays were shown to produce inconsistent and often unreliable results, particularly at the low testosterone concentrations observed in women and children. In a comprehensive evaluation by Taieb et al. [56] ten different testosterone immunoassays were compared with ID-GC/MS. The findings revealed that seven of the ten immunoassays overestimated testosterone levels in women, while most immunoassays underestimated these levels in men. These discrepancies highlight the limitations of traditional immunoassays, which do not always ensure the accuracy required for proper diagnostic and therapeutic decisions.

Taieb et al.'s report led to an editorial by Herold and Fitzgerald [57], who critiqued the efficacy of testosterone immunoassays for female patients. Citing Taieb et al.'s study, they argued that the measured values were frequently inaccurate, with deviations so substantial that they were rendered practically meaningless. Their analysis suggested that estimating testosterone levels would be nearly as accurate and significantly more cost-effective. They expressed concerns about the implications for epidemiologic research and advocated for the adoption of mass spectrometry techniques, which have demonstrated superior accuracy in measuring low-abundance steroids in clinical specimens from women.

The ongoing debate over the reliability of testosterone assays underscores the need to select appropriate and validated methods for both clinical and research applications. The future of testosterone measurement lies in the continued advancement and validation of mass spectrometry as a reference method, ensuring precise and reliable data across diverse patient populations.

Analytes Measured by LC-MS/MS

Mass spectrometry is a versatile analytical technique that can be used to measure a wide variety of analytes. Analytes that are measured by MS are typically categorized into two broad groups: small molecules and larger molecules.

Based on clinical utility, small molecules analyzed by mass spectrometry fall into two broad categories: exogenous and endogenous compounds. Exogenous compounds include therapeutic drugs and their metabolites, drugs of abuse, environmental toxins such as pesticides and volatile compounds. Small endogenous compounds include certain hormones, amino acids, organic acids, fatty acids, vitamins and cofactors, neurotransmitters, and bile acids. Commonly measured small molecules in a clinical laboratory are listed in Tables 1.1 and 1.2.

Similarly, large molecules analyzed by mass spectrometry can be divided into two broad categories: exogenous and endogenous compounds. Exogenous large molecules typically include therapeutic agents such as antibodies and peptide hormones. Endogenous compounds include peptide hormones, tumor markers, and other proteins. Commonly measured large molecules in a clinical laboratory are listed in Table 1.3.

Considerations for Implementing LC-MS/MS

The application of LC-tandem mass spectrometry (LC-MS/MS) is rightly hailed as a great advance for laboratory medicine. However, no analytical technique is perfect, and this also applies to diagnostic analyses that are used for patient care. This is because not only are there difficulties, uncertainties, and limitations on the analytical side, but the interpretation of analytical results can sometimes be compounded by uncertainties in how the analytical results are to be interpreted for

Table 1.1 Examples of exogenous small molecules measured by MS

Category	Examples
Therapeutic drugs	
Antibacterial	Sulfonamides, Trimethoprim
Anticoagulants	Dabigatran, Rivaroxaban, Apixaban, Warfarin
Anticonvulsants	Lamotrigine, Levetiracetam, 10-Hydroxycarbazepine, Topiramate, Zonisamide
Antidepressants	Tricyclics and Selective Serotonin Reuptake Inhibitors
Antifungals	Fluconazole, Ketoconazole, Voriconazole
Antihypertensives	Atenolol, Clonidine, Diltiazem, Labetalol, Verapamil
Antineoplastic drugs	Busulfan, Mercaptopurine and Metabolites, Methotrexate
Antipsychotics	Haloperidol, Fluphenazine, Perphenazine, Thiothixene
Antiviral	Acyclovir, Ganciclovir
Cardiac drugs	Flecainide, Mexiletine, Propafenone, Amiodarone
Immunosuppressants	Cyclosporine, Everolimus, Mycophenolic Acid, Sirolimus, Tacrolimus
Drugs of abuse	
Cannabinoids	Natural and Synthetic Cannabinoids such as K2, K3, JWH-018, JWH-073
Opioids	Natural and Synthetic Opioids such as Fentanyl, Acetylfentanyl, Carfentanil, Furanylfentanyl, U-47700, Nitazenes
Sedatives and hypnotics	Barbiturates and Benzodiazepines including Synthetics such as Etizolam, Flubromazolam, Diclazepam
Stimulants	Amphetamines (including synthetic such as MDMA), Cathinones (Methylenedioxypyrovalerone, Mephedrone, Methylone), Cocaine and Metabolites, NBOMe compounds

Table 1.2 Examples of endogenous small molecules measured by MS

Category	Examples
Acylcarnitines	Short, Medium and Long-Chain acylcarnitine
Amino Acids	Tyrosine, Glycine, Cystine, Phenylalanine, Homocystine, Leucine, Isoleucine, Valine, Methionine, Citrulline, Argininosuccinic Acid
Bile Acids	Cholic Acid, Chenodeoxycholic Acid, 7-Hydroxy-4-cholesten-3-one
Hormones	Testosterone, Aldosterone, 17-Hydroxyprogesterone, Androstenedione, Dehydroepiandrosterone, T4, T3
Neurotransmitters	Serotonin, Homovanillic acid, Methyl-Dopa
Organic Acids	Methylmalonic acid, Propionic Acid, Isovaleric Acid, Glutaric Acid
Vitamins and Cofactors	Vitamin D, Cobalamin (B12), Folate, Biotin, B6, Biopterin
Other	Creatine, Guanidinoacetate, Purines, Pyrimidines

patient care. There are numerous considerations to properly implement the platform in a clinical setting to serve patient needs.

From a technical viewpoint, the biggest advantage of LC-MS/MS is the very high degree of analytical specificity. Such high specificity can sometimes be a double-edged sword. For example, it may happen that two related compounds may be diagnostically relevant, but one may be detected in an MS-based assay while the

Table 1.3 Examples of large molecules measured by MS

Category	Examples
Hormones	Insulin, Parathyroid hormone (PTH)
Endogenous Proteins	Thyroglobulin, Hormone-Binding Globulin (SHBG), PTH-like protein, C-peptide, Albumin, Antibodies
Exogenous Proteins	Therapeutic antibodies, Insulin analogues, Vaccines, Bacterial Proteins, Viral Proteins

other may not because of the high analytical specificity of an LC-MS/MS method. This needs to be seriously considered during the assay development phase. A close interaction is required during the method development stage between the person on the diagnostic side of the method and the laboratory professional on the analytical side of the method.

25-OH Vitamin D assay is a great example where 25-OH Vitamin D_2 and 25-OH Vitamin D_3 are clinically important compounds and both should be measured. The way around this issue in the case of vitamin D is to design an LC-MS/MS method to measure the concentration of both analytes. This is technically fairly straightforward, as these compounds can be easily separated by LC. As with any human interaction, there is a possibility of miscommunication, and this could lead to the development of an inappropriate assay.

This issue of inadvertently missing a diagnostically relevant target may be more serious when one enters the realm of protein and peptide analysis (hereafter simply referred to as peptide analysis) because one must consider how to deal with both known and unknown peptide variants.

A successful LC-MS/MS method must target the "correct" *m/z* for the precursor ion. However, if a patient has a peptide sequence variant then the sequence variant is very likely to have a different mass, in which case the peptide is unlikely to be detected, possibly leading to an incorrect analysis and faulty interpretation of the patient's condition (unless the LC/MS–MS method is specifically designed to include the variant(s)).

This is complicated by the fact that a peptide is normally coded by two DNA strands, and unless a mutation occurs on both strands, then at least one of the peptides will have the expected mass, in which case one might expect the measured concentration to be approximately half of the total (normal plus variant) concentration.

A further complication depends on whether the variant form is biologically active or not. In addition, by the fact that not all sequence variants are necessarily known, if an unknown variant occurs, it is likely to be missed altogether. If the variant is from a form that is also active, then detecting only half of the peptide (or protein) may lead to an interpretation that the concentration is outside of the reference interval for the analyte, possibly leading to a faulty medical interpretation.

Another consideration is to avoid over-enthusiastic advocates of mass spectrometry, as there can be a temptation to unfairly denigrate more traditional methods used in the clinical chemistry lab, such as immunoassays. This consideration will ensure the labs to take best advantage of mass spectrometry and other analytical platforms for patient needs.

Testosterone is a case in point. LC-MS/MS has become a preferred method for the analysis of testosterone in patients who have low levels of testosterone in the blood, especially women and children. This application was to overcome the limitation of immunoassay at low concentrations for accurate results. However, an immunoassay is perfectly fine for patients such as male patients with high testosterone levels.

Another consideration of implementing mass spectrometry relates to cost. Mass spectrometry is often considered as a low-cost approach for day-to-day sample analysis due to its generic and low-cost consumables. However, the initial instrument capital cost is significant and so is the staffing requirements to develop the assay in assay and to operate the platform.

This points to a good strategy on how to use mass spectrometry in the clinical lab, which is to apply MS to problems that either have no other well-established solution or for which mass spectrometry provides a much better solution than other methods. For example, an important early driver for the adoption of mass spectrometry was the immunosuppressant drug sirolimus. When it was approved for patient use, there was no FDA approved method for this drug, so laboratories looked for other technologies to use as a basis for a laboratory-developed test. LC-MS/MS turned out to be very well suited for this task, and this in turn led to the application of MS for other immunosuppressant drugs, such as tacrolimus and others. Often, these analytes were combined into a single LC-MS/MS method, which in some ways can simplify the logistics of dealing with this class of drugs.

The "care and feeding" of mass spectrometers is also a challenge that needs to be considered. In particular, a good maintenance and servicing system is essential for a smooth-running lab, and because these instruments are generally not supplied by traditional vendors of clinical laboratory equipment, the laboratory will not be able to rely on those sources of maintenance and service. They will either have to depend on mass spectrometry vendors for those services, or third-party support, or they will need to develop those skills in-house, which usually means staff persons who are dedicated to those tasks rather than being directly involved in the day-to-day testing of patient samples. There is another issue that needs to be considered, and that is that mass spectrometers are inherently serial devices. Multiplexing technologies have made significant progress in the past decade, though the overall throughput is still limited.

In general, though a very powerful platform, implementing LC-MS/MS in the clinical laboratories has numerous considerations. A great deal of expertise and experience are needed to take the full advantage of LC-MS/MS to best serve clinical and patient needs. To advance the use of mass spectrometry in clinical diagnostics, several programs and organizations have emerged in the past couple of decades. In this regard, the 2007 Asilomar conference played a key role in the establishment of the Association for Mass Spectrometry & Advances in the Clinical Lab (MSACL) in 2009. Later, in 2013, the Association for Diagnostics & Laboratory Medicine (ADLM) created the mass spectrometry and separation sciences (MSSS) division.

These groups have collaborated to promote the applications of mass spectrometry platforms in clinical diagnostics for the betterment of patient care.

Looking to the Future

We can expect to see a greater degree of automation for methods that are LDTs. It also applies to a new class of products on the horizon, dedicated automated clinical mass spectrometers that operate much like automated analyzers typically found in core labs, except samples are prepared in a manner compatible with mass spectrometry, and mass spectrometers are used as detection devices [58–61]. It is to be anticipated that such instruments, and the methods targeted by those instruments, will go through FDA approval at the vendor level.

We can expect to see an expanded role for mass spectrometry in the analysis of biopolymers, particularly proteins and peptides. In the earliest stages, we can expect the analytical targets to be analytes that are well established, for which mass spectrometers provide an alternative means of analysis. This process has already started with mass spectrometry taking the place of immunoassays, either in part or in whole, for analytes such as thyroglobulin.

In other cases, proof-of-principle studies have been done using mass spectrometry to replace other means of analysis, an example being analysis of hemoglobinopathies and A1c. Although these capabilities have been shown in proof of principle R&D studies, widespread uptake is yet to occur.

In the more distant future, we may see newly discovered analytical targets that are brought into clinical practice using mass spectrometry analysis. Discoveries in "omics" fields (proteomics, metabolomics, lipidomics, etc.) come to mind. Interestingly, discovery studies in proteomics and metabolomics often make heavy use of mass spectrometry. So far, "omics" has had very little impact on diagnostics used for patient care because few, if any, omics-based discoveries have actually made their way into clinical diagnostic laboratories, but one can expect this to change in the future.

DNA/RNA are wild cards with more uncertain futures when it comes to the use of mass spectrometry for routine clinical analysis because it is hard to identify how mass spectrometry brings essential capabilities to the table that are not already met by other technologies, but only the future will tell.

Triple quadrupole mass spectrometry has so far dominated in the use of mass spectrometers for clinical applications. However, several other technologies provide advantages that may be useful in certain cases. Without going into details, a few examples include time-of-flight mass spectrometers (TOF), high-resolution mass spectrometry, quadrupole time-of-flight mass spectrometers, Fourier transform ion cyclotron resonance mass spectrometers, and Orbitrap mass spectrometers. These technologies may include advantages in higher throughput, multi-analyte analysis, higher resolution, or higher mass accuracy, depending on what technology is under consideration.

Point-of-care mass spectrometry may also have a future, and particularly as miniaturized mass spectrometers are being developed at several laboratories. These have the potential to be placed closer to the patient rather than at more distant centralized laboratories. An obvious application would be to use mass spectrometry for emergency toxicology, where time is often of the essence for receiving the analysis. Some work in this area has already been done. Looking even further into the future, one might envision the small bedside mass spectrometer in hospitals. Driving the field toward on-site mass spectrometers is not just miniaturization of the MS analyzers but also the development of new (so-called ambient) ion sources such as DESI and paper spray.

Imaging by mass spectrometry is rapidly developing at the R&D level. A potential advantage here is that the image can be specific for single analytes or specific to classes of analytes, and if the image is acquired in full mass spectrum mode the images at each *m/z* provides complementary chemical information in the images. One can think about this as being analogous to images acquired by histopathological staining methods, except that the MS-based imaging is potentially far more information-rich.

Overall, there are many potential exciting applications of mass spectrometry in clinical diagnostics. Taking advantage of these opportunities and implementing mass spectrometry are not necessarily straightforward. This book provides practical guidance to help more laboratories adopt this technology.

Overview of the Book Design

This book provides a comprehensive and practical guide to implementing liquid chromatography–mass spectrometry (LC-MS/MS) in clinical laboratories. It is designed for laboratory professionals, clinical chemists, and researchers who are either currently using or planning to adopt mass spectrometry for clinical applications.

The book begins with an introduction that offers essential background on mass spectrometry, including a brief history of the technology, its advantages in clinical laboratories, and the types of analytes it can measure. This section also addresses common challenges and limitations associated with LC-MS/MS implementation.

The core content of the book starts with *Fundamentals of Mass Spectrometry*, covering key principles such as ionization techniques, mass analyzers, and detectors. This chapter provides best practices for utilizing mass spectrometry to generate accurate and reliable patient results. Following this, the *Fundamentals of Liquid Chromatography* chapter introduces the principles and components of liquid chromatography, explaining how it supports mass spectrometry analysis.

A critical step in LC-MS/MS workflows is sample preparation, which is detailed in the *Sample Preparation for LC-MS/MS Analysis* chapter. This chapter offers practical strategies to optimize sample handling and preparation, ensuring precision and reproducibility. Next, the book explores *Specific Laboratory Techniques for*

LC-MS/MS Analysis, sharing expert insights and hands-on guidance to help laboratories avoid common pitfalls when developing assays.

With a strong foundation established, the book then delves into *Method Development and Validation*, providing a step-by-step approach to designing, optimizing, and validating LC-MS/MS assays to meet clinical and regulatory standards.

Once assays are developed, ongoing maintenance is critical to sustaining high-quality results. The *Instrument and Assay Maintenance* chapter outlines best practices for maintaining and servicing mass spectrometry instruments, including routine upkeep and troubleshooting strategies. This is followed by *Troubleshooting for LC-MS/MS Assays*, which offers expert approaches to diagnosing and resolving issues to ensure assay performance and reliability.

Interpreting mass spectrometry data is an essential skill, and *Data Analytics* provides foundational knowledge on processing, interpreting, and visualizing LC-MS/MS results.

To ensure accuracy and reliability in patient testing, a strong quality assurance program is necessary. *Quality Assurance for LC-MS/MS Assays* discusses quality control measures and best practices for maintaining robust assay performance.

Finally, the book addresses regulatory considerations in *Regulations and Laboratory-Developed Tests (LDTs) for LC-MS/MS Assays*. This chapter provides guidance on navigating regulatory requirements and compliance considerations for LC-MS/MS-based clinical tests.

Our goal is to provide practical guidance to those implementing LC-MS/MS in clinical laboratories to enhance patient care. The adoption of this technology is complex, requiring years of expertise and dedicated effort to ensure success. By sharing the collective experience of leaders in the field, this book aims to bridge knowledge gaps and support laboratories in leveraging LC-MS/MS for high-quality, patient-centered diagnostics. We hope that readers will gain the knowledge and confidence needed to successfully implement and optimize LC-MS/MS in their laboratories.

References

1. Ettre LS, Sakodynskii KIMS. Tswett and the discovery of chromatography I: early work (1899–1903). Chromatographia. 1993;35:223–31. https://doi.org/10.1007/BF02269707.
2. Novakova L, Vlckova H. A review of current trends and advances in modern bio-analytical methods: chromatography and sample preparation. Anal Chim Acta. 2009;656:8–35. https://doi.org/10.1016/j.aca.2009.10.004.
3. Robards K, Ryan D. Principles and practice of modern chromatographic methods. Elsevier Science & Technology; 2021.
4. Horvath CG, Preiss BA, Lipsky SR. Fast liquid chromatography: an investigation of operating parameters and the separation of nucleotides on pellicular ion exchangers. Anal Chem. 1967;39:1422–8. https://doi.org/10.1021/ac60256a003.
5. Colin H, Guiochon G. Introduction to reversed-phase high-performance liquid chromatography. J Chromatogr A. 1977;141:289–312. https://doi.org/10.1016/s0021-9673(00)93537-4.
6. Hirata Y, Novotny M. Techniques of capillary liquid chromatography. J Chromatogr A. 1979;186:521–8. https://doi.org/10.1016/s0021-9673(00)95272-5.

7. Novotny MV. Development of capillary liquid chromatography: a personal perspective. J Chromatogr A. 2017;1523:3–16. https://doi.org/10.1016/j.chroma.2017.06.042.
8. Jorgenson JW. Capillary liquid chromatography at ultrahigh pressures. Annu Rev Anal Chem. 2010;3:129–50. https://doi.org/10.1146/annurev.anchem.1.031207.113014.
9. Guillarme D, Schappler J, Rudaz S, Veuthey J-L. Coupling ultra-high-pressure liquid chromatography with mass spectrometry. TrAC Trends Anal Chem (Regular ed.). 2010;29:15–27. https://doi.org/10.1016/j.trac.2009.09.008.
10. Budzikiewicz H, Grigsby RD. Mass spectrometry and isotopes: a century of research and discussion. Mass Spectrom Rev. 2006;25:146–57. https://doi.org/10.1002/mas.20061.
11. Griffiths IWJJ. Thomson – the centenary of his discovery of the electron and of his invention of mass spectrometry. Rapid Commun Mass Spectrom. 1997;11:2–16. https://doi.org/10.1002/(SICI)1097-0231(19970115)11:1<2::AID-RCM768>3.0.CO;2-V.
12. Munro, G. C. The theory of the modified Aston-type mass-spectrometer, (1933).
13. Aston FW. Mass-spectra and the atomic weights of the elements. Sci Prog Twent Century (1919–1933). 1920;15:212–22.
14. Cotter RJ. Time-of-flight mass spectrometry for the structural analysis of biological molecules. Anal Chem (Washington). 1992;64:1027A–39A. https://doi.org/10.1021/ac00045a002.
15. Mamyrin BA. Time-of-flight mass spectrometry (concepts, achievements, and prospects). Int J Mass Spectrom. 2001;206:251–66. https://doi.org/10.1016/S1387-3806(00)00392-4.
16. Finnigan RE. Quadrupole mass spectrometers. Anal Chem (Washington). 1994;66:969A–75A. https://doi.org/10.1021/ac00091a002.
17. Dawson PH. Quadrupole mass spectrometry and its applications. Elsevier Scientific Pub. Co.; 1976.
18. Cooks RG, Glish GL, McLuckey SA, Kaiser RE. Ion trap mass spectrometry. Chem Eng News. 1991;69:26–41. https://doi.org/10.1021/cen-v069n012.p026.
19. March RE. An introduction to quadrupole ion trap mass spectrometry. J Mass Spectrom. 1997;32:351–69. https://doi.org/10.1002/(SICI)1096-9888(199704)32:4<351::AID-JMS512>3.3.CO;2-P.
20. Fenn JB, Mann M, Meng CK, Wong SF, Whitehouse CM. Electrospray ionization for mass spectrometry of large biomolecules. Science. 1989;246:64–71. https://doi.org/10.1126/science.2675315.
21. Fenn JB, Mann M, Meng CK, Wong SF, Whitehouse CM. Electrospray ionization-principles and practice. Mass Spectrom Rev. 1990;9:37–70. https://doi.org/10.1002/mas.1280090103.
22. Sekiya S, Wada Y, Tanaka K. Derivatization for stabilizing sialic acids in MALDI-MS. Anal Chem (Washington). 2005;77:4962–8. https://doi.org/10.1021/ac050287o.
23. Berkenkamp S, Kirpekar F, Hillenkamp F. Infrared MALDI mass spectrometry of large nucleic acids. Science. 1998;281:260–2. https://doi.org/10.1126/science.281.5374.260.
24. Hillenkamp, F. & Peter-Katalinić, J. MALDI MS: a practical guide to instrumentation, methods and applications. (2007).
25. Bahr U, Karas M, Hillenkamp F. Analysis of biopolymers by matrix-assisted laser desorption/ionization (MALDI) mass spectrometry. Fresenius J Anal Chem. 1994;348:783–91. https://doi.org/10.1007/BF01780979.
26. Zytkovicz TH, et al. Tandem mass spectrometric analysis for amino, organic, and fatty acid disorders in newborn dried blood spots: a two-year summary from the New England newborn screening program. Clin Chem (Baltimore, Md.). 2001;47:1945–55.
27. Rashed MS, Ozand PT, Bucknall MP, Little D. Diagnosis of inborn errors of metabolism from blood spots by acylcarnitines and amino acids profiling using automated electrospray tandem mass spectrometry. Pediatr Res. 1995;38:324–31. https://doi.org/10.1203/00006450-199509000-00009.
28. Covey TR, Lee ED, Bruins AP, Henion JD. Liquid chromatography/mass spectrometry. Anal Chem (Washington). 1986;58:1451A–61A. https://doi.org/10.1021/ac00127a001.
29. Pitt JJ. Principles and applications of liquid chromatography-mass spectrometry in clinical biochemistry. Clin Biochem Rev. 2009;30:19–34.

30. Pesce A, et al. An evaluation of the diagnostic accuracy of liquid chromatography-tandem mass spectrometry versus immunoassay drug testing in pain patients. Pain Physician. 2010;13:273–81.
31. Maralikova B, Weinmann W. Confirmatory analysis for drugs of abuse in plasma and urine by high-performance liquid chromatography–tandem mass spectrometry with respect to criteria for compound identification. J Chromatogr B Analyt Technol Biomed Life Sci. 2004;811:21–30. https://doi.org/10.1016/j.jchromb.2004.04.039.
32. Fitzgerald RL, Rivera JD, Herold DA. Broad spectrum drug identification directly from urine, using liquid chromatography-tandem mass spectrometry. Clin Chem (Baltimore, Md.). 1999;45:1224–34. https://doi.org/10.1093/clinchem/45.8.1224.
33. Dams R, Murphy CM, Lambert WE, Huestis MA. Urine drug testing for opioids, cocaine, and metabolites by direct injection liquid chromatography/tandem mass spectrometry. Rapid Commun Mass Spectrom. 2003;17:1665–70. https://doi.org/10.1002/rcm.1098.
34. Henion JD. Drug analysis by continuously monitored liquid chromatography/mass spectrometry with a quadrupole mass spectrometer. Anal Chem (Washington). 1978;50:1687–93. https://doi.org/10.1021/ac50034a029.
35. Taylor PJ, Tai C-H, Franklin ME, Pillans PI. The current role of liquid chromatography-tandem mass spectrometry in therapeutic drug monitoring of immunosuppressant and antiretroviral drugs: mass spectrometry in laboratory medicine. Clin Biochem. 2011;44:14–20.
36. Taylor PJ. Therapeutic drug monitoring of immunosuppressant drugs by high-performance liquid chromatography-mass spectrometry. Ther Drug Monit. 2004;26:215–9. https://doi.org/10.1097/00007691-200404000-00023.
37. McShane AJ, Bunch DR, Wang S. Therapeutic drug monitoring of immunosuppressants by liquid chromatography–mass spectrometry. Clin Chim Acta. 2016;454:1–5. https://doi.org/10.1016/j.cca.2015.12.027.
38. Kushnir MM, et al. Liquid chromatography tandem mass spectrometry for analysis of steroids in clinical laboratories: mass spectrometry in laboratory medicine. Clin Biochem. 2011;44:77–88.
39. Vogeser M, Parhofer KG. Liquid chromatography tandem-mass spectrometry (LC-MS/MS)—technique and applications in endocrinology. Exp Clin Endocrinol Diabetes. 2007;115:559–70. https://doi.org/10.1055/s-2007-981458.
40. Kushnir MM, Rockwood AL, Bergquist J. Liquid chromatography-tandem mass spectrometry applications in endocrinology. Mass Spectrom Rev. 2010;29:480–502. https://doi.org/10.1002/mas.20264.
41. Siekmann L, Hoppen H-O, Breuer H. Determination of steroid hormones in body fluids by gas chromatography-mass spectrometry, using a multiple ion detector. Anal Bioanal Chem. 1970;252:294–8.
42. Chapman JR, Bailey E. Determination of plasma testosterone by combined gas chromatography-mass spectrometry. J Chromatogr A. 1974;89:215–24. https://doi.org/10.1016/S0021-9673(01)99396-3.
43. Dehennin L, Reiffsteck A, Scholler R. A quantitative method for the estimation of testosterone and progesterone in human plasma, using the gas chromatograph/mass spectrometer combination with single ion monitoring. J Steroid Biochem. 1974;5:81–6. https://doi.org/10.1016/0022-4731(74)90032-6.
44. Björkhem I, Lantto O, Svensson L. Serum testosterone determination by mass fragmentography. Clin Chim Acta. 1975;60:59–66. https://doi.org/10.1016/0009-8981(75)90180-1.
45. Siekmann L. Determination of steroid hormones by the use of isotope dilution--mass spectrometry: a definitive method in clinical chemistry. J Steroid Biochem. 1979;11:117–23. https://doi.org/10.1016/0022-4731(79)90285-1.
46. Finlay EM, Gaskell SJ. Determination of testosterone in plasma from men by gas chromatography/mass spectrometry, with high-resolution selected-ion monitoring and metastable peak monitoring. Clin Chem. 1981;27:1165–70.
47. Salerno R, et al. Simultaneous determination of testosterone, dihydrotestosterone and 5 alpha-androstan-3 alpha,-17 beta-diol by isotopic dilution mass spectrometry in plasma and prostatic

tissue of patients affected by benign prostatic hyperplasia. Effects of 3-month treatment with a GnRH analog. J Androl. 1988;9:234–40. https://doi.org/10.1002/j.1939-4640.1988.tb01043.x.
48. Furuta T, Kusano K, Kasuya Y. Simultaneous measurements of endogenous and deuterium-labelled tracer variants of androstenedione and testosterone by capillary gas chromatography-mass spectrometry. J Chromatogr. 1990;525:15–23. https://doi.org/10.1016/s0378-4347(00)83376-9.
49. Legrand C, Dousset B, Tronel H, Belleville F, Nabet P. Measurement of plasma testosterone by gas chromatography-negative-ion mass spectrometry using pentafluoropropionic derivatives. J Chromatogr B Biomed Appl. 1995;663:187–92. https://doi.org/10.1016/0378-4347(94)00461-d.
50. Fitzgerald RL, Herold DA. Serum total testosterone: immunoassay compared with negative chemical ionization gas chromatography-mass spectrometry. Clin Chem. 1996;42:749–55.
51. Wians FH Jr, Stuart J. Ciba corning ACS:180 direct total testosterone assay can be used on female sera. Clin Chem. 1997;43:1466–8.
52. Fitzgerald RL, Herold DA. Ciba corning ACS:180 direct total testosterone assay can be used on female sera: reply. Clin Chem. 1997;43:1467–8.
53. Stanczyk FZ. Reliability of extraction/chromatography RIAs. Clin Chem. 2004;50:778. https://doi.org/10.1373/clinchem.2004.031492.
54. Herold DA, Fitzgerald RL. Reliability of extraction/chromatography RIAs: response. Clin Chem. 2004;50:778. https://doi.org/10.1373/clinchem.2004.032128.
55. Stanczyk FZ. Extraction/chromatographic testosterone RIA can be used as the "gold standard" for determining the reliability of direct testosterone immunoassay measurements. Clin Chem. 2004;50:2219–2220; author reply 2220–2211. https://doi.org/10.1373/clinchem.2004.038505.
56. Taieb J, et al. Testosterone measured by 10 immunoassays and by isotope-dilution gas chromatography-mass spectrometry in sera from 116 men, women, and children. Clin Chem. 2003;49:1381–95. https://doi.org/10.1373/49.8.1381.
57. Herold DA, Fitzgerald RL. Immunoassays for testosterone in women: better than a guess? Clin Chem. 2003;49:1250–1. https://doi.org/10.1373/49.8.1250.
58. Zhang YV, Rockwood A. Impact of automation on mass spectrometry. Clin Chim Acta. 2015;450:298–303. https://doi.org/10.1016/j.cca.2015.08.027.
59. Salvagno GL, Danese E, Lippi G. Mass spectrometry and total laboratory automation: opportunities and drawbacks. Clin Chem Lab Med. 2020;58:994–1001. https://doi.org/10.1515/cclm-2019-0723.
60. Gqamana PP, Militello L, McMaster JM, Daley SJ, Zhang YV. Analytical concordance of total vitamin D on a fully automated random-access LC–MS/MS platform. J Appl Lab Med. 2023;8:940–51. https://doi.org/10.1093/jalm/jfad036.
61. Mathieu E, Duterme C, Fage D, Cotton F. Cascadion™ SM clinical analyzer: evaluation of the whole blood immunosuppressants quantification and routine usability. Clin Chim Acta. 2023;539:97–104. https://doi.org/10.1016/j.cca.2022.11.029.

Fundamentals of Mass Spectrometry

2

Cody Orahoske, Hanna Lusk, Shanel C. Pickard, and Alan H. B. Wu

Introduction

The history of mass spectrometry (MS) dates back to the turn of the twentieth century when physicist John Thomson and his team constructed an instrument that could measure mass as a ratio of charge [1]. During the first few decades, most of the work involving mass spectrometry was conducted on isotope research of elements. These studies were important in the Manhattan Project, where ^{235}uranium and ^{239}plutonium were combined to produce the first atomic bomb. Chemists initially utilized this powerful new tool to determine the structures of newly synthesized organic compounds, but its application was limited to pure samples or simple, well-characterized mixtures. This changed in the early 1950s when Fred McLafferty and Roland Gohlke, then of Dow Chemical Co., coupled gas chromatography (GC) as a means of separation of complex mixtures and thereby greatly expanded MS as a detection method for unknown compounds [2]. Within a few years, GC/MS was adopted into routine clinical practice, especially for qualitative urine drug confirmations and later for quantitative therapeutic drug monitoring [3]. The utility of GC–MS, however, was primarily limited to small, non-volatile compounds and required a laborious pre-analytical step involving chemical derivatization to render them volatile compounds suitable for analysis.

The more widespread clinical implementation of mass spectrometry came in the 1980s, with several key developments significantly expanding its capabilities. First, the

C. Orahoske
Department of Laboratory Medicine, University of California, San Francisco, CA, USA

Lab Corp, Calabasas, CA, USA
e-mail: cody.orahoske@labcorp.com

H. Lusk · S. C. Pickard · A. H. B. Wu (✉)
Department of Laboratory Medicine, University of California, San Francisco, CA, USA
e-mail: hanna.lusk@ucsf.edu; shanel.pickard@ucsf.edu; alan.wu@ucsf.edu

Y. V. Zhang, U. Garg (eds.), *Practical Guide to Implementing Liquid Chromatography Mass Spectrometry in Clinical Laboratories*,
https://doi.org/10.1007/978-3-032-03852-4_2

development of soft ionization techniques, particularly electrospray ionization (ESI) and matrix-assisted laser desorption/ionization (MALDI), made it possible to analyze large biomolecules like proteins and peptides without the excessive fragmentation caused by hard ionization methods. Equally important, these novel ionization techniques expanded the sample types that could be compatible with mass spectrometry; ESI allowed for liquid-phase samples to be directly introduced into the mass spectrometer, eliminating the need to volatilize the sample and making it feasible to interface liquid chromatography as a pre-analytical step to efficiently separate unknown liquid mixtures [4]. In contrast, MALDI uses laser energy to ionize solid-phase samples, allowing for the direct analysis of crystallized specimens [5]. The impact of these ionization techniques was recognized by awarding the 2002 Nobel Prize in Chemistry to John Fenn, Koichi Tanaka, and Kurt Wüthrich for their contributions.

Clinical laboratories have long relied on immunoassays as the gold standard for hormone analysis, therapeutic drug monitoring, and biomarker detection. While effective, immunoassays inherently suffer from cross-reactivity, particularly in steroid hormone analysis and drug screening [6]. Furthermore, the immunoassays rely on the isolation of high-affinity antibodies through a scalable process to make commercial kits feasible and cost-effective. In other words, developing an assay for each target analyte is a process engineering challenge—ultimately limiting which analytes can be affordably targeted. Conversely, MS does not rely on affinity-based targeting paradigms. It uses unique mass-to-charge (*m/z*) signatures to identify and quantify analytes, thus allowing MS to distinguish between structurally similar compounds with high accuracy. Liquid chromatography–tandem mass spectrometry (LC-MS/MS) emerged in the 1990s that combines liquid chromatography for analyte separation with tandem mass spectrometry for highly specific identification and quantification. The tandem mass spectrometers work sequentially, with the first MS selecting for precursor ions of interest based on their mass-to-charge (*m/z*) ratio. Collision-induced dissociation (CID) or other fragmentation techniques further break the precursor ions to product ions that feed into the second MS for detection, making these systems a powerful alternative to immunoassays in complex biological matrices. In the microbiology laboratory, MALDI-TOF MS has revolutionized microbiology, replacing time-consuming culture-based identification methods with rapid microbial detection in minutes.

Additionally, improvements in mass analyzers—such as quadrupoles, time-of-flight (TOF), and Orbitraps—enhanced sensitivity and specificity, making MS more reliable for clinical diagnostics. These technological advancements positioned MS as an attractive alternative to traditional clinical methods, which often struggled with specificity, sensitivity, and turnaround time. For example, immunoassays, a mainstay in clinical testing, suffer from cross-reactivity, leading to inaccurate hormone and drug measurements. Similarly, conventional microbiological culture methods require extended incubation periods, whereas MALDI-TOF MS can identify pathogens in minutes. As a result, mass spectrometry emerged as a powerful solution to fill these critical gaps, offering precise, high-throughput analysis for modern clinical laboratories.

While mass spectrometry has addressed many limitations of traditional techniques—and, in some cases, replaced them—full reliance on MS in clinical laboratories still faces challenges. The technique lacks full automation and requires expertise for data interpretation and method development [3]. Standardization across laboratories remains an ongoing challenge, with regulatory bodies providing slow guidance on appropriate compliance and quality control measures. Despite these challenges, MS continues to have an expanding role in diagnostics across the spectrum of human disease. Advancements in automation, miniaturization, and bioinformatics will further solidify it in the modern clinical laboratory.

Basic Components and Concepts

While modern mass spectrometry workflows can be highly complex, the core analysis relies on three main components: the ion source, mass analyzer, and detector, each playing a crucial role in the identification and quantification of analytes. Figure 2.1 shows a prototypical MS workflow, including example pre-analytical

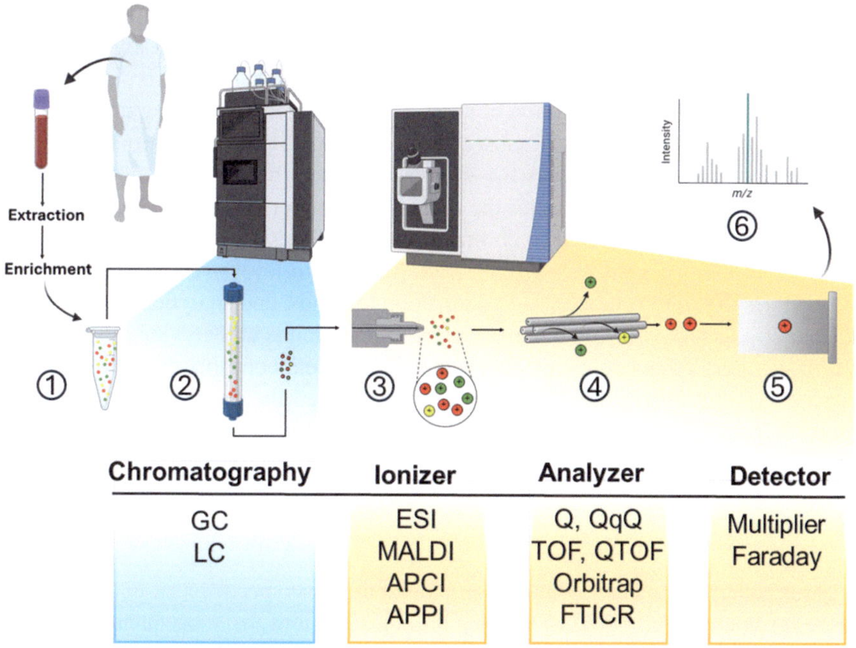

Fig. 2.1 A schematic of a typical mass spectrometry process flow, illustrating key steps from sample preparation to data analysis (1). A biological sample (e.g., blood) is collected and processed (2). The sample undergoes chromatographic separation via chromatography, such as liquid chromatography (LC) or gas chromatography (GC) to better separate constituents of the mixture (3). The analytes are ionized which can be done with varying types of ionization techniques, such as electrospray ionization (ESI), matrix-assisted laser desorption/ionization (MALDI), atmospheric pressure chemical ionization (APCI), or atmospheric pressure photoionization (APPI) (4). The mass analyzer separates ions based on their mass-to-charge ratio (m/z), using instruments such as quadrupole (Q, triple quadrupole: QqQ), time-of-flight (TOF, quadrupole-TOF: Q-TOF), Orbitrap, or Fourier transform ion cyclotron resonance (FTICR) (5). The ions are detected using devices like an electron multiplier or Faraday cup (6). The resulting mass spectrum displays the detected m/z values, enabling analyte identification and quantification

Table 2.1 High-level comparison of LC-MS and GC–MS, highlighting key differences in sample compatibility, ionization techniques, and analytical applications

	LC-MS		GC–MS	
Mobile phase	Liquid		Inert gas	
Ionization methods	Soft ionization techniques [11]: ESI APCI		Hard ionization techniques [11]: EI CI	
Applications	Non-volatile Thermally labile Polar Large (proteins and peptides) [11] Metabolic [12]	Qualitative [11] Quantitative [11]	Volatile Thermally stable Non-polar Small organic molecules Forensic toxicology	Qualitative [11] Quantitative [11]
Throughput	Slower		Faster	
Automation Capabilities	High [11]		Low-moderate [11]	

steps that may be incorporated into the processing of a sample. For example, patient samples may undergo extraction and dilution depending on the matrix; enrichment aims to increase the concentration of target analytes while minimizing matrix interference to improve sensitivity in subsequent steps (Fig. 2.1, step 1). Chromatography (Fig. 2.1, step 2) further refines the sample by separating complex mixtures such that the various constituents enter the mass spectrometer at distinct times. While a separate chapter is dedicated to chromatography, a brief table comparing LC-MS and GC–MS is provided here primarily to offer a high-level overview of their key differences in sample compatibility, ionization methods, and analytical applications (Table 2.1). Of interest to the remainder of this section is an overview of the spectrometer's core components and a review of high-yield concepts that will help the reader to better appreciate distinctions made between the compared technologies (see Table 2.2 for key definitions that will be seen in this chapter).

Ion Sources

The ion source is the first critical component of the mass spectrometer and is responsible for converting neutral molecules into charged ions, as subsequent MS steps rely on using charge to differentiate species and isolate targets (Fig. 2.1, step 3). In this configuration of LC-MS/MS, the eluent coming from the chromatography separation is in the liquid phase as it reaches the ion source. Due to this, the source must be able to convert the liquid into a gas phase to allow for the ions to travel into the mass analyzer. As far as clinical mass spectroscopy, atmospheric pressure ionization (API) is the predominant ion source type, which can be further subdivided into three different classifications: electrospray ionization (ESI), atmospheric pressure chemical ionization (APCI), and atmospheric pressure photoionization (APPI) [1, 2].

Table 2.2 Key mass spectrometry definitions

Concept	Component	Definition
Isotope	–	Variants of an element with the same number of protons but different numbers of neutrons
Ion	Ionizer	A charged particle formed when a molecule gains or loses electrons during ionization
Mass-to-charge ratio (*m/z*)	Analyzer	Fundamental measurement used to differentiate ions based on their charge state
Resolution	Analyzer	The degree by which two closely spaced peaks in a spectrum can be distinguish with less than a defined overlap [7–9].
Resolving power	Analyzer	"Ability to distinguish between peaks differing in the *m/z* by an increment $\Delta(m/z)$ given by $(m/z)/\Delta(m/z)$. The value of $\Delta(m/z)$ is obtained from the peak width at a specified fraction of the peak height or from the valley between two peaks of specified height" [9, 10]
Accurate mass	Analyzer	The deviation between the measured and actual mass [8]
Mass range	Analyzer	The span of m/z values that the analyzer can detect [9]
Fragmentation	Analyzer	The process where precursor ions break apart into two or more fragment, and at least one fragment is an ion [9]
Mass spectrum	Detector	Graphical representation of detected ions, displaying their mass-to-charge ratio (*m/z*) on the x-axis and relative abundance on the y-axis [9]
Isotope patterns	Detector	A series of peaks of relative abundance of ions with the same chemical formula but different isotopic composition [9]
Deconvolution	Analysis	A computational method used to resolve overlapping peaks in a mass spectrum [9]

This table outlines essential concepts in mass spectrometry, categorizing them by their corresponding components and definitions

More recently, research has explored ionization techniques that eliminate the need for LC, allowing direct ionization of the sample into the mass spectrometer. Matrix-assisted laser Desorption/Ionization (MALDI) has become an integrated instrument within microbiology for the identification of bacterial cultures [3]. Newer ionization methods in the past two decades belong to a class of ionization sources called ambient ionization mass spectrometry (AIMS), some highlighted, coated blade spray (CBS), desorption electrospray ionization (DESI), direct analysis in real time (DART), and rapid evaporative ionization mass spectrometry (REIMS) [4–7].

Electrospray Ionization

As the field of clinical mass spectrometry matures, one of the most widely used ion sources belongs to ESI [6, 8–10]. The technique involves applying a high voltage to a flowing stream of liquid eluent, which results in the production of a fine mist of charged droplets at atmospheric pressure [10, 11]. These droplets undergo gradual solvent evaporation, assisted by heat and the electric field, leading to a progressive reduction in droplet size. As the droplets shrink, their surface charge density increases until they reach a critical point known as the Rayleigh limit, where coulombic repulsion causes them to undergo fission or emit ions directly into the gas phase [12]. A major advantage of ESI is its ability to generate multiply charged ions. In this process of imparting multiple charges to peptides, proteins, and biomolecules, ESI reduces their mass-to-charge ratio (*m/z*), bringing otherwise high-molecular-weight compounds within the operational limits of most instruments [13, 14].

Discovered in the 1980s, ESI technology has diversified into two main categories based on liquid flow rates: low-flow systems, such as nano-electrospray ionization (nano-ESI), and high-flow systems, such as pneumatically assisted electrospray or ion spray sources. Nano-ESI operates at flow rates in nL/min, often used in proteomics and biomarker discovery, where sample volumes are limited [10, 11]. By generating smaller droplets, nano-ESI enhances ionization efficiency and minimizes sample consumption. Pneumatically assisted electrospray or ion spray functionality was designed to meet the needs of high-throughput testing. These systems typically operate at flow rates of μL/min, compatible with most HPLC platforms [10, 11].

The ionization mechanisms of both low- and high-flow ESI systems are fundamentally similar they both require droplet formation, charging, and solvent evaporation to produce gas-phase ions. However, they differ in droplet generation strategies. In nano-ESI, droplets are formed primarily through the electrical forces at the tip of a fine emitter, while in pneumatically assisted systems, nebulizing gases provide additional shear forces to aid droplet formation and stabilize the spray under a broader range of conditions [1, 10, 11]. Both approaches have been optimized over the past two decades to enhance ionization efficiency, minimize ion losses, and maximize the number of ions sampled into the mass spectrometer's vacuum system [6, 15]. A review of ESI's development, including adaptations to overcome its limitations, was provided by Meher and Chen, highlighting the historical evolution of the technique [16]. Their work outlines not only the foundational discoveries of ESI but also the innovations that have expanded its utility in clinical mass spectrometry, such as improved emitter designs, optimized flow rates, and better integration with chromatographic systems.

ESI does have some limitations, including sensitivity to mobile phase composition, flow rate stability, and matrix effects that can lead to ion suppression in complex samples. However, ongoing advancements in source design, interface technology, and data processing algorithms continue to improve their robustness and reliability in clinical diagnostic testing. To address some of the disadvantages associated with ESI, other ion sources can be substituted depending on the analyte.

Atmospheric Pressure Chemical Ionization

Since its introduction in the 1970s and commercial implementation in the 1980s, APCI has found widespread use in the analysis of pharmaceutical compounds, ste roids, fat-soluble vitamins, and therapeutic drugs in clinical and forensic toxicology laboratories [8, 9]. APCI remains a complementary technique to ESI, particularly favored for the analysis of small-to-medium-sized, relatively nonpolar, or moderately polar compounds [17, 18]. APCI in clinical laboratories is mainly used when ESI fails to ionize the target analyte, due to its ability to efficiently ionize neutral and low-polarity molecules while tolerating complex biological matrices and high flow rates [6, 8, 19]. Unlike ESI, which produces ions directly from charged droplets in the liquid phase, APCI operates as a gas-phase ionization technique. This makes APCI less susceptible to ion suppression from salts, buffers, and other matrix components frequently encountered in clinical and environmental sample analysis.

The APCI process begins with the introduction of the liquid chromatography effluent, typically at flow rates ranging from 200 μL/min up to 2000 μL/min, into a pneumatic nebulizer. The eluent is then sprayed as fine droplets into a heated vaporization chamber, where it is rapidly desolvated and vaporized by temperatures often exceeding 400 °C [1]. The resulting gas-phase analyte molecules are carried by a nebulizing gas, commonly nitrogen, toward a corona discharge electrode positioned at atmospheric pressure. The corona discharge generates a plasma that ionizes the vaporized solvent molecules, producing reactant ions. These reactant ions subsequently ionize the analyte molecules via chemical ionization mechanisms, primarily through proton transfer or charge exchange reactions. For example, in positive ion mode, solvent ions ([S + H]+) can transfer a proton to the analyte (M) to form protonated molecular ions ([M + H]+), while in negative ion mode, deprotonation or anion attachment can occur, depending on analyte chemistry [1, 20]. As a result, APCI does not produce multiply charged ions; instead, it yields predominantly singly charged species. This makes APCI ideal for small molecules but limits its utility for the analysis of large biomolecules, which typically require the multiple charging capabilities of ESI to bring them within the *m/z* detection range of most mass spectrometers.

Modern APCI sources have been refined to improve desolvation efficiency and minimize thermal degradation. Innovations include zoned heating of the vaporization tube, optimized nebulizer design for better droplet impact and evaporation, and precise control of corona discharge current to maintain stable ionization conditions [18, 21, 22]. Despite these improvements, APCI remains best suited for analytes that can withstand the thermal energy required for vaporization. APCI does have limitations. It is less effective for highly polar or ionic compounds that are more readily ionized by ESI. Additionally, analytes sensitive to high temperatures may degrade during the vaporization step, reducing assay sensitivity or requiring alternative approaches [1, 20].

Atmospheric Pressure Photoionization

Roughly two decades after the advent of both ESI and APCI, a new ionization source was described, APPI [23]. Fundamentally, APPI was a modified form of APCI, where the corona discharge electrode was replaced by a photon-emitting lamp. As the eluent reaches the source, the sample is first vaporized using a heated nebulizer, which generates gas-phase molecules of both the analyte and solvent. These gas-phase molecules then interact with photons emitted from a discharge lamp, usually a krypton lamp, leading to ion formation. The photons emitted have energies of approximately 10.0 eV, which are optimal for ionizing analytes that have ionization energies lower than the photon energy but higher than those of the solvent or air molecules [1, 20, 23]. This selective ionization process helps APPI to be less prone to ion suppression and matrix effects compared to ESI and APCI, making it particularly advantageous for analyzing complex biological or environmental samples with high concentrations of salts or buffers [20, 24].

APPI is particularly advantageous for ionizing nonpolar and low-polarity compounds that are challenging to ionize using ESI or APCI, such as polycyclic aromatic hydrocarbons, lipids, and other nonpolar biomolecules [24–26]. It has demonstrated superior sensitivity, signal intensity, and signal-to-noise ratio when analyzing nonpolar lipids compared to ESI and APCI [24]. APPI works via two ionization mechanisms: direct and indirect. In direct ionization, analytes with ionization energies lower than the photon energy are directly ionized by absorbing photons, forming radical cations. In indirect ionization, a dopant such as acetone or toluene absorbs the photon energy, forming a radical cation that then ionizes the analyte via proton transfer or charge exchange [20, 24, 27].

Although APPI offers significant advantages, particularly for nonpolar analytes, it is not as efficient as ESI or APCI for highly polar compounds. While ESI excels in ionizing polar analytes and APCI is effective for semi-polar compounds, APPI's range is limited to specific types of molecules. Furthermore, APPI's ionization efficiency depends heavily on the energy of the emitted photons, and if the photon energy is too high or too low, ionization may not occur or lead to fragmentation. However, its ability to reduce matrix effects and provide high sensitivity makes it a valuable tool in specific applications such as the analysis of steroids, lipids, and environmental pollutants [24, 25].

In summary, APPI is a powerful ionization technique that excels in the analysis of nonpolar and low-polarity compounds, offering advantages in sensitivity and reduced matrix effects compared to ESI and APCI. However, its application is generally limited to nonpolar analytes, and its ionization efficiency is highly dependent on the photon energy.

Matrix-Assisted Laser Desorption/Ionization

MALDI is a soft ionization technique that enables the analysis of large biomolecules, including proteins, peptides, nucleotides, and polymers, with minimal fragmentation [20, 28, 29]. Unlike ESI, which generates multiply charged ions in the liquid phase, MALDI primarily produces singly charged ions in the gas phase. The MALDI process involves three key steps: sample preparation, laser desorption/ionization, and ion detection. In the first step, the sample is co crystallized with an organic matrix that absorbs laser energy, typically using compounds such as α-cyano-4-hydroxycinnamic acid, sinapinic acid, or 2,5-dihydroxybenzoic acid [29, 30]. The matrix serves several crucial functions: it absorbs the laser energy, assists in desorption of the sample from the solid phase into the gas phase, and facilitates protonation or deprotonation, leading to ion formation with minimal fragmentation [29, 30].

During the laser desorption/ionization step, a pulsed laser, often in the ultraviolet range (e.g., nitrogen laser at 337 nm or Nd:YAG laser at 355 nm), is used to excite the matrix molecules [29, 30]. This energy is rapidly transferred to the embedded analyte molecules, causing them to be ejected into the gas phase in an ionized state [30]. The desorbed ions are then accelerated into a mass analyzer, commonly a time-of-flight system, where their *m/z* is determined based on the time taken to reach the detector.

MALDI-TOF MS has become a critical tool in clinical microbiology, where it enables rapid identification of bacterial and fungal pathogens directly from culture plates [3, 31]. The technique has been integrated into automated diagnostic workflows, significantly reducing turnaround times compared to traditional biochemical identification methods. Beyond microbiology, MALDI has been applied in various clinical and biomedical fields, including tissue imaging MALDI Imaging Mass Spectrometry (MALDI-IMS), biomarker discovery, and pharmaceutical analysis [32, 33]. MALDI-IMS enables spatially resolved detection of biomolecules within tissue sections, providing insights into disease pathology, tumor heterogeneity, and drug distribution at the molecular level [32]. In proteomics, MALDI is used for peptide mass fingerprinting and top-down protein sequencing, facilitating the study of post-translational modifications and protein–protein interactions and providing MASS-fix an alternative for immunofixation [34, 35].

Despite its many advantages, MALDI has some limitations. One of the primary challenges is the need for careful sample preparation, as inconsistent crystallization of the matrix can lead to signal variability and poor reproducibility. Additionally, while MALDI excels in the analysis of large biomolecules, its sensitivity for small molecules is often lower than that of ESI or APCI, due to ion suppression effects from the matrix. To address these limitations, alternative approaches such as surface-assisted laser desorption/ionization (SALDI) and high-mass MALDI are beyond the scope of this chapter [36].

Ambient Ionization Methods

AIMS has the potential to significantly shift clinical mass spectrometry by allowing direct ionization of analytes in ambient conditions, often with minimal sample preparation. Unlike conventional ion sources that typically require chromatographic separation or specialized matrices, AIMS approaches facilitate rapid analysis of unprocessed samples or mildly treated samples, which can substantially reduce turnaround times in clinical settings [37]. These techniques capitalize on mechanisms such as plasma discharge, thermal desorption, or solvent-assisted extraction at the sample surface, enabling researchers and clinicians to perform rapid assays for diagnostic and research purposes without compromising analytical specificity [5, 38, 39]. Briefly, four different AIMS techniques will be highlighted as these techniques, over the past two decades, have demonstrated clinical utility and have the potential to become used routinely.

Among the plasma-based AIMS techniques, a clinically relevant technique called DART was discovered and introduced back in 2002, and since then, it has found utilization in various fields [39–41]. Briefly, a stream of gas, commonly helium, passes through a glow discharge to generate metastable neutral species. These species help with the desorb process of the analyte on the surface [40]. DART has been successfully employed for detecting small-molecule analytes in biological specimens, screening drug metabolites, and rapidly identifying unknowns in toxicology [42, 43]. In a recently published article by Choucair et al., they demonstrate that DART could be implemented in the clinical setting, with a turnaround time of 10 min to provide urine drug definitive testing [42].

CBS, a relatively newer technique, was described in 2014, and it takes a different approach to sample preparation and ionization [44]. In CBS, a thin, blade-like substrate with a specialized sorbent coating is dipped or swabbed in the sample, enabling analyte adsorption onto the blade surface. Then, the blade is configured in front of the mass spectrometer; an applied voltage and a micro-volume of solvent elute the analytes from the blade, generating an electrospray directly into the instrument [44]. The streamlined design and reduced sample handling allow rapid therapeutic drug monitoring or toxicology screening in blood or other bodily fluids, rendering CBS a particularly promising application [45–47]. Recently, CBS has found use in tissue analysis and was even able to differentiate meningiomas based on the acylcarnitine profile [48, 49].

DESI is a widely adopted solid–liquid extraction-based approach that was introduced to the field in 2004, and since its introduction, it has found wide application in clinical research [38, 50–53]. In DESI, a charged solvent spray is directed at the sample surface, extracting viable analytes and subsequently transferring them into the gas phase via electrospray-like ionization processes [52]. This facilitates rapid molecular imaging of tissues, allowing researchers to map lipid, metabolite, or drug distributions without matrix application. DESI-based imaging has proven valuable for characterizing diseased tissues and correlating molecular signatures with histopathological features [51–54].

A final noteworthy technique is REIMS, developed in 2009, which leverages electrosurgical or ultrasonic energy to thermally ablate tissue, generating a vapor that is channeled into a secondary ionization assembly before mass spectrometric detection [55]. After the development of REIMS in 2013, the term "iKnife" was introduced into the literature, which demonstrated REIMS could identify cancerous tissue from many different organs by profiling different glycerophospholipids [56].

In the following years researchers used this technique during surgery as well as ex vivo tissue analysis of biopsies for stratification and identification of cancer [57–59]. A review recently highlighted the last 15 years of REIMS technology beyond clinical use; in this review, the authors highlighted different sampling devices, applications, cancer diagnosis, food analysis, and other applications [60].

Mass Analyzers

After ionization, ions are directed to the mass analyzer, where they are separated based on their mass-to-charge ratio (*m/z*) [61]. The mass analyzer serves as the primary component of the mass spectrometer, allowing the user to determine the mass of analytes based on their *m/z* and isotope pattern. Various types of mass analyzers exist which utilize distinct methods of ion separation, each with its own advantages and limitations. Factors including resolution, sensitivity, and speed differ among mass analyzers, making specific MS systems more suitable for specific clinical applications [62]. For instance, quadrupole mass analyzers can function as mass filters, allowing only selected *m/z*'s to pass through to the detector, which results in high sensitivity, making them ideal for targeted applications. In contrast, time-of-flight mass analyzers measure all ions in a sample with high resolution, making them well-suited for untargeted applications.

Beyond stand-alone mass analyzers, hybrid MS systems combine multiple mass analyzers to enhance performance and enable ion fragmentation for structural identification. Tandem MS (MS/MS) improves specificity by selecting, fragmenting, and analyzing product ions, making it invaluable for both clinical and research applications. The choice of an MS system depends on factors such as the required *m/z* range, resolution, sensitivity, and cost. Since no single analyzer meets all needs, laboratories commonly use multiple mass spectrometers with different analyzers and ionization sources [62] (Table 2.3).

Quadrupole (Q)

Quadrupole mass analyzers consist of four parallel cylindrical rods with applied radio frequency (RF) and direct current (DC) potentials (Fig. 2.2), creating an oscillating electric field that stabilizes ions of a specific *m/z*, allowing them to reach the detector, while unstable ions are filtered out [63]. Their ability to function as mass filters yields high sensitivity, and they are widely used in clinical settings due to their affordability, compact size, and durability [64]. Quadrupoles can also operate in RF-only mode to transfer ions between different regions of the mass spectrometer, such as from the ionization source to another analyzer, or serve as collision cells for fragmentation [65].

The main limitations of quadrupole mass analyzers include a restricted mass range and low resolution. Consequently, they are not well suited for untargeted applications or detecting high-molecular-weight compounds (>3000 Da) that do not

Table 2.3 Summary comparison of mass analyzers in mass spectrometry

	Quadrupole	QqQ-MS	TOF-MS	Q-TOF	Orbitrap-MS	FTICR-MS
Resolution	Low	Low	Moderate—high	High	Very high	Ultra-High [19]
Mass resolving power			1×10^4 [8]	1×10^4 [15]	$1–2 \times 10^5$ [15, 16]	1×10^6 [8]
Mass accuracy	Low	Low	Moderate to high	High [15]	Very High [15]	Ultra-High [19]
Quantitation	Yes	Yes	Limited	Yes [15]	Yes	Limited
Fragmentation capability	No	Yes	No	Yes	Yes	Yes [19]
Mass range	Low—moderate	Low—moderate	Wide	Wide	Wide	Ultra-Wide [19]
Speed	Fast	Fast	Very fast	Moderate—fast [15]	Moderate	Slow
Common applications	Drug testing Clinical assays	Drug monitoring Biomarker validation	Fast screening Proteomics	Structural analysis Proteomics	Metabolomics Proteomics	Complex molecular analysis
Typical cost	Low-moderate	Moderate	High	High	Very high	Extremely high

These factors may influence the choice of analyzer for various analytical applications in the clinical setting

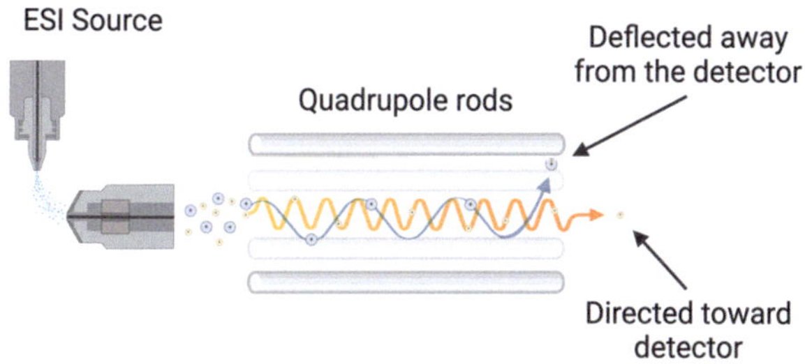

Fig. 2.2 A quadrupole mass analyzer uses four metal rods with applied RF and DC potentials. Ions oscillate as they pass through, and only those with stable paths reach the detector; unstable ions collide with the rods and are filtered out

carry multiple charges [62]. Quadrupoles integrate seamlessly with ESI ionization sources; however, their fast duty cycles and reliance on a continuous flux of ions make them less suitable for use with pulsed ion sources like MALDI [62, 66, 67].

Ion Trap (TRAP)

Ion traps function similarly to quadrupoles but can trap ions before selectively ejecting them. They enhance sensitivity by accumulating ions over time, making them effective for detecting low-abundance analytes. There are two main types: three-dimensional (3D) ion traps (Paul traps) and two-dimensional (2D) linear ion traps. While 3D ion traps were widely used historically, 2D ion traps are now preferred due to their greater ion storage capacity and faster scan rates [68]. Like quadrupoles, ion traps use an oscillating RF field combined with a superimposed DC field to retain ions. By adjusting the RF potential, ions of different *m/z* are selectively ejected [62]. Like quadrupole analyzers, ion traps are compact and relatively inexpensive, making them a cost-effective choice for many applications.

The main drawback of ion traps is low resolution, as they provide only unit mass accuracy. With the development of faster, higher-resolution, and more accurate mass analyzers, ion traps have become less commonly used. Nevertheless, 2D ion traps are still used in many hybrid MS systems, where their geometry makes them well-suited for use as precursor mass filters in tandem workflows.

Time-of-Flight (TOF)

TOF analyzers determine *m/z* by measuring ion flight times in a vacuum tube (Fig. 2.3). Ions with the same kinetic energy travel at different velocities based on their *m/z*, allowing accurate mass determination using the TOF. Many modern TOF instruments include a reflectron, which redirects ions to correct kinetic energy variations, improving resolution [69, 70]. Delayed extraction can also be used to enhance resolution by allowing ions to equilibrate before acceleration [71, 72].

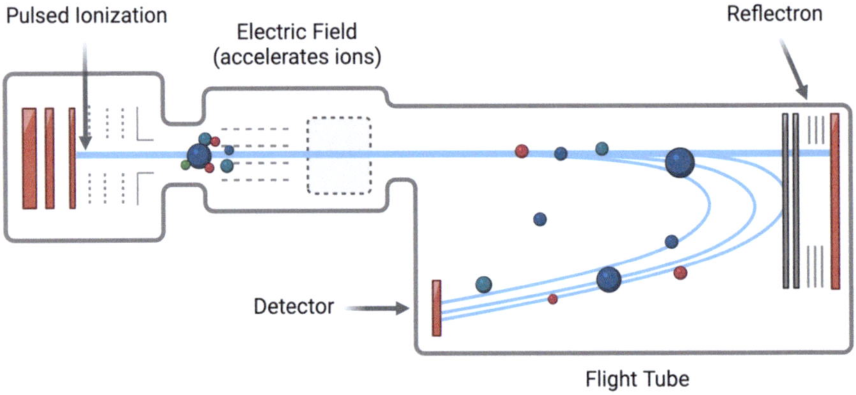

Fig. 2.3 In a TOF mass analyzer, ions from the source are accelerated by a pulsed electric field and enter a flight tube. They are separated by *m/z*, with heavier ions traveling more slowly. The detector records arrival time, which is proportional to *m/z*

Fig. 2.4 In an Orbitrap analyzer, ions enter tangentially through the outer electrode and orbit the central electrode under an applied voltage. They also oscillate along its axis, and this motion is detected and converted into a mass spectrum using a Fourier transform

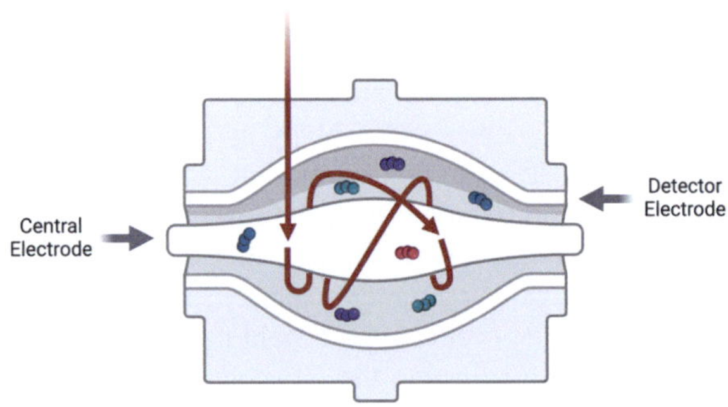

Initially limited to pulsed ion sources like MALDI, advances in tandem configurations have enabled TOF-MS to integrate with continuous ion sources, thereby expanding its applications. TOF analyzers offer a broad mass range and high resolution, making them particularly effective for proteomics, peptide mass fingerprinting, and microbial identification, in addition to untargeted applications [73].

Orbitrap

Orbitrap mass analyzers use electrostatic fields to trap ions in oscillatory motion around a central electrode, generating an image current on two outer electrodes (Fig. 2.4). This signal is processed via Fourier transformation to determine *m/z* and produce a mass spectrum with high accuracy and resolution [74–76].

Orbitrap mass analyzers are known for their excellent resolving power, which makes them particularly valuable for proteomics and top-down protein analysis [62]. However, they are costly and slower than other analyzers, limiting their use in high-throughput applications. They are also not ideal for analyzing small molecules or low-molecular-weight compounds. While not yet widespread in clinical settings, ongoing technological improvements may expand their potential for use in clinical workflows in the coming years.

Tandem Mass Spectrometers

In tandem mass spectrometry (MS/MS), the first analyzer selects ions based on their mass-to-charge ratio (*m/z*), and these ions are fragmented using collision-induced dissociation (CID) or another fragmentation technique (Fig. 2.5). The resulting product ions are analyzed by a second mass analyzer. By leveraging fragmentation patterns, MS/MS improves specificity and aids in compound identification.

Fragmentation Methods

CID fragments ions by colliding them with a chemically inert gas (argon or nitrogen) at low pressure. The collision transfers energy to the analyte ion, leading to bond breakage and the formation of product ions that provide important structural information. Other fragmentation methods include higher-energy collisional dissociation (HCD), a high-energy variant of CID that improves peptide sequencing and protein identification [77]. Electron capture dissociation (ECD) and electron transfer dissociation (ETD) both induce fragmentation by electron interaction with multiply charged cations, preserving labile modifications and making them ideal for top-down proteomics [21]. More specialized techniques, such as infrared multiphoton dissociation (IRMPD) and ultraviolet photodissociation (UVPD), provide unique fragmentation patterns for structural elucidation, but are mainly used in research [78, 79]. Each fragmentation technique has unique advantages, and the optimal choice depends on the analytical requirements and the desired structural information.

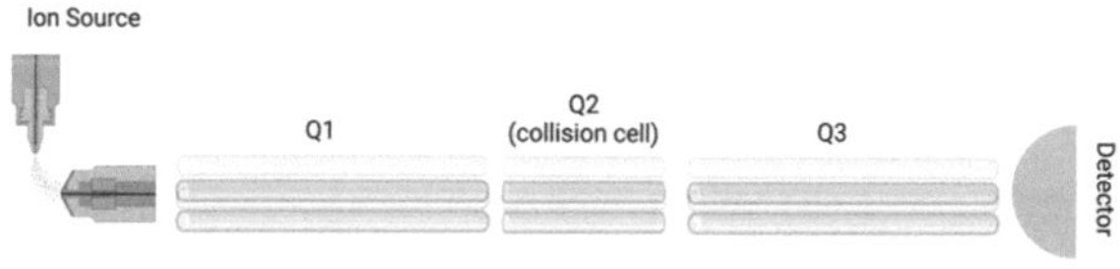

Fig. 2.5 Triple quadrupole mass spectrometers consist of three quadrupoles in tandem. Ions enter Q1 then move into Q2 where they are fragmented, and product ions are separated in Q3

Triple Quadrupole (QQQ)

QQQ mass spectrometers are widely used in clinical and research settings, exemplifying the power of MS/MS. [80] These systems consist of three quadrupoles: Q1 acts as a mass filter, Q2 serves as a collision cell for fragmentation, and Q3 analyzes the resulting product ions. Q1 and Q3 can either scan across a mass range or target specific ions, enabling both comprehensive and highly targeted analyses [81, 82].

QQQ instruments are particularly well suited for quantitative workflows due to their high sensitivity and specificity. Their ability to filter both precursor and product ions reduces matrix effects and background noise, which makes them ideal for targeted applications such as therapeutic drug monitoring. However, with lower mass resolution than other systems like Q-TOF or Orbitrap, QQQs are less effective for untargeted analysis or structural characterization. As a result, they are primarily employed in studies where precise quantification of known analytes is the primary goal, rather than in discovery applications.

QQQ Scan Modes

Scan modes define how data is acquired and processed. Different QQQ scan modes optimize ion selection and fragmentation (Fig. 2.6):

Full Scan—Also called a survey scan, is an MS mode where the instrument scans across a broad *m/z* range, detecting and recording all ions present without selecting specific ions for fragmentation. In this mode, the mass spectrometer provides a comprehensive overview of the ions in a sample, generating a complete mass spectrum.

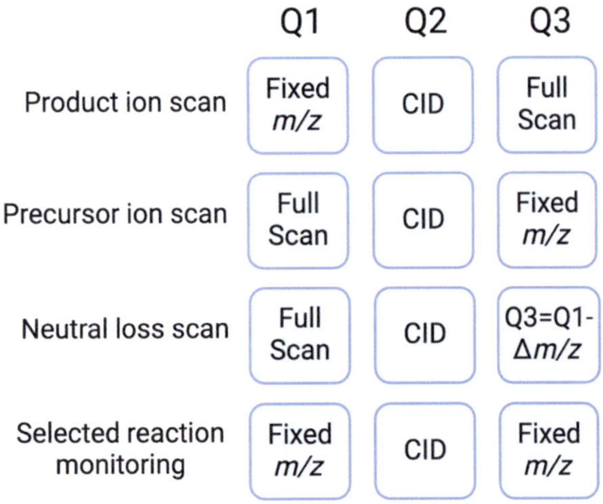

Fig. 2.6 Triple quadrupole scan modes

Product Ion Scan—Q1 filters ions of a specific *m/z*, which are fragmented in Q2, and all product ions are analyzed in Q3. This method is useful for obtaining fragmentation patterns for library building or structural elucidation.

Precursor ion scan—Q1 scans the entire *m/z* range while Q3 filters specific product ions. This method identifies precursor ions that produce the same product ion, which is valuable for identifying structurally similar compounds.

Neutral loss scan—Tracks ions before and after losing a neutral group. Both Q1 and Q3 scan the *m/z* range, with Q3 offset to detect the loss of a specific neutral fragment. This technique is useful for identifying modified peptides, like those with phosphorylation.

Selected Reaction Monitoring (SRM)—Q1 selects specific precursors, fragmentation occurs in Q2, and Q3 filters the resulting product ions. A known precursor-product ion transition is monitored. This allows monitoring of known compounds, though the *m/z* of product ions must be known ahead of time. When applied to multiple analytes simultaneously, it is referred to as multiple reaction monitoring (MRM).

Quadrupole Time-of-Flight (Q-TOF)

Quadrupole analyzers operate most efficiently with a continuous ion stream, whereas TOF analyzers require ion pulses. To integrate these two mass analyzers, the TOF analyzer is positioned after the quadrupole [83]. Ions filtered through the quadrupole are pulsed into the TOF analyzer in discrete packets using a set of pusher and puller plates [84]. Q-TOF systems offer several advantages over QQQ mass spectrometers, including superior mass accuracy, higher resolution, and faster scan speeds. These capabilities make Q-TOF instruments well-suited for untargeted applications.

Q-TOF Acquisition Methods

Different acquisition modes are used to optimize MS/MS data collection. Automatic switching between MS and MS/MS modes based on real-time data enhances the efficiency of ion selection and fragmentation.

Data-dependent acquisition (DDA)—The instrument selects the most abundant ions in the MS1 scan and performs MS/MS on those ions, optimizing data collection in complex samples.

Data-independent acquisition (DIA)—Ions within predefined *m/z* windows are fragmented, regardless of their intensity. This approach generates comprehensive fragment spectra across the selected range, enhancing the detection and identification of low-abundance analytes.

TOF/TOF

TOF/TOF mass spectrometry utilizes 2 TOF analyzers in tandem, with fragmentation occurring between them [85]. This setup enables rapid tandem MS analysis of biological compounds, which are commonly ionized using MALDI, such as peptides and oligonucleotides [86]. The high-speed nature of TOF analyzers allows for efficient precursor ion selection and fragmentation, making TOF/TOF systems well-suited for peptide analysis from tryptic digests.

Future Directions in MS for Clinical Use

MS continues to evolve as a powerful tool in clinical diagnostics, offering unparalleled sensitivity and specificity. However, its widespread adoption has been hindered by challenges such as high complexity, automation limitations, and workflow integration. Recent advancements aim to bridge these gaps, making MS more accessible and practical for routine clinical use. Innovations in automation, point-of-care applications, and emerging analytical techniques are paving the way for a more streamlined, efficient, and impactful role for MS in clinical chemistry.

LC-MS/MS is recognized for its high specificity and sensitivity, with the potential to transform clinical chemistry if widely adopted. However, its implementation has traditionally been constrained by technical complexity and a lack of automation. Fortunately, advancements in laboratory automation are addressing these limitations. Automation not only expands the accessibility of LC-MS/MS in clinical diagnostics but also improves workflow efficiency and result consistency [87].

Roche Diagnostics is leading the charge with the development of the cobas® i601 Mass Spec solution, an automated LC-MS/MS system designed to streamline clinical workflows [88]. While previous attempts, such as the Thermo Cascadian system, failed due to reliability and workflow integration challenges [89, 90], Roche seeks to overcome these barriers. By transitioning from batch processing to a random-access testing model, this innovation provides laboratories with greater flexibility, allowing them to choose between immunoassay and mass spectrometry for a broader range of tests. With Roche setting a precedent, other major diagnostic companies that manufacture automated analyzer systems are likely to follow, further accelerating the integration of mass spectrometry into routine clinical diagnostics.

Advancements in Point-of-Care Mass Spectrometry

In addition to automation, miniaturized point-of-care (POC) mass spectrometry is emerging as a game changer in clinical diagnostics. One of the first ambient ionization techniques to be integrated into routine clinical use was rapid evaporative ionization mass spectrometry (REIMS). This technology laid the groundwork for intraoperative tissue analysis, leading to the development of devices like the iKnife and iEndoscope [91, 92]. These tools enable real-time, high-resolution molecular analysis during surgery, providing immediate diagnostic insights upon tissue contact.

A significant drawback of REIMS is its destructive nature, which can limit its applicability in certain clinical settings. In response, researchers have developed alternative point-of-care MS devices that offer non-destructive tissue analysis. One such innovation is the MasSpec Pen, a handheld tool that utilizes a single water droplet to extract analytes from tissue via liquid–solid chemical extraction. A pressurized vacuum system then transfers the droplet to a mass spectrometer for real-time analysis [93]. Unlike REIMS-based tools, the MasSpec Pen preserves tissue integrity, making it a safer and more versatile option for clinical applications. These innovations in point-of-care MS are transforming clinical diagnostics by enabling rapid, highly sensitive, and specific analyses directly at the bedside.

Emerging Technologies and Future Outlook

Beyond automation and point-of-care applications, emerging MS technologies are set to further revolutionize clinical diagnostics. One promising advancement is ion mobility spectrometry (IMS), which has the potential to replace time-consuming liquid chromatography (LC) by separating ions based on their size, shape, and charge in a gas-phase environment [94]. By offering faster separations, IMS could significantly enhance the throughput and efficiency of MS-based clinical assays.

Additionally, the integration of artificial intelligence (AI) and machine learning has the potential to improve automated data interpretation and seamless integration with laboratory information systems (LIS). AI-driven spectral analysis can reduce manual interpretation errors, increase diagnostic accuracy, and optimize workflow efficiency, making MS-based diagnostics more accessible and scalable in clinical settings [95].

As these innovations continue to develop, MS is poised to become an indispensable tool in modern clinical diagnostics. The combination of automation, point-of-care advancements, and AI-driven data analysis will drive greater adoption, improving speed, accuracy, and accessibility. With continued advancements, MS is set to redefine the future of precision medicine and laboratory diagnostics.

References

1. Covey TR, Thomson BA, Schneider BB. Atmospheric pressure ion sources. Mass Spectrom Rev. 2009;28:870–97.
2. Siuzdak G. An introduction to mass spectrometry ionization: an excerpt from the expanding role of mass spectrometry in biotechnology, 2nd ed.; MCC Press: San Diego, 2005. J Assoc Lab Autom. 2004;9:50–63.
3. Hou T-Y, Chiang-Ni C, Teng S-H. Current status of MALDI-TOF mass spectrometry in clinical microbiology. J Food Drug Anal. 2019;27:404–14.
4. Rankin-Turner S, Sears P, Heaney LM. Applications of ambient ionization mass spectrometry in 2022: an annual review. Anal Sci Adv. 2023;4:133–53.

5. Li L-H, Hsieh H-Y, Hsu C-C. Clinical application of ambient ionization mass spectrometry. Mass Spect. 2017;6:S0060.
6. Seger C, Salzmann L. After another decade: LC-MS/MS became routine in clinical diagnostics. Clin Biochem. 2020;82:2–11.
7. Fung AWS, Sugumar V, Ren AH, Kulasingam V. Emerging role of clinical mass spectrometry in pathology. J Clin Pathol. 2020;73:61–9.
8. Thomas SN, French D, Jannetto PJ, Rappold BA, Clarke WA. Liquid chromatography–tandem mass spectrometry for clinical diagnostics. Nat Rev Methods Primers. 2022;2:96.
9. Thomson BA, Iribarne JV. Field induced ion evaporation from liquid surfaces at atmospheric pressure. J Chem Phys. 1979;71:4451–63.
10. Ho CS, Lam CWK, Chan MHM, Cheung RCK, Law LW, Lit LC, Ng KF, Suen MWM, Tai HL. Electrospray ionisation mass spectrometry: principles and clinical applications. Clin Biochem Rev. 2003;24:3–12.
11. Wilm M. Principles of electrospray ionization. Mol Cell Proteomics. 2011;10:M111.009407.
12. Disintegration of water drops in an electric field. Proc R Soc Lond A Math Phys Sci. 1964;280:383–97.
13. Liuni P, Wilson DJ. Understanding and optimizing electrospray ionization techniques for proteomic analysis. Expert Rev Proteom. 2011;8:197–209. https://doi.org/10.1586/epr.10.111.
14. Fenn JB, Mann M, Meng CK, Wong SF, Whitehouse CM. Electrospray ionization for mass spectrometry of large biomolecules. Science. 1989;1979(246):64–71.
15. Himmelsbach M. 10 years of MS instrumental developments—impact on LC–MS/MS in clinical chemistry. J Chromatogr B. 2012;883–884:3–17.
16. Meher AK, Chen Y-C. Electrospray modifications for advancing mass spectrometric analysis. Mass Spect. 2017;6:S0057.
17. Thurman EM, Ferrer I, Barceló D. Choosing between atmospheric pressure chemical ionization and electrospray ionization interfaces for the HPLC/MS analysis of pesticides. Anal Chem. 2001;73:5441–9.
18. Rebane R, Kruye A, Liigand PL, Liigand J, Herodes K, Leito I. Establishing atmospheric pressure chemical ionization efficiency scale. Anal Chem. 2016;88:3435–9.
19. Kamel A, Prakash C. High performance liquid chromatography/atmospheric pressure ionization/tandem mass spectrometry (HPLC/API/MS/MS) in drug metabolism and toxicology. Curr Drug Metab. 2006;7:837–52.
20. Awad H, Khamis MM, El-Aneed A. Mass spectrometry, review of the basics: ionization. Appl Spectrosc Rev. 2015;50:158–75.
21. Strmeň T, Vrkoslav V, Bosáková Z, Cvačka J. Atmospheric pressure chemical ionization mass spectrometry at low flow rates: importance of ion source housing. Rapid Commun Mass Spectrom. 2020;34:e8722.
22. Strmeň T, Vrkoslav V, Pačes O, Cvačka J. Evaluation of an ion source with a tubular nebulizer for microflow atmospheric pressure chemical ionization. Monatshefte für Chemie – Chemical Monthly. 2018;149:987–94.
23. Robb DB, Covey TR, Bruins AP. Atmospheric pressure photoionization: an ionization method for liquid chromatography−mass spectrometry. Anal Chem. 2000;72:3653–9.
24. Kauppila TJ, Syage JA, Benter T. Recent developments in atmospheric pressure photoionization-mass spectrometry. Mass Spectrom Rev. 2017;36:423–49.
25. Gaudin M, Imbert L, Libong D, Chaminade P, Brunelle A, Touboul D, Lapreyote O. Atmospheric pressure photoionization as a powerful tool for large-scale lipidomic studies. J Am Soc Mass Spectrom. 2012;23:869–79.
26. Cai S-S, Syage JA. Comparison of atmospheric pressure photoionization, atmospheric pressure chemical ionization, and electrospray ionization mass spectrometry for analysis of lipids. Anal Chem. 2006;78:1191–9.
27. Marchi I, Rudaz S, Veuthey J-L. Atmospheric pressure photoionization for coupling liquid-chromatography to mass spectrometry: a review. Talanta. 2009;78:1–18.
28. Stump MJ, Fleming RC, Gong WH, Jaber AJ, Jones JJ, Surber CW, Wilkins CL. Matrix-assisted laser desorption mass spectrometry. Appl Spectrosc Rev. 2002;37:275–303.

29. Zenobi R, Knochenmuss R. Ion formation in MALDI mass spectrometry. Mass Spectrom Rev. 1998;17:337–66.
30. Knochenmuss R. MALDI ionization mechanisms: an overview. In: Electrospray and MALDI mass spectrometry. Wiley; 2010. p. 147–83. https://doi.org/10.1002/9780470588901.ch5.
31. Santiago LS, Guerrero-Lopez A, Sevilla-Salcedo C, Rodriquez-Temporal D, Rodriguez-Sanchez B, Gomez-Verdejo V. Machine learning applied to MALDI-TOF data in a clinical setting: a systematic review. Lenguas Modernas. 2025:183–209. https://doi.org/10.1101/2025.01.25.634879.
32. Moore JL, Charkoftaki G. A guide to MALDI imaging mass spectrometry for tissues. J Proteome Res. 2023;22:3401–17.
33. Li D, Yi J, Han G, Qiao L. MALDI-TOF mass spectrometry in clinical analysis and research. ACS Meas Sci Au. 2022;2:385–404.
34. Mellors PW, Dasari S, Kohlhagen MC, Lourelis T, Go RS, Muchtar E, Gertz MA, Kumar SK, Baudi FK, Willrich MAB, Lust JA, Kapoor P, Lacy MQ, Dingli D, Hwa Y, Fonder A, Hobbs M, Hayman S, Warsame R, Leung NR, Lin Y, Gonsalves W, Sikddiqui M, Kyle RA, Rajkumar SV, Murray DL, Dispenzieri A. MASS-FIX for the detection of monoclonal proteins and light chain N-glycosylation in routine clinical practice: a cross-sectional study of 6315 patients. Blood Cancer J. 2021;11:50.
35. Kohlhagen M, Dasari S, Willrich M, Hetrick M, Netzel B, Dispenzieri A, Murray DL. Automation and validation of a MALDI-TOF MS (Mass-Fix) replacement of immunofixation electrophoresis in the clinical lab. Clin Chem Lab Med. 2020;59:155–63.
36. Müller WH, Verdin A, De Pauw E, Malherbe C, Eppe G. Surface-assisted laser desorption/ionization mass spectrometry imaging: a review. Mass Spectrom Rev. 2022;41:373–420.
37. Swiner DJ, Jackson S, Burris BJ, Badu-Tawiah AK. Applications of mass spectrometry for clinical diagnostics: the influence of turnaround time. Anal Chem. 2020;92:183–202.
38. Rankin-Turner S, Sears P, Heaney LM. Applications of ambient ionization mass spectrometry in 2022: an annual review. Analy Sci Adv. 2023;4:133–53.
39. Feider CL, Krieger A, DeHoog RJ, Eberlin LS. Ambient ionization mass spectrometry: recent developments and applications. Anal Chem. 2019;91:4266–90.
40. Cody RB, Laramée JA, Durst HD. Versatile new ion source for the analysis of materials in open air under ambient conditions. Anal Chem. 2005;77:2297–302.
41. Kuo T-H, Dutkiewicz EP, Pei J, Hsu C-C. Ambient ionization mass spectrometry today and tomorrow: embracing challenges and opportunities. Anal Chem. 2020;92:2353–63.
42. Choucair I, Shang E, Tran MN, Cassella-McLane G, El-Khoury JM. Direct analysis in real time mass spectrometry (DART-MS/MS) for rapid urine opioid detection in a clinical setting. Clin Chim Acta. 2025;564:119939.
43. Vasiljevic T, Gómez-Ríos GA, Li F, Liang P, Pawliszyn J. High-throughput quantification of drugs of abuse in biofluids via 96-solid-phase microextraction–transmission mode and direct analysis in real time mass spectrometry. R Comm Mass Spect. 2019;33:1423–33.
44. Gómez-Ríos GA, Pawliszyn J. Development of coated blade spray ionization mass spectrometry for the quantitation of target analytes present in complex matrices. Angew Chem Int Ed. 2014;53:14503–7.
45. Gómez-Ríos GA, Tascon M, Reyes-Garces N, Boyaci E, Pool JJ, Pawliszyn J. Rapid determination of immunosuppressive drug concentrations in whole blood by coated blade spray-tandem mass spectrometry (CBS-MS/MS). Anal Chim Acta. 2018;999:69–75.
46. Gómez-Ríos GA, Tascon M, Reyes-Garces N, Boyaci E, Pool JJ, Pawliszyn J. Quantitative analysis of biofluid spots by coated blade spray mass spectrometry, a new approach to rapid screening. Sci Rep. 2017;7:16104.
47. Zhou W, Nazdrajić E, Pawliszyn J. Rapid screening and quantitation of drugs of abuse by both positive and negative modes via coated blade spray–mass spectrometry. J Am Soc Mass Spectrom. 2022;33:1187–93.
48. Bogusiewicz J, et al. Determination of acylcarnitines in intact brain tumors using coated blade spray mass spectrometry (CBS-MS). Adv Sample Prep. 2025;13:100146.

49. Bogusiewicz J, Bojko B. Determination of endogenous metabolites in intact tissue in clinical settings using coated blade spray mass spectrometry (CBS-MS). Green Anal Chem. 2025;13:100244.
50. Takáts Z, Wiseman JM, Gologan B, Cooks RG. Mass spectrometry sampling under ambient conditions with desorption electrospray ionization. Science. 2004;1979(306):471–3.
51. Kumar BS. Desorption electrospray ionization mass spectrometry imaging (DESI-MSI) in disease diagnosis: an overview. Anal Methods. 2023;15:3768–84.
52. Morato NM, Cooks RG. Desorption electrospray ionization mass spectrometry: 20 years. Acc Chem Res. 2023;56:2526–36.
53. Ifa DR, Eberlin LS. Ambient ionization mass spectrometry for cancer diagnosis and surgical margin evaluation. Clin Chem. 2016;62:111–23.
54. Sans M, Jaroch K, Furtak J, Birski M, Soszynska K, Majdanska A, Ryfa A, Harat M, Bojko B. Performance of the masSpec pen for rapid diagnosis of ovarian cancer. Clin Chem. 2019;65:674–83.
55. Schäfer K-C, Denes J, Albrect K, Sxaniszlo T, Balog J, Skoumal R, Katona M, Toth M, Balogh L, Takats Z. In vivo, in situ tissue analysis using rapid evaporative ionization mass spectrometry. Angew Chem Int Ed Engl. 2009;48:8240–2.
56. Balog J, Sasi-Szabo L, Kinross J, Lewis R, Muirhead LJ, Veselkov K, Mirnezami R, Dezso B, Damjanovic L, Darzi A, Nicholson JK, Takas T. Intraoperative tissue identification using rapid evaporative ionization mass spectrometry. Transl Sci. 2013;5(194):194ra93.
57. St John ER, Balog J, McKenzie JS, Rossi M, Covington A, Muirhead L, Bodai Z, Rosini F, Speller AVM, Shousha S, Ramakrishnan R, Darzi A, Takats Z, Leff DR. Rapid evaporative ionisation mass spectrometry of electrosurgical vapours for the identification of breast pathology: towards an intelligent knife for breast cancer surgery. Breast Cancer Res. 2017;19:59.
58. Tzafetas M, Mitra A, Paraskevaidi M, Bodai Z, Kalliala I, Bowden S, Lathouras K, Rosini F, Szasz M, Savage A, Manoli E, Balog J, McKenzie J, Lyons D, Bennett P, MacIntyre D, Ghaem-Magham S, Takats Z, Kyrgiou M. The intelligent knife (iKnife) and its intraoperative diagnostic advantage for the treatment of cervical disease. Proc Nat Acad Sci. 2020;117:7338–46.
59. Phelps DL, et al. The surgical intelligent knife distinguishes normal, borderline and malignant gynaecological tissues using rapid evaporative ionisation mass spectrometry (REIMS). Br J Cancer. 2018;118:1349–58.
60. Cafarella C, Mangraviti D, Rigano F, Dugo P, Mondello L. Rapid evaporative ionization mass spectrometry: a survey through 15 years of applications. J Sep Sci. 2024;47:e2400155. https://doi.org/10.1002/jssc.202400155.
61. Jennings KR, Dolnikowski GG. Mass analyzers. Methods Enzymol. 1990;193(C):37–61. https://doi.org/10.1016/0076-6879(90)93410-M.
62. Lambris JD. Adv Exp Med Biol. http://www.springer.com/series/5584.
63. March RE. An introduction to quadrupole ion trap mass spectrometry. J Mass Spect. 1997;32:351–69. https://doi.org/10.1002/(SICI)1096-9888(199704)32:4<351::AID-JMS512>3.0.CO;2-Y.
64. Miller PE, Bonner Denton M. The quadrupole mass filter: basic operating concepts. UTC. 1986;63. https://pubs.acs.org/sharingguidelines
65. Hayes RN, Gross ML. Collision-induced dissociation. Methods Enzymol. 1990;193(C):237–63. https://doi.org/10.1016/0076-6879(90)93418-K.
66. Blakley CR, Vestal ML. Thermospray interface for liquid chromatography/mass spectrometry. Anal Chem. 1983;55(4):750–4. https://doi.org/10.1021/ac00255a036.
67. Arpino PJ, Guiochon G. LC/MS coupling. Anal Chem. 1979;51:7. https://doi.org/10.1021/ac50043a001.
68. Stafford GC, Kelley PE, Syka JEP, Reynolds WE, Todd JFJ. Recent improvements in and analytical applications of advanced ion trap technology. Int J Mass Spectrom Ion Process. 1984;60(1):85–98. https://doi.org/10.1016/0168-1176(84)80077-4.
69. Cotter RJ. The new time-of-flight mass spectrometry. Anal Chem. 1999;71(13):445A.
70. Mamyrin BA, Karataev VI, Shmikk DV, Zagulin VA. The mass-reflectron, a new nonmagnetic time-of-flight mass spectrometer with high resolution. Sov Phys JETP. 1973;37(1).

71. Juhasz P, Vestal ML, Martin SA. On the initial velocity of ions benerated by matrix-assisted laser desorption ionization and its effect on the calibration of delayed extraction time-of-flight mass spectra. J Am Soc Mass Spectrom. 1997;8(3):209–17. https://doi.org/10.1016/S1044-0305(96)00256-5.
72. Vestal ML, Juhasz P, Martin SA. Delayed extraction matrix-assisted laser desorption time-of-flight mass spectrometry. Rap Comm Mass Spect. 1995;9(11):1044–50. https://doi.org/10.1002/rcm.1290091115.
73. Karas M, Bahr U. Laser desorption ionization mass spectrometry of large biomolecules. Trends Anal Chem. 1990;9:321–5. https://doi.org/10.1016/0165-9936(90)85065-F.
74. Hu Q, Noll RJ, Li H, Makarov A, Hardman M, Cooks RG. The orbitrap: a new mass spectrometer. J Mass Spect. 2005;40(4):430–43. https://doi.org/10.1002/jms.856.
75. Perry RH, Cooks RG, Noll RJ. Orbitrap mass spectrometry: instrumentation, ion motion and applications. Mass Spect Rev. 2008;27(6):661–99. https://doi.org/10.1002/mas.20186.
76. Scigelova M, Hornshaw M, Giannakopulos A, Makarov A. Fourier transform mass spectrometry. Mol Cell Proteomics. 2011;10(7):M111.009431. https://doi.org/10.1074/mcp.M111.009431.
77. Qi Y, Volmer DA. Electron-based fragmentation methods in mass spectrometry: an overview. Mass Spect Rev. 2017;36(1):4–15. https://doi.org/10.1002/mas.21482.
78. Brodbelt JS, Morrison LJ, Santos I. Ultraviolet photodissociation mass spectrometry for analysis of biological molecules. Chem Rev. 2020;120(7):3328–80. https://doi.org/10.1021/acs.chemrev.9b00440.
79. Madsen JA, Cullen TW, Trent MS, Brodbelt JS. IR and UV photodissociation as analytical tools for characterizing lipid A structures. Anal Chem. 2011;83(13):5107–13. https://doi.org/10.1021/ac103271w.
80. Yost RA, E. C. G. Triple quadrupole mass spectrometry for direct mixture analysis and structure elucidation. Anal Chem. 1979;51(12):1251–64. https://doi.org/10.1021/ac50048a002.
81. Domon B, Aebersold R. Mass spectrometry and protein analysis. Science. 1979;2006(312):212–7. https://doi.org/10.1126/science.1124619.
82. Yost RA, E. C. G. Selected ion fragmentation with a tandem quadrupole mass spectrometer. J Am Chem Soc. 1978;100(7):2274–5. https://doi.org/10.1021/ja00475a072.
83. Morris HR, Paxton T, Dell A, Langhorne J, Berg M, Bordoli RS, Hoyes J, Bateman RH. High sensitivity collisionally-activated decomposition tandem mass spectrometry on a novel quadrupole/orthogonal-acceleration time-of-flight mass spectrometer. Rap Comm Mass Spect. 1996;10(8):889–96. https://doi.org/10.1002/(SICI)1097-0231(19960610)10:8<889::AID-RCM615>3.0.CO;2-F.
84. Chernushevich IV, Loboda AV, Thomson BA. An introduction to quadrupole-time-of-flight mass spectrometry. J Mass Spect. 2001;36(8):849–65. https://doi.org/10.1002/jms.207.
85. Medzihradszky KF, Campbell JM, Baldwin MA, Falick AM, Juhasz P, Vestal ML, Burlingame AL. The characteristics of peptide collision-induced dissociation using a high-performance MALDI-TOF/TOF tandem mass spectrometer. Anal Chem. 2000;72(3):552–8. https://doi.org/10.1021/ac990809y.
86. Vestal ML, Campbell JM. Tandem time-of-flight mass spectrometry. Methods Enzymol. 2005;402:79–108. https://doi.org/10.1016/S0076-6879(05)02003-3.
87. Vogeser M, Seger C. Pitfalls associated with the use of liquid chromatography-tandem mass spectrometry in the clinical laboratory. Clin Chem. 2010;56:1234–44. https://doi.org/10.1373/clinchem.2009.138602.
88. Vogeser M, Habler K, Reuter A, Schneider-Thauern C. Research Letter: Pilot study of a prototype fully automated mass spectrometry system for routine clinical laboratory use. J Mass Spect Adv Clin Lab. Elsevier B.V. 2024;34:44–5. https://doi.org/10.1016/j.jmsacl.2024.10.004.
89. Junger S, Hoene M, Shipkova M, Danzl G, Schöberl C, Peter A, Lehmann R, Wieland E, Braitmaier H. Automated LC-MS/MS: Ready for the clinical routine laboratory? J Mass Spect Adv Clin Lab. 2023;30:1–9. https://doi.org/10.1016/j.jmsacl.2023.07.001.
90. Benton SC, Tetteh GK, Needham SJ, Mücke J, Sheppard L, Alderson S, Ruppen C, Curti M, Redondo M, Milan AM. Evaluation of the 25-hydroxy vitamin D assay on a fully automated

liquid chromatography mass spectrometry system, the Thermo Scientific Cascadion SM clinical analyzer with the Cascadion 25-hydroxy vitamin D assay in a routine clinical laboratory. Clin Chem Lab Med. 2020;58(6):1010–7. https://doi.org/10.1515/cclm-2019-0834.
91. Alexander J, Gildea L, Balog J, Speller A, McKenzie J, Muirhead L, Scott A, Kontovounisios C, Rasheed S, Teare J, Hoare J, Veselkov K, Goldin R, Tekkis P, Darzi A, Nicholson J, Kinross J, Takats Z. A novel methodology for in vivo endoscopic phenotyping of colorectal cancer based on real-time analysis of the mucosal lipidome: a prospective observational study of the IKnife. Surg Endosc. 2017;31(3):1361–70. https://doi.org/10.1007/s00464-016-5121-5.
92. Golf O, Strittmatter N, Karancsi T, Pringle SD, Speller AVM, Mroz A, Kinross JM, Abbassi-Ghadi N, Jones EA, Takats Z. Rapid evaporative ionization mass spectrometry imaging platform for direct mapping from bulk tissue and bacterial growth media. Anal Chem. 2015;87(5):2527–34. https://doi.org/10.1021/ac5046752.
93. Zhang J, Rector J, Lin JQ, Young JH, Sans M, Katta N, Giese N, Yu W, Nagi C, Suliburk J, Liu J, Bensussan A, Dehoog RJ, Garza KY, Ludolph B, Sorace AG, Syed A, Zahedivash A, Milner TE, Eberlin LS. Nondestructive tissue analysis for ex vivo and in vivo cancer diagnosis using a handheld mass spectrometry system. Sci Transl Med. 2017;9(406):eaan3968. https://doi.org/10.1126/scitranslmed.aan3968.
94. Cumeras R, Figueras E, Davis CE, Baumbach JI, Gràcia I. Review on ion mobility spectrometry. Part 1: current instrumentation. Analyst. Royal Society of Chemistry; 2015. p. 1376–90. https://doi.org/10.1039/c4an01100g.
95. Beck AG, Muhoberac M, Randolph CE, Beveridge CH, Wijewardhane PR, Kenttämaa HI, Chopra G. Recent developments in machine learning for mass spectrometry. ACS Meas Sci Au American Chemical Society. 2024;4:233–46. https://doi.org/10.1021/acsmeasurescia u.3c00060.

Fundamentals of Liquid Chromatography

3

David S. Hage

Introduction

Analysis of the contents of complex clinical samples often requires the use of a chemical separation step. *Liquid chromatography* (*LC*) is one common approach used for this purpose. LC is a form of chromatography, which is a separation method based on the different interactions of applied compounds with a mobile phase vs a stationary phase [1–4]. In LC, the mobile phase is a liquid solvent or solution. LC is often used in modern clinical laboratories in combination with mass spectrometry (MS) or tandem mass spectrometry (MS/MS). These combinations are referred to as liquid chromatography-mass spectrometry (LC–MS) or liquid chromatography-tandem mass spectrometry (LC-MS/MS), respectively [5, 6].

The general principle behind LC is illustrated in Fig. 3.1 In this example, a sample containing a mixture of compounds is applied at one end of a tube or column that contains a support material and an interacting surface or fixed chemical layer that acts as the stationary phase. A liquid is then applied as the mobile phase and allowed to pass through the column, carrying the sample components with it. The compounds in the sample that interact the most with the stationary phase will take the longest time to pass through the column, after which they will be detected or collected. The result is a separation of the sample components based on these interactions and the relative amount of time each component spends in the mobile phase compared to the stationary phase [2].

LC is like gas chromatography (GC) in that both techniques use a stationary phase and a mobile phase to separate the components of an applied sample. However, LC uses a liquid as the mobile phase while GC employs a gas [1–3]. This change in

D. S. Hage (✉)
Department of Chemistry, University of Nebraska-Lincoln, Lincoln, NE, USA
e-mail: dhage1@unl.edu

Y. V. Zhang, U. Garg (eds.), *Practical Guide to Implementing Liquid Chromatography Mass Spectrometry in Clinical Laboratories*,
https://doi.org/10.1007/978-3-032-03852-4_3

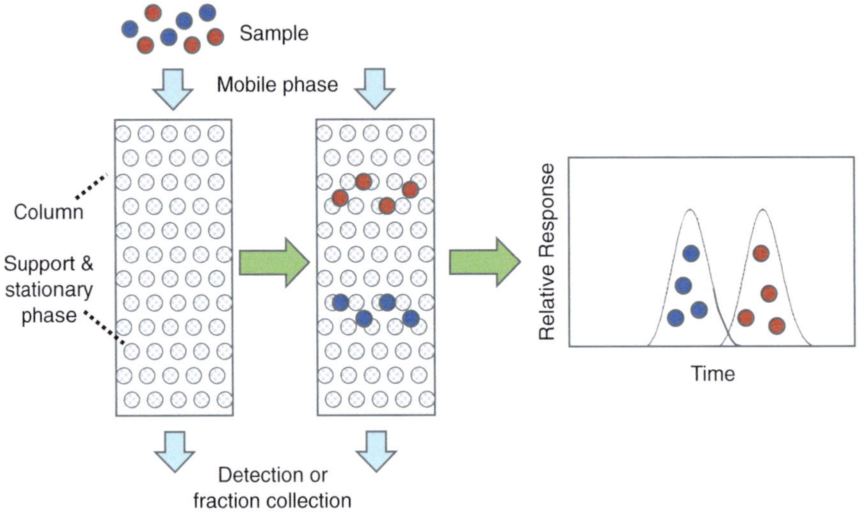

Fig. 3.1 Principles underlying the separation of chemicals by liquid chromatography, as illustrated here for a mixture of two components that are passed in a mobile phase and through a column that contains a support with a stationary phase that has different degrees of interactions with these components

mobile phase means these two methods differ in their advantages or limitations. For instance, the faster diffusion of chemicals in gases compared to liquids means peaks in GC tend to be much sharper than in LC; this also means more compounds can usually be separated in GC in a shorter time than in LC. A significant limitation of GC is that it requires the chemicals in the injected samples to be either sufficiently volatile to enter the gas phase passing through the column or capable of being converted into a volatile derivative before they are injected and separated. This is a much stricter requirement than LC, where sample components must only be soluble in a liquid. This difference means LC can be used with many chemicals that cannot be examined by GC, including large biomolecules (e.g., proteins or nucleic acids) or organic polymers. The lower temperatures that are used in LC compared to GC also make LC a better choice for the separation of chemicals that may be thermally unstable. Finally, the mobile phase in GC typically has little or no interactions with the applied chemicals, due to the low density of gases. In contrast to this, the mobile phase in LC can play a role in affecting chemical retention. This provides an additional parameter in LC that can be used to adjust the separation of a sample mixture.

The earliest columns used in LC were packed with large and irregular particles as the support. The use of such a support resulted in separations that had broad peaks with low resolution. This form of LC is sometimes referred to as "column chromatography" or "classical liquid chromatography" and is still often used for the pretreatment of samples. However, smaller and more uniform supports for LC columns began to appear in the 1960s. These supports made it possible to obtain sharper peaks that provided separations with higher resolutions and shorter run times. This development resulted in a form of LC now called *high-performance liquid chromatography* (*HPLC*). HPLC is the most common form of LC that is used in chemical analysis [2]. Further decreases in the size and increases in the efficiencies of supports for LC over the last few decades have resulted in a subcategory of HPLC known as *ultrahigh-performance liquid chromatography* (*UPLC* or *UHPLC*), in which even sharper peaks and faster separations are possible [7]. Both HPLC and UPLC are now used with MS and MS/MS for the analysis of clinical and biological samples.

Description of Separations in Liquid Chromatography

General Description of a Chromatographic Separation

The result of a separation in LC and other types of chromatography is often represented by a plot showing the detector response for compounds leaving the system over time or as the volume of applied mobile phase is increased. This plot is known as a *chromatograph* and is illustrated in Fig. 3.2 [2, 3]. Such a plot can be used to identify an eluting compound by using the response obtained by the detector and the time or mobile phase volume the compound requires to exit the chromatographic system. The amount or concentration of this compound in the injected sample can also be determined from the area or height of the compound's peak if this compound is well resolved from other eluting components in the same chromatogram.

Figure 3.2 illustrates several terms that can be used to describe the position and shapes of peaks in a chromatogram [1, 3]. First, there is the column *void time*, as represented by t_M. The void time is the average time it takes the mobile phase or a compound that is completely non-retained by the stationary phase to pass through the column. The *void volume* (V_M) represents the corresponding volume of mobile phase that is present in the column, as well as the volume of mobile phase that is needed to carry a non-retained substance through this column. If a compound does have interactions with the stationary phase, this chemical will take longer to pass

Fig. 3.2 Plot of response vs. time obtained for a separation in liquid chromatography

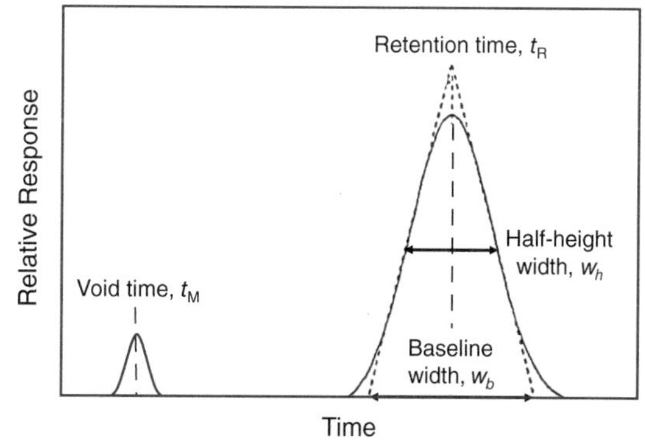

through the column than a non-retained substance. The average time it takes this retained compound to elute is called the *retention time* (t_R). The volume of mobile phase that is needed to move this retained compound through the column is the *retention volume* (V_R). The terms t_R and V_R, as well as t_M and V_M, are related to each other through the flow-rate (F) of the mobile phase, where $V_R = F\, t_R$ and $V_M = F\, t_M$.

Describing Retention and Efficiency

The values of t_R and V_R increase as an injected compound has stronger interactions with the stationary phase in an LC column. This retention in LC will depend on the structure of the compound and the type of stationary phase that is present, along with the type of mobile phase that is being used. This relationship can be represented by a parameter known as the *retention factor* (k). The retention factor can be calculated by comparing t_R to t_M through the use of the following equation [1, 3].

$$k = \left(t_R - t_M\right) / t_M \tag{3.1}$$

The value of k can also be determined by using V_R and V_M in the equivalent relationship $k = (V_R - V_M)/V_M$. The retention factor not only provides an overall measure of compound retention in chromatography but it also gives a way of determining how various properties of the system affect this retention. For example, Eq. 3.2 indicates the general factors that affect retention and the value of k for a compound that partitions between the mobile phase and the stationary phase in a column.

$$k = K_D \left(V_S / V_M\right) \tag{3.2}$$

This equation shows that the level of retention in this type of system is related to both the distribution equilibrium constant (K_D) for the compound in going from the mobile phase to the stationary phase and to the ratio of the volumes of the stationary phase (V_S) vs mobile phase (V_M, the void volume) in this system [2].

Another important feature of each peak in a chromatogram is its width. As is shown in Fig. 3.2, two ways of describing this feature are by using the width of a peak at its baseline (w_b) or the width of the peak at its half-height (w_h) [3]. These widths are determined by the processes that lead to broadening of a peak as its corresponding compound passes through the column. These processes are listed below [2].

- Movement of a compound around particles through multiple paths (eddy diffusion).
- Movement between particles (mobile phase mass transfer).
- Diffusion into and out of the particles (stagnant mobile phase mass transfer).
- Movement between the mobile phase and the stationary phase (stationary phase mass transfer).
- Diffusion along the length of the column (longitudinal diffusion).

Together, these processes lead to peak-broadening and, along with retention, determine the overall separation that is obtained between compounds in chromatography.

The values w_b and w_h for a given peak are both affected by the retention time or retention volume for this peak. It is possible to compare the peak-broadening, or column "efficiency," for compounds with different levels of retention by instead using the *number of theoretical plates* (*N*), or the *plate number* [1–3]. Equation 3.3 shows how *N* can be determined by using the values of t_R and w_b or w_h for a peak with a Gaussian shape.

$$N = 16\left(t_R / w_b\right)^2 \quad \text{or} \quad N = 5.545\left(t_R / w_h\right)^2 \tag{3.3}$$

A chromatographic system with a large value for *N* will tend to have narrow peaks, making it easier to use this system for the separation of injected compounds. The term *N* can be viewed as the number of times a compound is able to reach a local equilibrium in a column as this compound transfers between the mobile phase and the stationary phase. As the number of these steps increases, it becomes easier for a column to separate substances with small differences in their retention.

The expression in Eq. 3.3 assumes the peaks that are obtained in a chromatographic separation have a symmetrical, Gaussian shape. However, non-symmetrical peaks can also be obtained due to factors such as overloading a column, slow rates of binding or dissociation of compounds within the column, and the presence of multiple forms of interactions between a compound and the stationary phase. These effects can result in either *peak tailing* or *peak fronting* (i.e., peaks with a broader tailing edge than front or peaks with a sharper back than front, respectively). The extent to which a peak may be non-uniform in shape can be determined by measuring its *A/B ratio*, or *asymmetry factor* [2]. As shown in Fig. 3.3, the asymmetry factor can be found by comparing, at a given height of the peak, the distance from the peak maximum to the tail of the peak (A) and the distance from the peak maximum to the front of the peak (B). This measurement is often made at a height that is either one-half or one-tenth the distance between the baseline and the peak maximum. A symmetrical, Gaussian-shaped curve will give a ratio for *A* vs *B* that is equal to one. Peak tailing will give a value for *A/B* that is greater than one, and peak fronting will give a *A/B* value that is less than one.

One problem with *N* is that it depends on the length of a chromatographic column. A more general way of comparing peak-broadening and efficiency between columns is to use the *height equivalent of a theoretical plate*, or *plate height* (H or HETP). The value of *H* is found by using Eq. 3.4 along with values of *N* and the length of the column (*L*) [1–3].

$$H = L / N \tag{3.4}$$

The plate height represents the distance along the column that is needed for one theoretical equilibration step (or "plate") for an injected compound as it moves between the mobile phase and the stationary phase. Just as a large value for *N* is

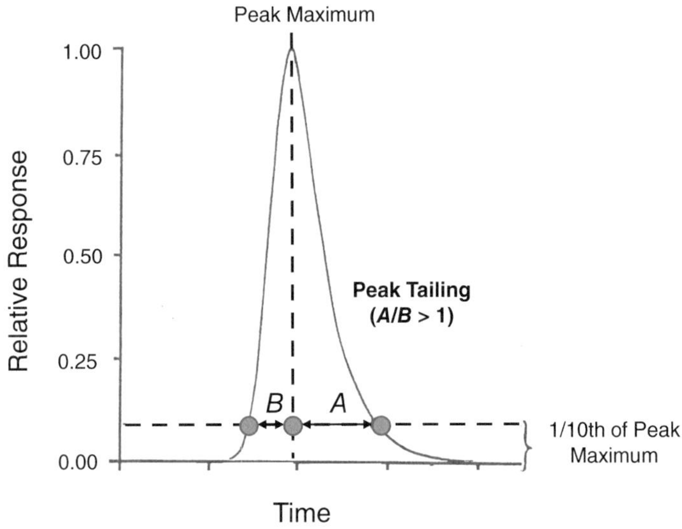

Fig. 3.3 Describing the asymmetry of a chromatographic peak

ideally needed to produce a chromatographic separation with narrow peaks, a small value for H is desirable. Another useful feature of H is that it can be used to see how changing a parameter such as flow rate will affect the overall peak-broadening that is obtained in a chromatographic separation. The *van Deemter equation*, as given in Eq. 3.5, is one example of such a relationship [2, 4]. This equation shows how H changes as the flow rate or linear velocity u, which is directly proportional to flow rate, is varied for a chromatographic separation.

$$H = A + B / u + Cu \tag{3.5}$$

In the van Deemter equation, A, B, and C are constants that represent the various processes that lead to the broadening of peaks in chromatography. For instance, the A term gives the contributions to peak-broadening from eddy diffusion and mobile phase mass transfer; the B term shows the effects of longitudinal diffusion; and the C term provides the combined effects of stagnant mobile phase mass transfer and stationary phase mass transfer. A plot made of Eq. 3.5 will ideally give a "U"-shaped curve in which the plate height will have its lowest value, and the column will have its best efficiency, at some optimum flow-rate.

Evaluating Compound Separations in Chromatography

There are several ways of evaluating the overall extent to which two peaks are separated by chromatography (see Fig. 3.4) [1, 2]. The first term that is used for this purpose is the *separation factor* (α) [3]. This value provides a measure of the relative retention of one compound compared to another in a chromatographic system.

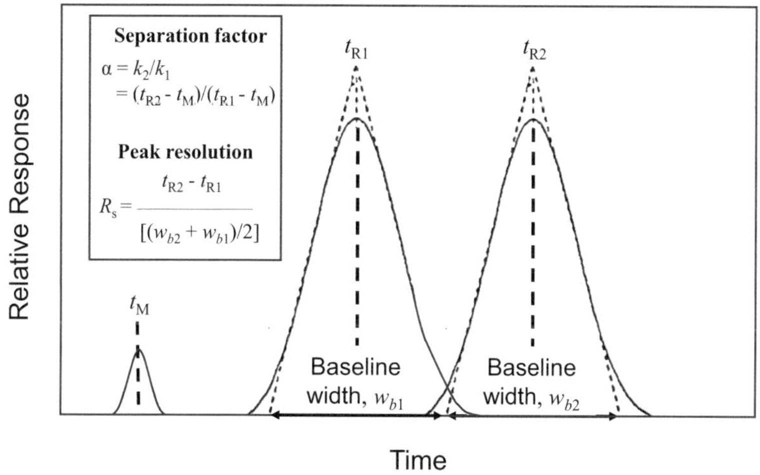

Fig. 3.4 Use of retention times and peak widths to describe the separation between two compounds in chromatography, such as through the separation factor (α) and peak resolution (R_s)

Equation 3.6 is used to calculate the value of α by taking the ratio of the retention factors for the second eluting compound (k_2) vs the first eluting compound (k_1), where k_2 will have a value that is greater than or equal to k_1. An equivalent expression can be written in which α is found by taking the ratio of ($t_{R2} - t_M$) vs ($t_{R1} - t_M$).

$$\alpha = k_2 / k_1 \qquad \text{or} \qquad \alpha = \left(t_{R2} - t_M\right) / \left(t_{R1} - t_M\right) \tag{3.6}$$

For two compounds to be separated by chromatography, it is necessary that their separation factor be greater than one. The peaks for these compounds will become better separated as the size of α is increased. However, one problem with the separation factor is it only considers the difference in retention for the eluting compounds and not the widths of their peaks.

The *peak resolution* (R_s) is another term that can be used to evaluate the extent of separation between two peaks in chromatography [1–3]. The resolution between the peaks for two compounds (1 and 2) can be found by using Eq. 3.7 along with the retention times and baseline widths for these peaks.

$$R_s = \frac{t_{R2} - t_{R1}}{\left[\left(w_{b2} + w_{b1}\right)/2\right]} \tag{3.7}$$

This term considers both the difference in retention of the two compounds and their peak widths in describing the extent of their separation. A value of zero for R_s represents no degree of separation, and R_s increases as the two peaks become better resolved [2]. A value of 1.5 or greater for R_s is often seen as representing *baseline resolution*; this level of peak resolution is sufficient for most applications of chromatography and provides separations that can be used in either peak height or area measurements. In some situations, an R_s value between 1.0 and 1.5 may be acceptable, such as when only the heights of peaks are to be used for compound quantitation and the peaks being separated are similar in size.

The general factors that affect peak separations in chromatography can be illustrated by using the following alternative equation for the peak resolution, R_s [2].

$$R_s = \left[(\mathrm{N})^{1/2}/4\right]\left[(\alpha-1)/\alpha\right]\left[k_2/(1+k_2)\right] \tag{3.8}$$

In this equation, N is again the number of theoretical plates that are obtained in the separation, α is the separation factor between two neighboring peaks, and k_2 is the retention factor for the most strongly retained of these two peaks. The relationship in Eq. 3.8 is known as the *resolution equation*. This equation shows that there are three ways to improve or alter a separation in chromatography.

- Changing factors that affect peak-broadening in the column (N).
- Adjusting the selectivity of the chromatographic system for retaining one compound compared to the other (α).
- Increasing the overall extent of retention for the compounds (k_2).

For instance, peak-broadening can be improved by using a longer or more efficient column, while retention or selectivity in LC can be adjusted by changing the mobile or stationary phase of the system [2].

Mobile Phases and Elution Methods in Liquid Chromatography

The mobile phase in LC plays an important role, along with the stationary phase, in determining the retention that is obtained for a given compound in a column. This means it is necessary to have a means of describing the extent to which a particular mobile phase will affect this retention. This is done by using the general terms *strong mobile phase* and *weak mobile phase* [2]. A strong mobile phase in LC is a liquid or solution that causes a compound to have low retention and to quickly elute from a column. Such low retention will occur when the mobile phase has similar types of interactions with the compound vs interactions involving the stationary phase, thus causing the compound to spend more time in the mobile phase and to elute sooner. A weak mobile phase represents the opposite situation, in which a compound will have strong interactions with the stationary phase and will take a long time to elute from a column. In this case, the mobile phase is quite different from the stationary phase in its interactions, allowing the compound to have its best retention on the stationary phase and the column. Whether a given liquid or solution is a strong or weak mobile phase will depend on the type of stationary phase that is present in the system. As an example, a polar liquid like water will be a weak mobile phase for a stationary phase that is non-polar but a strong mobile phase with a polar stationary phase.

If a complex mixture of compounds is present in a sample, it may be difficult to find one set of a mobile phase and stationary phase that will give good resolution between all these peaks and lead to their elution from the system in a reasonable amount of time. This situation can occur when a single mobile phase is used during a separation in chromatography, an approach known as *isocratic elution* [1–3]. A common way in LC to overcome the poor resolution or long elution of some sample components in this situation is to instead change the mobile phase that is passed through the column over time. The process of changing any chromatographic condition over time is called *gradient elution*. The use of gradient elution to change the mobile phase is known as *solvent programming* [1, 2, 4]. Examples of solvent programming and isocratic elution, the latter in which the mobile phase composition is not changed but kept constant, are shown in Fig. 3.5.

Solvent programming begins by first passing a weak mobile phase through a column. A weak mobile phase (i.e., often referred to as solvent "A") is used to allow the best retention and resolution of compounds that may have only low-strength interactions with the stationary phase. The composition of the mobile phase is then changed to a strong mobile phase (i.e., solvent "B"). The rate of this change is selected to allow compounds with moderate or strong interactions with the stationary phase to also be well separated. The final strength of the mobile phase is further selected to allow the sample components with the highest retention to leave the column in a reasonable amount of time. After all the sample components have been eluted, the mobile phase composition is changed back to the original weak mobile phase A and the process is repeated for the next injection. Solvent programming can be carried out in one step or many steps and may use either a linear change in mobile phase composition or a non-linear change over time. A linear change from solvent A to B is the most common format.

Along with the type of stationary phase that is being used, there are additional items to consider when selecting a mobile phase for LC. For instance, the sample

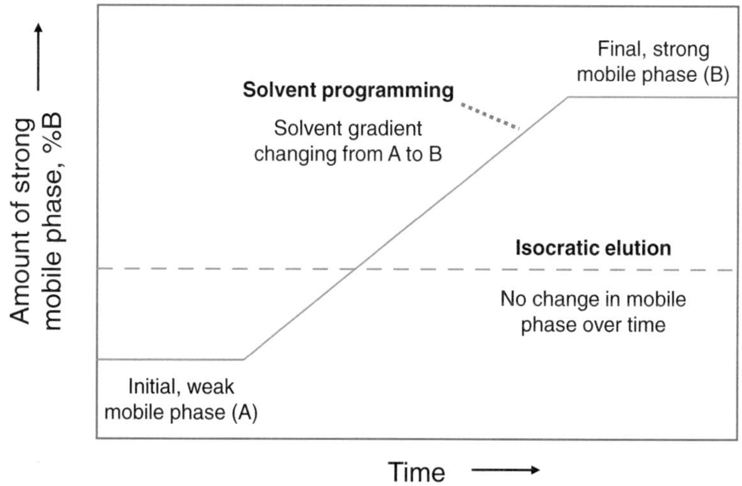

Fig. 3.5 Examples of solvent programming (solid line) and isocratic elution (horizontal dashed line) in liquid chromatography

components should be soluble in the mobile phases that will be used for applying these chemicals to the column. If solvent programming is to be used, the weak and strong mobile phases need to be fully miscible with each other at the ratios over which they will be combined. The background signal and purity of the mobile phase are important to consider as well if a detector is being used may have a response to this mobile phase or trace contaminants in this liquid.

Other parameters can also be varied as part of gradient programming in LC. For example, temperature programming is sometimes used to improve LC separations based on size-exclusion chromatography or ion-exchange chromatography, two methods discussed later in this chapter. However, temperature programming is much less common in LC than in GC. The flow rate may also be varied in LC to adjust the retention of compounds. One issue with this latter approach is that the pressure across the column will increase as the flow rate is increased, so care must be taken to avoid exceeding the pressure limits of the chromatographic system.

Stationary Phases in Liquid Chromatography

Partition Chromatography

There are five categories of LC based on the stationary phase that is present in the column, as listed below [1–3].

- Partition chromatography.
- Ion-exchange chromatography.
- Size-exclusion chromatography.
- Adsorption chromatography.
- Affinity chromatography.

A summary of these categories is provided in Table 3.1. Further details on each method are given in the following sections.

The first type of LC is *partition chromatography*. In this method, compounds are separated as they pass through a column by partitioning and moving between the mobile phase and a coating or layer of a stationary phase. Most modern LC systems use chemically bonded layers of the stationary phase for this method rather than liquid coatings. This stationary phase layer can be either non-polar or polar, which will then have its strongest retention for non-polar or polar compounds, respectively.

Reversed-phase liquid chromatography (*RPLC*) is the most common form of partition chromatography and of LC that is used in clinical and pharmaceutical applications [8, 9]. This type of partition chromatography uses a non-polar stationary phase. The most common stationary phases in RPLC are bonded phases based on octyl (C_8) or octadecyl (C_{18}) chains (see Fig. 3.6). Because RPLC has a non-polar stationary phase, the weak mobile phase for this method will be polar, such as water or an aqueous buffer. The strong mobile phase will be a less polar liquid, such as an organic solvent (e.g., methanol or acetonitrile) or a mixture of water with this organic

Table 3.1 Types of liquid chromatography based on the separation mechanism and stationary phase

LC method	Stationary phase
Partition chromatography	Liquid coating or bonded phase into which compounds can partition
Reversed-phase liquid chromatography	Non-polar coating or bonded phase
Normal-phase liquid chromatography	Polar coating or bonded phase
Ion-exchange chromatography	Fixed charges on a support that retain ions of the opposite charge
Cation-exchange chromatography	Fixed negatively-charged groups to bind cations
Anion-exchange chromatography	Fixed positively-charged groups to bind anions
Size-exclusion chromatography	Porous support that can separate compounds based on size
Gel filtration chromatography	Porous support that can be used with an aqueous mobile phase
Gel permeation chromatography	Porous support that can be used with an organic mobile phase
Other LC methods	Various stationary phases, depending on the method
Adsorption chromatography	Support with polar or non-polar surface that can adsorb chemicals
Affinity chromatography	Biologically-related agent that can specifically retain target compounds
Ion-pair chromatography	Non-polar phase that is used with ion-pairing agent to retain ions

Reversed-Phase Liquid Chromatography (RPLC)

Stationary Phase	Structure
Octyl Phase (C_8)	*Support*-$(CH_2)_7CH_3$
Octadecyl Phase (C_{18})	*Support*-$(CH_2)_{17}CH_3$

Normal-Phase Liquid Chromatography (NPLC)

Stationary Phase	Structure
Aminopropyl Phase (NH_2)	*Support*-$CH_2CH_2CH_2NH_2$
Diol Phase (Diol)	*Support*-$(CH_2)_3OCH_2CH(OH)CH_2(OH)$
Cyanopropyl Phase (CN)	*Support*-$CH_2CH_2CH_2CN$

Fig. 3.6 Common stationary phases used in reversed-phase liquid chromatography (RPLC) and normal-phase liquid chromatography (NPLC)

solvent. The fact that water is a weak mobile phase, as would be used for sample injections, and the fact that separations in this method are based on the general property of polarity make RPLC valuable in separating compounds that are present in clinical samples. In addition, RPLC is easy to combine with MS, so it is often the type of liquid chromatography that is used in LC-MS or LC-MS/MS [5, 6, 9].

Normal-phase liquid chromatography (*NPLC*) is another form of partition chromatography. This method uses a polar coating or bonded phase as the stationary phase, giving it retention properties that are opposite those of RPLC [1, 2]. Examples of stationary phases that are utilized in NPLC are bonded phases that contain aminopropyl, diol or cyanopropyl groups (Fig. 3.6). These are all polar phases that will have their strongest interactions with polar compounds. The fact that the stationary phase is polar in NPLC means that a nonpolar solvent will be the weak mobile phase, and the strong mobile phase will be a more polar liquid. The need for a nonpolar liquid as the weak mobile phase and for sample injections has made NPLC less common than RPLC in clinical and pharmaceutical applications. This method is sometimes employed, however, for compounds of clinical interest that have both a few polar functional groups and good solubility in organic solvents. Examples of such compounds are lipids and steroids [8, 9].

Another type of partitioning LC that uses a polar stationary phase is *hydrophilic interaction liquid chromatography* (*HILIC*). This method separates compounds based on their partitioning between an organic solvent in the mobile phase and a water-enriched layer near the surface of a polar support [8]. Gradient elution in HILIC begins with a weak mobile phase that is an organic solvent such as acetonitrile that contains a small amount of water. The water content of this mixture is then increased as a switch is made to a strong mobile phase that promotes compound elution. The support in HILIC may contain either a noncharged polar surface, as is found on underivatized silica, or a surface that contains polar bonded phases (i.e., like those used in traditional NPLC). The surface of the support may also have charges based on carboxylic acids, protonated amines, or zwitterionic groups. HILIC is complementary to RPLC in that it can retain polar or charged compounds that may have only weak retention on a RPLC column. Examples of compounds of clinical interest that have been separated by this method are amino acids, small organic acids, sugars, nucleosides, and phosphate-containing agents [8, 9]. Another valuable feature of HILIC is that it can be used in LC-MS [9].

Ion-Exchange Chromatography

Ion-exchange chromatography (*IEC*) is a second type of LC based on the stationary phase and separation mechanism. This method employs the adsorption of ionic compounds to a support that contains complementary fixed charges, which acts as the stationary phase [1–3]. Examples of ionic substances in clinical samples that can be separated and analyzed by this approach are small inorganic and organic ions, amino acids, peptides, proteins and nucleic acids [8, 9].

Cation-Exchange Chromatography

Stationary Phase	Structure
Sulfonic Acid (Strong Acid)	*Support*-$SO_3^-H^+$
Carboxylic Acid (Weak Acid)	*Support*-COO^-H^+

Anion-Exchange Chromatography

Stationary Phase	Structure
Quaternary Amine (Strong Base)	*Support*-$CH_2N(CH_3)_3^+Cl^-$
Diethylaminoethyl (Weak Base)	*Support*-$O(CH_2)_2NH^+Cl^-$ with two CH_2CH_3 groups on N

Fig. 3.7 Examples of stationary phases used in cation-exchange chromatography and anion-exchange chromatography

IEC can be divided into two types based on the charge that is present as the stationary phase: *cation-exchange chromatography* and *anion-exchange chromatography* (see Fig. 3.7) [1–3]. Cation-exchange chromatography is used to retain and separate positively-charged compounds, or cations. This type of IEC uses a column that contains negatively-charged groups (i.e., an anion-exchange column). For instance, the stationary phase in cation-exchange chromatography may use the ionized form of a strong acid, such as a negative sulfonate group, or the conjugate base of a weak acid, such as a carboxylate group. Anion-exchange chromatography retains negatively-charged compounds, or anions, and uses a column that contains positively-charged groups (i.e., a cation-exchange column). Examples of stationary phases in anion-exchange chromatography are the protonated forms of quaternary amines and tertiary amines (i.e., the conjugate acids of strong and weak bases). Supports that may be used in IEC with these stationary phases are polystyrene (e.g., as used in work with small organic and inorganic ions), carbohydrate-based materials like agarose or cross-linked dextran and cellulose gels (e.g., for work with large and ionic biological molecules) and silica (e.g., for use in some HPLC-based applications).

The mobile phase strength in IEC is usually controlled by altering the concentration of ions that are added to compete with ions in the sample for the charged groups on the stationary phase [2]. A strong mobile phase in IEC will be a solution that has a high concentration of these competing ions, and a weak mobile phase will have a low concentration of these ions. Another factor that can be varied to adjust retention in IEC is the pH, which may cause a change in retention when the charges on either the sample ions or the stationary phase are pH-dependent. Changing the type of competing ions or adding complexing agents that can alter the charges on sample components can also be used to adjust retention in IEC.

In a special type of IEC known as *ion chromatography* (*IC*), a stationary phase with a small amount of charged sites is used along with a low concentration of competing ions in the mobile phase. A second suppressor column or membrane is also utilized to lower the background conductivity of the mobile phase [2, 10]. These changes are made to the system to allow coupling of the IEC column with a conductivity detector, as described later, that can then monitor ions after they are separated. One benefit of IC is it can be coupled with MS through the suppressor system to convert the final mobile phase to an aqueous solution that has only a small level of competing ions. This eluent may then be further combined with an organic solvent for use in electrospray ionization and LC-MS.

Size-Exclusion Chromatography

The third form of LC, based on the stationary phase and separation mechanism, is *size-exclusion chromatography* (*SEC*). This LC technique is used to separate compounds according to their size and ability to enter the various mobile phase regions within a porous support [1–3]. In this situation, the mobile phase in the support's pores is what acts as the stationary phase. As components in the sample travel through a column in SEC, small compounds will be able to enter more pores than larger compounds. This will cause the larger compounds to elute first and produce a separation that is based on the size or mass of components in the sample.

There are two types of SEC based on the solvent and support that are being used [2]. If an aqueous mobile phase and water-compatible support are used in SEC, this method is known as *gel filtration chromatography*. This is the form of SEC that is employed with biological molecules and aqueous samples, such as for removing salts or small solutes from proteins [8]. The supports in this approach are often carbohydrate-based materials like agarose and dextran or hydrophilic polymers like polyacrylamide. If an organic solvent is used as the mobile phase in SEC, along with an organic-compatible support, the resulting method is called *gel permeation chromatography*. This type of SEC is utilized in separating and characterizing organic polymers and often has polystyrene or a related material as the porous support [2].

Other Chromatographic Methods

There are also other forms of LC based on the stationary phase and separation mechanism. One of these other methods is *adsorption chromatography*, in which compounds are separated through their differences in adsorption to a support's surface [1–3, 11]. Another name that is sometimes used for this technique is "liquid-solid chromatography". This method has the same material acting as both the support and, at its surface, the stationary phase.

The supports used in adsorption chromatography can have either a polar or non-polar surface. Common supports used for this purpose and that have polar surfaces include silica and alumina. Both these materials have their strongest retention for polar compounds and have a non-polar organic solvent as the weak mobile phase. Adsorption chromatography based on silica or alumina can be useful in isolating compounds like steroids that contain some polar groups but also dissolve well in nonpolar solvents. Silica and alumina supports are also commonly used in separating geometrical and structural isomers of organic compounds. Charcoal is an example of a non-polar support that can be utilized in adsorption chromatography. This non-polar support will have its strongest binding to non-polar compounds and with a polar solvent such as water acting as the weak mobile phase.

Affinity chromatography is a type of LC in which the separation employs a biological-related interaction [1, 12]. A common example is the binding that occurs between an antibody and its target, or antigen. The stationary phase in this method is an immobilized binding agent, called the affinity ligand, which can bind the desired compounds but not with many other components in the sample. The weak mobile phase in affinity chromatography is a buffer or solution that promotes strong binding between the desired compounds and the affinity ligand. The strong mobile phase is a solution or buffer that weakens or disrupts this binding to promote elution of the retained substances. Antibodies and related binding agents are the most common stationary phases used in affinity chromatography, although many other biological substances can be used for this purpose [12]. These other binding agents may include enzymes, antibody- or carbohydrate-binding proteins, dyes, boronates, aptamers, and molecularly imprinted polymers. These binding agents may be attached to supports that range from carbohydrate gels (e.g., agarose) to a polymeric material or silica support that contains a hydrophilic coating [2, 12].

Affinity chromatography is often used in sample pretreatment to isolate a compound or group of related substances from a sample prior to their analysis by a second method, such as LC–MS. This is often done by using immobilized antibodies as the stationary phase, giving a method known as *immunoaffinity chromatography* or *immunoextraction* [12]. As an analytical tool, affinity chromatography has been used with boronate columns in clinical laboratories for the measurement of glycated hemoglobin in diabetes [8]. Columns containing *chiral stationary phases*, as are frequently used to separate the stereoisomers of drugs in clinical or pharmaceutical samples, are another set of important tools that are based on affinity chromatography [8, 13, 14].

Ion-pair chromatography (*IPC*) is a separation method for ionic compounds that combines features of IEC and RPLC [8]. This method uses a non-polar column for RPLC with an additive to the mobile phase that is an ion-pairing agent for charged compounds. The ion-pairing agent usually contains a charged group at one end and a non-polar tail at the other. Examples of ion-pairing agents are sodium dodecyl sulfate, perchlorate, and *t*-butyl ammonium. The charged portion of this agent will interact with ionic compounds that have the opposite charge. This interaction either produces a neutral complex that can be retained on an RPLC column or a complex that is formed between the ions and the ion-pairing agent that is already retained by the RPLC stationary phase. IPC is useful in separating charged compounds that are weakly retained by RPLC or poorly resolved by IEC. Examples of clinical applications for IPC are the separations of catecholamines, nucleic acids, and various drugs [8, 9].

General Instrumentation for LC

A typical system for LC, in the form of HPLC, is shown in Fig. 3.8. The main components of this system include the following [2, 15].

- A source for the liquid mobile phase.
- A pumping system for the mobile phase.
- An injection system to apply the samples.
- A column that contains the stationary phase and support.
- A detector.

More advanced systems may contain multiple columns, more than one detector, a system for mobile phase recycling, or a fraction collector.

The mobile phase for HPLC is usually placed into one or more solvent reservoirs, such as bottles or flasks. Feed lines are inserted into these containers to take the mobile phase to the pumps. Usually, filters are put on the feed lines to keep particles in the mobile phase from entering the pumps and the remainder of the chromatographic system. The mobile phase container may also have helium or nitrogen passing through it, in a process known as *sparging*, to remove any dissolved air and oxygen from the mobile phase. Gas filters can also be used to remove these dissolved gases from the mobile phase [8].

The columns used in HPLC require pumps that can be used to deliver the mobile phase at pressures of several hundred to several thousand psi [8]. Most prior applications of HPLC have used systems with an upper pressure limit of 5000–6000 psi (34–41 MPa). Commercial instrumentation of UPLC is designed to go up to even higher pressures of 15,000 psi (103 MPa). The mobile phase pressures needed in HPLC and UPLC can be reached by using reciprocating pumps or syringe pumps. Reciprocating pumps are employed in HPLC and can be used to deliver the mobile

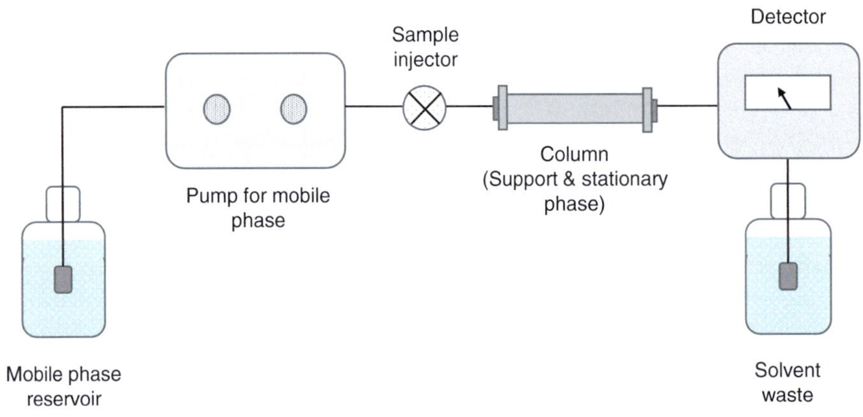

Fig. 3.8 General design of a system used in high-performance liquid chromatography (HPLC)

phase at flow-rates usually around the mL/min range. In this type of pump, a piston moving into and out of a solvent chamber is used with check valves to pressurize the mobile phase and flow it towards the column. A syringe pump also uses check values but instead acts by pushing a syringe head into the solvent chamber to pressurize and move the mobile phase to the column [8, 15]. An advantage of a syringe pump is it can deliver the mobile phase at lower flow-rates than reciprocal pumps (e.g., flow-rates down to the μL/min range), as may be required in UPLC.

The mobile phase can be changed during solvent programming by using either low- or high-pressuring mixing. In low-pressure missing, the contents of two or more mobile phase reservoirs are connected to a valve that alters the amount of each liquid that passes over time into a mixing chamber and through a single pump. In high-pressure mixing, one pump is used for each type of mobile phase. The liquids are each pressurized and mixed in this second method after they pass through the pumps by varying the flow-rate that is used to deliver each corresponding mobile phase.

Samples are typically applied to an HPLC column by using an injection valve that is either operated manually or as part of an automated injection system [8, 15]. This may involve the use of a fixed or variable injection volume. Some automated systems can inject several portions of the same sample or combine a sample and reagent for compound derivatization before injection. This type of pre-column derivatization can be used to improve the response of some compounds in LC to detectors that are based on absorbance, fluorescence, or an electrochemical response. The combination of eluting compounds with a reagent after a column can be used in a similar manner in post-column derivatization to enhance or change a compound's response on a detector.

Other than the column and detector (see following sections), there are several other instrumental components that may be present in an HPLC system [15]. For instance, a means of temperature control is often present for the column and/or samples. If post-column derivatization is to be utilized, separate pumps will be needed to apply the reagents for this process and a mixer plus reaction chamber will be required to combine the eluting components with these reagents. In some systems, a fraction collector may be included to obtain eluting components for use in other applications.

Columns and Supports for LC

Various types of columns and related components are used in LC for clinical analysis. An inlet filter is often used before the column in HPLC to prevent particles in the samples or mobile phase from entering and plugging the column. A small guard column that has the same support and stationary phase as the longer analytical column in the system may also be used to protect this second column and extend the time over which it can be utilized. Small LC columns may be employed if they are being used for only sample pretreatment, as may be carried out off-line based on separation methods such as size-exclusion, reversed-phase, ion-exchange or affinity chromatography. The housing for analytical columns that are used in HPLC systems is often made of stainless steel or a high-pressure resistant polymer. The internal diameters of analytical columns for HPLC are often in the range of 4–5 mm and their lengths are typically 5–30 cm, although narrow diameters and other lengths can be used. Examples of these other sizes include narrow-bore columns (with inner diameters of 2–3 mm) and microbore columns (with inner diameters of 1–2 mm). In addition, capillary columns are sometimes employed in LC, although these are not as common as packed columns [8, 15].

A packed bed of particles is the most common support format used for LC. In HPLC, this support often consists of porous particles with diameters of 1.8–10 μm, with typical diameters of 3–5 μm [8]. The particles at the lower end of this range are those that are used in UPLC, as these particles make it possible to obtain sharper peaks and better separations but also require the use of instrumentation that can work at higher pressures than traditional HPLC. LC columns that are used only for off-line sample preparation usually contain much larger particles that provide less resistance to flow. These latter types of columns can be used when the mobile phase is to be applied through the column by a low-pressure pump, gravity, or a centrifuge.

Other supports that are used in LC are those based on non-porous or pellicular media and perfusion or monolithic materials [8, 9]. In a porous support for LC, the mobile phase flows around the support but not through the particle. This creates a situation in which the movement of compounds into and out of the pores of the support is an important source of peak-broadening. Two ways around this issue are to use a nonporous support or pellicular beads (i.e., a particle with a thin, porous layer) to reduce the distance compounds must travel as part of this process. Perfusion particles also reduce this type of peak-broadening by providing both small pores to contain most of the stationary phase and larger through-pores that allow the mobile phase to travel both through and around the support. Another type of material in which the mobile phase can flow through the support is a monolith, which consists of a single porous bed made from an organic or inorganic polymer (e.g., silica). Both perfusion and monolithic materials help to reduce peak-broadening while producing lower back pressures than normal packed bed columns [8].

Detectors for Liquid Chromatography

There are many approaches by which compounds can be detected as they elute from an LC column (see Table 3.2). For example, MS can be used for this purpose, as occurs in LC–MS and LC-MS/MS. These two methods have been used in clinical and biomedical laboratories in fields such as pharmaceutical testing, metabolomics, and proteomics [8, 16]. There are many ionization approaches and mass analyzers that can be utilized in LC–MS. One common combination is the use of electrospray ionization with a quadrupole mass analyzer. Examples of other ionization methods that may be used with LC–MS are photoionization or chemical ionization [16]. It is necessary in these systems to use solvents and buffers for LC that are volatile so that they can be readily removed at the interface between the LC and MS systems. It

Table 3.2 Detectors for liquid chromatography[a]

Detector type	Compounds detected	Detection level
Mass spectrometry	Full-scan mode—general for compounds with ions in selected mass range	0.1–1 ng
	Selected-ion monitoring—specific for compounds that produce given ions	≤1 pg
UV/vis absorbance detector	Compounds with groups that can absorb light at selected wavelengths	0.1–1 ng
Refractive index detector	Compounds with refractive index different from the mobile phase	0.1–1 μg
Fluorescence detector	Compounds that both absorb and give off light at selected wavelengths	1 pg–1 ng
Evaporative light scattering detector	Compounds that form particles, after solvent evaporation, which can scatter light	1 ng
Electrochemical detector	Compounds with groups that can be reduced or oxidized under selected conditions	10 pg–1 ng
Conductivity detector	Ions that create a change in conductivity in the mobile phase	1 ng

[a]The approximate detection limits are from Hage [8] and Poole and Poole [17]

may also be necessary in some methods to use a switching valve to prevent nonvolatile sample components or salts from entering the MS system [8].

A valuable feature of LC–MS methods is they may be used in either a general or selective detection mode [2, 16]. This can be accomplished by using LC-MS to detect compounds by using either their molecular ions or fragment ions. When spectra are acquired throughout a separation and over a broad mass range, as is done in a full-scan mode, the MS component of the system is being used as a general detector. If the MS component is instead used to look at specific ions, this is then utilized as a selective detector. More details on MS are provided in Chap. 2.

Along with MS, there are many other detectors that are employed in LC. Examples of these other detectors are those based on absorbance, refractive index, fluorescence, evaporative light scattering, and electrochemical or conductivity measurements [2, 15]. Many of these non-MS detectors have a flow cell that allows the mobile phase and compounds eluting from the column to pass through the detector during the separation process. Most LC detectors are nondestructive, which means they can be used either alone or combined with another detector, such as MS. These detectors can also be employed with post-column derivatization to provide some eluting compounds with better responses and lower detection limits.

One type of detector that is often used in LC and in association with LC-MS is a *UV/vis absorbance detector*. This detector monitors the ability of eluting compounds to absorb UV or visible light at a given wavelength or wavelength range [2, 15]. There are three general types of UV/vis absorbance detectors: fixed-wavelength, variable wavelength and photodiode array detectors. A *fixed-wavelength absorbance detector* is designed to always monitor eluting compounds at a single wavelength, such as 254 nm. The design of a *variable-wavelength absorbance detector* is more complex and can use wavelengths that may vary over a broad range, such as 190–900 nm. A *photodiode array detector*, or *PDA*, monitors absorbance over a broad range of wavelengths at the same time, allowing the collection of an entire UV/vis spectrum for each eluting compound. A PDA does this by using a large set of diodes that each examines a small set of wavelengths within the overall spectral range that is monitored [15]. Absorbance detectors can be used for compounds with groups that can absorb UV/vis light or that can be derivatized to contain such groups. In addition, absorbance detectors can be utilized with solvent programming if the mobile phase does not have any appreciable absorbance at the wavelength(s) being monitored.

Another general means for monitoring eluting compounds in LC and LC–MS is to use a *refractive index (RI) detector*. An RI detector monitors the change in refractive index (i.e., a measure of the ability of matter to bend or "refract" light) as compounds elute from the column and change the composition of the mobile phase [2, 15]. All chemicals may refract light, so this device can give a signal for any eluting compound that is present at a sufficiently high concentration and differs from the mobile phase in its refractive index. This feature makes the RI detector a good choice to monitor the elution of compounds that have unknown structures or that may not produce good signals on absorbance detectors. This is also another example of a non-destructive detector that can be combined with other detection systems, such as LC–MS. One limitation of an RI detector is its detection limit, which is several orders of magnitude higher than when using MS or absorbance for monitoring eluting compounds (see Table 3.2). This detector can also give a change in background response during solvent programming as the composition, and corresponding refractive index, of the mobile phase is varied.

A *fluorescence detector* can be used in LC and LC–MS to monitor compounds that both absorb light and reemit light at different wavelengths. Fewer chemicals have strong fluorescence than good absorbance of light, which makes fluorescence a much more selective means of detecting compounds with this ability [2, 15]. The selectivity and low background that are usually associated with fluorescence measurements further means this type of detector will tend to provide much lower detection limits than when using UV/vis absorbance, as shown in Table 3.2. A fluorescence detector is non-destructive and can be readily used with gradient elution if the mobile phases have high purity and contain no significant amounts of fluorescing impurities. The selectivity of fluorescence does limit the types of chemicals that can be detected by this approach. However, even compounds that are not originally fluorescent can be first converted into a fluorescent derivative through pre-column or post-column derivatization. This derivatization is commonly used for the analysis of alcohols, amino acids, and proteins by fluorescence.

Several other types of detectors may be used in LC. An *evaporative light scattering detector (ELSD)* is a general way of monitoring compounds based on the conversion of the mobile phase and its contents into a spray of small droplets [2]. As the solvent evaporates from these droplets, less volatile components from the sample remain and form particles that can scatter light. An ELSD can be used with gradient elution and with compounds that do not absorb UV/vis light. In addition, this device has a better detection limit than an RI detector. LC systems may also contain a *conductivity detector*, which can be used for the general monitoring of ionic compounds. A conductivity detector monitors the ability of the mobile phase and eluting ions to conduct a current in the presence of an electrical field. *Electrochemical detectors* that employ compound oxidation or reduction to produce a current as the measured signal may be used to monitor chemicals that can undergo such reactions [2]. The combination of LC with electrochemical detection (EC) is sometimes known as *LC–EC*. This method can be used to provide sensitive and selective measurements for chemicals containing aldehydes, ketones, esters, unsaturated or aromatic groups, phenols, aromatic amines, purines, and compounds such as carbohydrates with neighboring alcohol groups.

Conclusions

LC is an important method for chemical separations for clinical and pharmaceutical testing that is often used in combination with MS and other means of detection. This method offers several advantages over GC, including its ability to work directly with liquid-phase samples and with a much larger range of compounds than can be examined by GC. Terms and parameters that can be used to describe the separation of compounds by LC were examined, such as ways of describing compound retention, peak-broadening, and the separation of two peaks. The role of the mobile phase in LC and the use of solvent programming were also discussed. The types of LC methods based on the stationary phase and method of compound retention were considered as well.

Some common forms of LC that are used with clinical and biological samples are RPLC, HILIC, cation- or anion-exchange chromatography, and size-exclusion chromatography. Other forms of LC methods that are sometimes used in these fields are NPLC, adsorption chromatography, and affinity chromatography. In addition, information was provided on the instrumentation, detectors, and types of supports that are used with LC in systems for HPLC. Given the wide range of separation and detection modes with which LC can be used, it is not surprising that LC and methods based on LC-MS have become popular for clinical testing and biomedical research.

Acknowledgments This work was supported, in part, by the National Science Foundation under grants CHE 2108881, CHE 2404209 and CHE 2320239 and by the University of Nebraska Research Council.

References

1. Ettre LS. Nomenclature for chromatography. Pure Appl Chem. 1993;65:819–72. https://doi.org/10.1351/pac199365040819.
2. Hage DS, Carr JD. Analytical chemistry and quantitative analysis. Pearson; 2011.

3. Inczedy J, Lengyel T, Ure AM. International Union of Pure and Applied Chemistry: compendium of analytical nomenclature: definitive rules 1997. Blackwell Science; 1997. p. Chap. 9.
4. Miller JM. Chromatography: concepts and contrasts. 2nd ed. Wiley-Interscience; 2009.
5. Shushan B. A review of clinical diagnostic applications of liquid chromatography-tandem mass spectrometry. Mass Spectrom Rev. 2010;29:930–44. https://doi.org/10.1002/mas.20295.
6. Vogeser M, Seger C. A decade of HPLC-MS/MS in the routine clinical laboratory: goals for further developments. Clin Biochem. 2008;41:649–62. https://doi.org/10.1016/j.clinbiochem.2008.02.017.
7. Wu N, Clausen AM. Fundamental and practical aspects of ultrahigh pressure liquid chromatography for fast separations. J Sep Sci. 2007;30:1167–82. https://doi.org/10.1002/jssc.200700026.
8. Hage DS. Chromatography. In: Rifai N, Chiu RWK, Young I, et al., editors. Tietz textbook of laboratory medicine. 7th ed. Elsevier; 2023. p. 241.
9. Ovbude ST, Sharmeen S, Kyei I, et al. Applications of chromatographic methods in metabolomics: a review. J Chromatogr B. 2024;1239:124124. https://doi.org/10.1016/j.jchromb.2024.124124.
10. Haddad PR, Nesterenko PN, Buchberger W. Recent developments and emerging directions in ion chromatography. J Chromatogr A. 2008;1184:456–73. https://doi.org/10.1016/j.chroma.2007.10.022.
11. Hurtubise RJ. Adsorption chromatography. In: Cazes J, editor. Encyclopedia of chromatography, vol. 2. 2nd ed. Taylor & Francis; 2005. p. 21.
12. Rodriguez EL, Poddar S, Iftekhar S, et al. Affinity chromatography: a review of trends and developments over the past 50 years. J Chromatogr B. 2020;1157:122332. https://doi.org/10.1016/j.jchromb.2020.122332.
13. Allenmark S. Chromatographic enantioseparations: methods and applications. 2nd ed. Ellis Horwood; 1991.
14. Armstrong DW. Direct enantiomeric separations in liquid chromatography and gas chromatography. In: Issaq HJ, editor. A century of separation science. Marcel Dekker; 2002. p. Chap. 33.
15. Ewing GW, editor. Analytical instrumentation handbook. 2nd ed. Marcel Dekker; 1997.
16. Kushnir MM, Rockwood AL, Clarke NJ. Mass spectrometry. In: Rifai N, Chiu RWK, Young I, et al., editors. Tietz textbook of laboratory medicine. 7th ed. Elsevier; 2023. p. 270.
17. Poole CF, Poole SK. Chromatography today. Elsevier; 1991.

Sample Preparation

4

Jacqueline A. Hubbard, Judith A. Stone,
and J. Grace van der Gugten

Abbreviations

ACP	AC plate (Tecan)
ALH	Automated liquid handling
DBS	Dried blood spots
D&S	Dilute and shoot sample preparation
ESI	Electrospray ionization
IP	Immunopurification
I.S.	Internal standard
LC	Liquid chromatography
LC-MSMS	Liquid chromatography–tandem mass spectrometry
LLOQ	Lower limit of quantitation
MS	Mass spectrometry (generically or denoting single stage)
MSMS	Tandem mass spectrometry (QqQ = triple quadrupole unless otherwise specified)
PLD	Phospholipid depletion media
PPT	Protein precipitation sample preparation
QqQ	Triple quadrupole or tandem mass spectrometry in space (versus tandem in time)

J. A. Hubbard
Department of Pathology, Beth Israel Deaconess Medical Center, Harvard Medical School, Boston, MA, USA
e-mail: jhubbar4@bidmc.harvard.edu

J. A. Stone (✉)
Clinical Chemist (Retired), Oakland, CA, USA

J. G. van der Gugten
BC Provincial Toxicology Centre, Vancouver, BC, Canada

Y. V. Zhang, U. Garg (eds.), *Practical Guide to Implementing Liquid Chromatography Mass Spectrometry in Clinical Laboratories*,
https://doi.org/10.1007/978-3-032-03852-4_4

Rs	LC resolution
SPE	Solid phase extraction
SST	System suitability test
ULF	Ultrafiltration

Introduction

Prior to analysis by liquid chromatography tandem mass spectrometry (LC-MSMS), the measurand(s), commonly referred to as analyte(s) of interest, must be separated from the rest of the sample—that is, the biological matrix. There are several reasons why this is necessary, including longer instrument maintenance-free intervals and optimizing analytical performance. The quest for a robust method that minimizes imprecision, achieves reproducible limits of quantification, and maximizes selectivity must also consider the higher cost and increased time/labor typical of more extensive sample cleanup.

The optimal medical laboratory sample preparation (prep) method will deplete sufficient sample matrix and reliably meet analytical goals, not only during validation, but such that sustained use over months to years is feasible. The extent and method of cleanup required depends on sample type, the measurand(s), and desired analytical performance. Choosing an LC-MSMS sample prep protocol can be complex. There are many options and multiple selection criteria, including aspects of analytical chemistry, medical laboratory cost analysis, and extraction workflows. This chapter describes sample prep methods for LC-MSMS analysis of small molecules, peptides/proteins, DBS samples, and strategies for selecting the best fit for purpose protocol.

Matrix Removal

Sample matrix itself may have co-eluting compounds that simultaneously ionize at the source with the measurand(s) of interest and subsequently interfere with its detection. This phenomenon is called "matrix effect" and may result in ion suppression (most common) or ion enhancement. The amount of matrix effect observed partially depends on the ionization source used. For example, electrospray ionization (ESI) typically exhibits more matrix effect than atmospheric pressure chemical ionization (APCI) because ESI generates ions directly from the liquid sample, including matrix components, whereas APCI introduces fewer matrix components during the ionization process [1, 2]. Thus, more extensive matrix depletion can provide improvements in the lower limit of quantitation (LLOQ) and assay linearity.

Matrix removal prolongs the lifespan of the LC-MSMS system. Removing macromolecules, cellular components, and salts avoids precipitation into the LC system and clogging of the LC column [3, 4]. When the column is exposed to proteins and other matrix components over time, it will degrade the stationary phase and subsequently lead to increased pressure, poor peak shapes, and shifting retention times.

Phospholipids are notorious for causing extreme ion suppression and may contaminate the mass spectrometer. An efficient sample preparation leads to longer maintenance-free intervals and minimizes instrument downtime. As a result, the assay will likely exhibit a lower background noise, better signal-to-noise ratio, more efficient chromatography, less variability in LC peak shape, and subsequently will lead to a more precise, analytically sensitive, and selective method.

Achieving better LLOQs is often accomplished by using a cleanup method that concentrates the sample without concentrating the matrix, such as liquid-liquid or solid phase extraction. A common approach is to dry down the extracted sample, after much of the matrix has been removed, and reconstitute it in a smaller volume. Conversely, for measurands that are commonly present in high concentrations, samples may be diluted to achieve the desired analytical measuring range. Prior to LC-MSMS analysis, the sample must be compatible with the LC method starting conditions [3]. Generally, in reversed-phase chromatography, the sample should be equally or slightly more aqueous than the LC starting conditions. If there is too much organic solvent present, it may lead to split or wider chromatographic peaks.

Basic Measurand Chemistry

Measurand chemistry can be exploited during sample prep to improve extraction efficiency as well as chromatographic retention and resolution [4]. Prior to developing a method, the ionization state of functional groups (pKa), polarity (i.e., log P), and molecular interactions should be considered. Simple modifications to parameters such as buffer composition or pH can have profound effects on extraction efficiency.

The tendency of a measurand to partition between the aqueous and organic phase can be predicted by its log P. Nonpolar measurands will more readily partition into the organic phase, whereas polar measurands are partial to the aqueous phase. Taking advantage of log P can help eliminate salts, proteins, waste products, and endogenous metabolites from a sample, leaving the unwanted compounds in the aqueous phase, while extracting measurand(s) of interest into the organic solvent phase. Extraction yield of some measurands can be improved by adding alcohols to promote hydrogen bonding with drugs [5]. Amphipathic drugs pose a challenge as they may partition into both phases, so buffer composition and other measurand properties must be considered.

Modification of pH is a common way to alter measurand chemistr,y but is only applicable to measurands with ionizable functional groups. At a low pH ($pH < pKa$), measurands are protonated, acidic compounds become uncharged and partition into the organic fraction, whereas basic compounds become positively charged. Conversely, acidic compounds lose a proton at a high pH ($pH > pKa$) and have a negative charge, whereas basic compounds become uncharged and partition into the organic fraction. Extreme pH conditions may cause measurand instability, emulsification of the sample, and degradation of the silica backbone in LC columns. At two pH units above or below the pKa, the ratio of uncharged to charged species (or vice versa) is 100:1. Therefore, adjustment well beyond two pH units of the pKa will not substantially increase the extraction yield [5]. Amphoteric drugs, such as morphine, will perform best when the pH is equivalent to the isoelectric point, but functional groups will still be charged, and this may decrease extraction efficiency into an organic solvent. Neutral (nonpolar) measurands, such as testosterone, will be unaffected by pH and can be extracted at any pH value.

Description of Small Molecule Sample Preparation Methods

Common Sample Prep Techniques with No Commercial Media Required

Dilute and Shoot (D&S) is arguably the simplest form of sample cleanup. After the sample is pipetted into a well or vial, internal standard(s) (I.S.) and a favorable diluent are added ("dilute"), and it is then loaded onto the instrument and injected ("shoot"). To further simplify D&S, the I.S. may be made and stored, if stable, in that favorable diluent, limiting the assay to a single addition step. After mixing, centrifugation or filtration may be performed to minimize particulates that enter the LC system. D&S has the benefits of being fast, cost-effective, and an incredibly streamlined workflow.

While this technique is highly recognized for its ease of use, it is not a true extraction and therefore all constituents of the matrix, including potential interferents, are still present in the sample. It may exhibit a noisier baseline and is more susceptible to matrix effects than other cleanup methods. In addition, the introduction of a "dirty" sample onto the instrument can increase turnover rates of consumables and require more frequent maintenance to clean the instrument, leading to increased cost and downtime, respectively. D&S is most commonly used with matrices that are low in protein, phospholipids, and cellular components, such as urine, CSF, and breath [3, 6]. D&S would be insufficient for "dirtier" matrices, such as serum, plasma, whole blood, and tissue, or with measurands that require high analytical sensitivity, such as testosterone in women and children. While D&S is widely used across clinical labs, careful monitoring of the assay should be conducted to ensure reproducibility over time.

Protein precipitation (PPT) is a simple sample cleanup technique designed to remove proteins from a sample. Therefore, it is most appropriately used in protein-rich matrices such as serum, plasma, and whole blood. Typically, sample and I.S. are added to a vial, followed by a precipitation solution. The precipitation solution is most commonly an organic solvent (acetonitrile, methanol, isopropanol, or acetone) or zinc sulfate in methanol, but perchloric acid, trichloroacetic acid, sodium tungstate with sulfuric acid, and ammonium sulfate with hydrochloric acid may also be used [5, 7–11]. The solution causes proteins to rapidly precipitate out of the sample, which is why this technique is frequently referred to as a "protein crash." In some instances, the use of an ice-cold solvent, especially when added slowly, can improve the cleanliness and efficiency of precipitation [5, 12]. Next, the sample is either centrifuged to pellet the protein or filtered to remove the precipitate. The extracted sample (supernatant) or filtrate may be transferred to a new vial or well. If the assay is automated, the pipette may be set to only transfer the upper portion of the sample.

The sample can then be introduced to the instrument, or it may be subjected to further cleanup to improve analytical sensitivity.

The benefits of PPT are similar to those of D&S—it is a simple workflow and cost-effective, with the added benefit of removing proteins from more complicated matrices. However, it produces a "dirty" sample with risk of matrix effect (due to phospholipids), a noisier baseline, the need for more regular instrument maintenance, and consequently the potential for increased downtime. To combat this, many labs opt to combine this technique with other cleanup methods, such as an online extraction (see the Online SPE paragraph in the section Common Sample Prep Techniques Using Commercial Media of this chapter).

Liquid–liquid extraction (LLE) is a sample prep technique commonly used with reversed-phase chromatography to separate measurands based on their relative solubilities in two immiscible liquids, typically an aqueous phase and an organic solvent. In a typical LLE preparation, the sample (serum, plasma, urine, etc.) is added to a vial along with I.S. It is then mixed with an organic solvent combination in which measurand(s) of interest are more soluble. Common organic extraction solvents used include hexane, ethyl acetate, ethyl ether, methyl-butyl ether (MTBE), butanol, isopropanol, acetone, and acetonitrile [5, 13]. The preferential solvent to sample ratio is 5:1–10:1 [5]. In addition, buffering or pH adjustments may be used to increase selectivity for ionizable measurands. After adding the solvent, the sample is mixed vigorously, and the nonpolar measurands partition into the organic phase while other matrix components, such as salts and proteins, remain in the aqueous phase. Sequential extraction steps may be used to separate measurands with different chemical properties. This may increase the purity of the extract, but each additional step adds complexity to the method and will result in recovery loss. After centrifugation, the organic solvent layer is then transferred to a new vial. Finally, the organic supernatant is typically concentrated with an evaporation step and reconstituted in an injection matrix compatible with the LC-MSMS starting conditions.

LLE is considered "cleaner" than D&S and PPT, particularly with respect to phospholipid removal [14], so it may result in longer maintenance-free intervals and less matrix effect compared to those simpler cleanup methods. Disadvantages of LLE include the variability introduced by the manual transfer step and the time-consuming nature of the technique, which is challenging to automate. LLE is not suitable for all measurands, especially polar ones, and may lead to incomplete extractions for measurands that partition equally between the two phases. In samples containing high proteins or lipids, emulsions may form and prevent complete separation between the layers. In light of the complexity of LLE, methods should be optimized to balance cost and ease of use against sensitivity and efficiency.

Common Sample Prep Techniques Using Commercial Media

Supported liquid extraction (SLE) builds on the principles of LLE but incorporates a solid support material, such as diatomaceous earth, to facilitate the separation between the aqueous and organic phases. Specialized cartridge or plate-based consumables are readily available, and they efficiently remove proteins, lipids, surfactants, enzymes, and other interferences. In a typical method preparation, the sample and I.S. are added to the support material and allowed to absorb onto the solid phase. Similar to LLE, a solvent to elute the nonpolar measurands from the solid support is added. The solvent can pass through the solid phase cartridge by gravity, but a vacuum or positive pressure (PP) is commonly used to facilitate elution into a collection vial or plate. The sample can then undergo evaporation and reconstitution.

SLE reduces matrix effect, particularly via phospholipid removal, compared to PPT. The use of the solid phase enhances the contact between the sample and the solvent, resulting in a more efficient partitioning of measurands into the organic phase compared to LLE. This also helps avoid emulsion formation, resulting in a cleaner and more consistent extraction. Because the organic phase does not need to be manually transferred with a pipette, SLE can easily be automated to improve throughput. SLE often requires smaller volumes of organic solvent compared to LLE, however, the maximum sample volume that can be used is dictated by the bed mass of the plate or cartridge used. This will affect the achievable LLOQ. Not all organic solvents are compatible with the solid support materials used in SLE, potentially limiting the solvent types that may be used for specific measurands. SLE has a higher per-sample cost compared to LLE due to the need for specialized plates or cartridges. The overall cost increase can be offset by the increased productivity (higher throughput and reduced hands-on time), reduced solvent cost, and potentially longer maintenance-free intervals of the LC-MS/MS. SLE is often preferred over LLE, despite the additional cost, especially for high-volume labs that require automation to meet throughput demands.

Solid phase extraction (SPE) is a low-resolution chromatographic process across a small sorbent bed contained by frits in a cartridge/96 well plate. Over the last 10–20 years, SPE options have expanded dramatically (stationary supports [polymer vs silica]; formats, e.g., dispersive [d-SPE], pipet-tip-SPE [PT-SPE], microelution-[μ-SPE]; multiple sorbents within one well [e.g., ISOLUTE® HYDRO DME+, Biotage]; retention mechanisms [selective sorbents]) [15]. Conventional SPE and updates are discussed here.

Steps for conventional reversed-phase (RP)/mixed-mode SPE are:

1. Mix I.S. with sample/application buffer (SPE reagents may need pH control to optimize retention or elution)
2. Activate the SPE stationary phase with methanol/acetonitrile
3. Equilibrate the bed with aqueous buffer/water
4. Load diluted sample at the vendor-recommended flow rate, measurands retain on the stationary phase, and sample flows to waste
5. Flush one/more wash solutions through the SPE bed to waste, removing matrix while retaining measurands
6. Dry the SPE bed with heated air/nitrogen to remove residual water/solvent
7. Replace the waste container with a collection plate or vials
8. Elute measurands with a solvent/mixture
9. Evaporate the eluate
10. Reconstitute/concentrate with an LC-compatible solution
11. Cap vials/seal plates and mix
12. Centrifuge to sediment particulate (optional) [16].

Slow SPE flow, e.g., 20 drops/min, is used to equilibrate fluids and optimize interaction of measurands with all retention mechanisms. Vacuum or positive pressure (PP) and evaporator manifolds are necessary for conventional SPE. PP moves fluids through SPE beds more reliably than does vacuum. Recent trends are towards eco-friendly options that consume less solvent/plastic. Reductions in housing size/bed mass also permit smaller sample volumes. SPE plates with smaller bed mass/hold-up volume (e.g., Waters µElution plate) can be eluted with <50 µL, so evaporation becomes optional. A reduced volume alternative is dispersive-solid phase extraction (d-SPE) sorbent within pipet tips (pipet tip-solid phase extraction [PT-SPE], multiple vendors) [16, 17].

SPE media vendors typically offer polymer (polystyrene/divinylbenzene: PS-DVB) and silica stationary supports for sorbents. Unmodified PS-DVB also functions by itself as an RP. Unlike silica-bonded phases, PS-DVB does not necessarily require activation, saving time/solvent. PS-DVB tolerates a wider pH range (1–14 vs 2–10 for silica). Drying of PS-DVB while processing does not alter measurand retention, unlike silica. PS-DVB has a higher loading capacity, but silica typically has a broader sorbent menu available [18].

SPE sorbent categories for biofluids include RP, weak/strong ion-exchange, mixed mode, Hydrophilic-Lipophilic Balanced (HLB), and Hydrophilic Interaction Liquid Chromatography (HILIC). RP (e.g., unmodified PS-DVB or C18-silica) is less selective than mixed-mode SPE. RP is primarily useful to retain nonpolar measurands and remove salts/polar matrix components. Mixed mode can be highly effective for matrix depletion and very selective for weak acids/bases as both RP functionality and weak anion or cation exchangers are bonded to the stationary support. HLB polymers are designed to retain both nonpolar and polar compounds, useful to extract a broad Log P spectrum of measurands. HILIC is less commonly described for biofluid extraction, but applications combining PPT/HILIC-SPE have been developed for strongly polar oligonucleotides/peptides [19, 20] A wide range of SPE sorbent selectivity is now available (e.g., amino, aminopropyl, C2, C4, C8, C18, C30, cyano, cyclohexyl, diol, diphenyl, phenyl, polyamide). Several vendors offer media with a range of sorbents across different wells of a single 96-well plate to accelerate/reduce costs of method development (Oasis Method Development µElution Plate, Waters; Versaplate, Agilent; TELOS neo MicroPlate Method Development, Kinesis). There is abundant literature, many application notes, and strong support from media vendors to optimize SPE. First steps for SPE method development are to consult vendor application chemists as well as the scientific literature. Questions to ask for newer formats (d-SPE, PT-SPE, µ-SPE) include: is there a) documented robustness in a medical laboratory production environment? b) are a wide range of sorbents available? c) Is ancillary equipment needed and is the format compatible with standard ALH?

SPE advantages include high selectivity and the option to concentrate, deplete matrix and adjust injection solutions. SPE is straightforward to automate with vacuum/PP on an ALH deck [21]. Disadvantages include cost, complexity (optimization and production), and longer TAT. SPE in 96-format is easier to automate than LLE, so to handle large numbers of samples, SPE is preferred over LLE.

Online SPE works by first retaining measurands on an LC trap column while LC flow with unbound matrix goes to waste. Then the flow path, mobile phase(s), and in some cases, flow direction are switched. Measurands are eluted from the trap column to then be retained and separated on an analytical LC column, or to flow directly to the MS [22].

In-house designed online SPE is less expensive than commercial systems and simple or highly complex separations can be customized with design of experiments (DOE) [22]. Additional LC pumps, switching valves, and appropriate software are used to control flows/timing. Stationary phases are typically coordinated so that measurands have a lower/higher affinity for trap/analytical columns, respectively [22]. Inline mobile phase modification (pH, additives, solvents) via switching valves between trap/analytical columns can be used to maximize elution recovery from the trap column. Measurands must be refocused on the analytical column for the best peak shape via mobile phase gradients designed to optimize both analytical separation and ionization at the MS source [22].

Commercial online SPE systems may be significantly more expensive than in-house development, but should include vendor design, installation, and application support, with higher throughput if LC multiplexing is included. Vendors selling online SPE systems in 2024 include Agilent Technologies, Gerstel GmbH & Co. KG, Spark Holland BV (multiple resellers, supported by Axelsemrau), and Thermo Fisher Scientific. Transcend™ TLX Systems with turbulent flow LC (TFLC) columns are patented/commercially available from Thermo Fisher Scientific. TFLC characteristics and retention mechanisms are fundamentally different from standard LC [23]. With large (50–100 mm) particles, high flow rates (5–8 mL/min) and short, narrow columns (1 × 50 mm) LC laminar flow becomes turbulent and highly chaotic, yielding faster mass transfer and higher efficiency. For small molecule analysis, slower diffusing macromolecules (proteins) are excluded from, while small molecules can still interact with, TFLC stationary phases. This allows direct injection of high protein matrices (serum/plasma). After extraction on a TFLC trap column, LC flow is switched, and separation occurs on an analytical column [23].

Advantages of online SPE are minimal hands-on time, optional direct sample injection, compatibility with thermally labile measurands/limited sample volumes (entire sample can be injected). Disadvantages are greater complexity, expertise needed for method development, troubleshooting, and maintenance, higher cost of capital equipment, and increased risk for carryover.

Phospholipid depletion (PLD) media development was driven by the major matrix effect problem seen with PPT of serum/plasma/whole blood, that is ion suppression due to phospholipids [14, 24]. PLD that retains blood phospholipids and precipitated proteins but not measurands has been commercially available since the mid-2000s [25]. The workflow is mixing of I.S., patient sample, and a precipitating reagent in a PLD plate/cartridge. The media bed retains >95% of blood phospholipids, commonly through binding of the polar phosphate group to zirconium or titanium [26]. Vacuum/positive pressure is applied, precipitated proteins are retained above the bottom filter/frit and filtrate containing measurands flows through to a collection plate. Precipitation with two different reagents and mixing *before* addition to the PLD plate improved flow-through characteristics in one high-throughput use case [27]. Constraints specific to each vendor include the nature of the precipitation reagent, the ratio of serum to precipitant volume, and the potential for nonspecific binding of measurands [25]. Like PPT, PLD is simple with few method development steps to optimize, but is limited by dilution of measurands and an injection matrix dominated by the precipitation reagent (typically 3:1 of methanol or acetonitrile with 1% formic acid:serum). Advantages compared to PPT include a major reduction in matrix effect and prolongation of both LC column lifetimes and maintenance-free intervals for the MS instruments [24–26].

Less Commonly Used Sample Prep Techniques with Commercial Media

Dual mode extraction (DME) uses both liquid partitioning and scavenging techniques and is available in column or plate format. One of the examples is Biotage ISOLUTE HYDRO dual mode extraction (DME) + that is primarily designed for urine toxicology assays. The composition of the support material from top to bottom includes a HYDRO frit, scavenging sorbent, a middle frit, hygroscopic sorbent, and finally a lower frit [28–30]. The frit technology holds the sample above the sorbent bed and allows for in-situ hydrolysis during the incubation process, thus eliminating the need for a post-hydrolysis transfer step. The scavenging layer is designed to remove the biological matrix, including salts, urea, and creatinine in urine. Combined, it potentially eliminates >90% of the matrix [29].

A general method workflow would include adding the patient sample (urine), I.S., and any other reagents to each well or individual column. A hydrolysis step can then occur in the well itself. After an incubation period, acetonitrile is added, and a positive pressure manifold is used to elute the extracted samples. Depending on the sensitivity needs and desired LC starting conditions, evaporation and reconstitution steps may be required. DME technology provides a simple pass-through workflow, without the need for a transfer or plate swap step, that achieves higher sensitivity compared to D&S. However, it does require ancillary equipment, is more expensive than D&S, and is dependent on the availability of the DME products, making it vulnerable to supply chain issues.

Immunopurification (IP) uses immobilized, measurand specific, antibodies to bind the measurand of interest during an incubation step with the biological sample. The residual matrix is washed away, and the measurand is eluted from the antibody for LC-MSMS analysis. Antibodies are typically attached to a solid particle support such as agarose or magnetic beads. Removal of residual matrix, washing, and elution can be done using filtration or magnets. See Fig. 4.1 for a workflow summary.

The use cases of IP for small molecules in medical LC-MSMS are few [31, 32], primarily due to ease of use and cost considerations. The only application of IP for small molecules in use in medical LC-MSMS known by the authors at the time of print is for 1,25-dihydroxyvitamin D (^{125}D) [33, 34].

Magnetic microparticles (MMP) linked to a reversed phase for HPLC–UV online plasma itraconazole extraction was reported more than 15 years ago [35]. Despite this early proof of concept, as of 2024, MMP linked to extraction phases (e.g., C18, HILIC, SAX) are promoted by vendors for research proteomics but not for small molecule sample prep (e.g., Thermo Fisher Scientific, Inc., Waltham, MA; Resyn

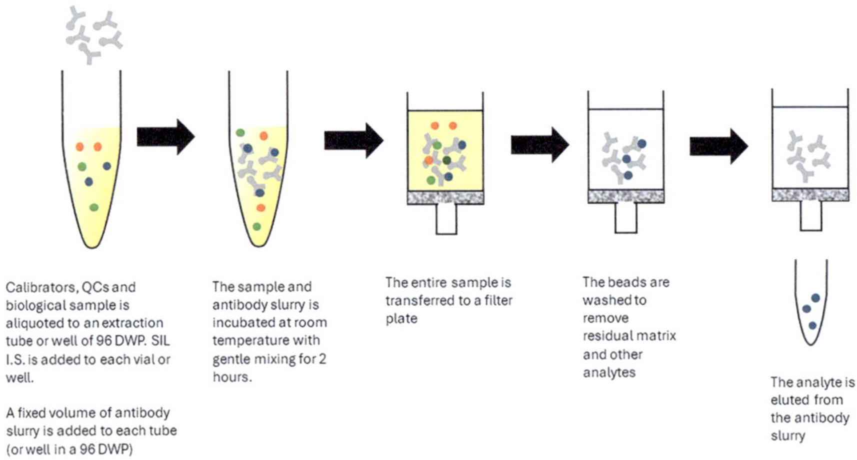

Fig. 4.1 Graphical summary of the IP sample prep process using IDK antibody slurry (Immundiagnostik AG/KM1022)

Biosciences, Edenvale, Gauteng, South Africa). MMP-SPE automation has been described for LC-MSMS sample prep of metanephrines and gastrin (GBI EX-48; Beijing BGI-GBI Biotech Co., Ltd., Beijing, China) but is not US-FDA or EU-CE mark approved as of 2024 [36, 37]. An alternative use case, MMP matrix depletion of biofluids rather than MMP-SPE of measurands, could have broader application for medical LC-MSMS. Konig et al. validated a MMP matrix depletion workflow followed by online SPE and LC-MSMS analysis of amiodarone. Good agreement was found between MMP protein depletion and organic solvent precipitation protocols [38]. A MMP matrix depletion kit was validated for direct coagulation factor inhibitor drugs in plasma [39]. However, the kit described by Konig and Weisen (Magtivio, The Netherlands) appears to have been discontinued. MMP theoretically could save time and labor using ALH compared to the centrifugation or filtration steps needed for solvent/acid-based PPT. However, like IP, routine use of MMP for small molecule medical LC-MSMS appears to be infrequent, likely due to cost and unfamiliarity.

QuEChERS stands for Quick, Easy, Cheap, Effective, Rugged, and Safe, the target attributes of a sample prep method extensively optimized to measure pesticides in vegetables and fruit but potentially of interest for medical laboratory LC-MSMS users [40–42]. The first step is the partitioning of measurands and I.S.s from the sample into acetonitrile, facilitated by salting-out and mixing [40]. After centrifugation, the second step is mixing of the decanted acetonitrile with dispersive (d-)SPE media (Primary and Secondary Amine exchanger + $MgSO_4$) to adsorb out the sample matrix interferences onto the dispersed solid phase [43]. Use of d-SPE means that vacuum/positive pressure modules are unnecessary, and flow errors (channeling, clogging) are avoided. After a second centrifugation, the acetonitrile phase is ready for injection or evaporation to concentrate measurands and/or swap injection solutions to improve LC compatibility and peak shape [41]. QuEChERS is widely used for pesticide/ veterinary drug testing of food; there are now three officially standardized versions—the original unbuffered and two buffered [41–44]. Variants include miniaturization and an update by the original authors, adding Efficient and Robust features (QuEChERSER) [41]. QuEChERS salts and d-SPE media are available commercially from many sample prep vendors. Most described use cases are for solid, non-medical samples, but the technique has been applied with LC-MSMS for medical body fluid and post-mortem toxicology [44–47]. Advantages include measurand recovery across a wider range of polarity compared to simple LLE, due to salting out of the initial liquid extraction step, improved matrix depletion through incorporation of the second, orthogonal extraction mode (d-SPE), and technical simplicity [41, 43, 44]. The low complexity steps of the original protocol are suitable for small manual batches but are cumbersome with increased sample numbers and not easily automatable with standard ALH (need for centrifugation, additions of powered salts, and d-SPE). Automated systems for QuEChERS and QuEChERSER sample prep are available [48, 49].

AC Plate (ACP) media consists of a reversed-phase extraction coating (TICE™) immobilized within 96-well plates [50]. ACP was released by Tecan in 2014. The principle is essentially a stationary phase liquid-liquid extraction that can be performed manually, but is optimal with ALH automation [51]. The workflow is

(a) Measurands and I.S. partition into the nonpolar coating on the plate wells from body fluids added in a relatively polar application reagent
(b) The application reagent containing matrix residue is discarded
(c) Interferences can be depleted by flushing the wells with wash reagents designed to retain measurands but remove matrix residue from the immobilized extraction phase
(d) A more nonpolar solution, such as water:acetonitrile (pH modified if necessary) is used to partition the measurand back out of the nonpolar coating [50].

An orbital shaker is required on the ALH deck to accelerate mass transfer of measurands, but vacuum/positive pressure modules are not needed. Tecan recommends the use of the ACP for compounds with a log D > 3, and published applications are for steroid hormones and drugs [51–53]. Advantages of ACP are ease of automation, effective matrix depletion, avoiding the flow-through issues of packed media, and the option to bypass an evaporation step due to small elution volumes. Disadvantages are cost and minimal concentrating ability/lower recovery for relatively polar measurands.

Ultrafiltration (ULF) sample prep is the use of molecular weight cutoff (MWCO) filters with centrifugation to deplete macromolecules from serum/plasma (e.g., Amicon® Centrifree Ultra Centrifugal filters, 30 kDa MWCO). The resulting filtrate is typically defined as "protein-free" for quantification of unbound measurands (e.g., free phenytoin). To evaluate whether ULF may have sufficient measurand recovery and matrix depletion for a specific medical LC-MSMS sample prep application, review the MWCO of the device (e.g., <5 vs <30 kDa), predicted ultrafiltrate composition, expected percentage of unbound measurand(s) in serum/plasma, and consider the following:

- Will loss of measurand occur through nonspecific adsorption to filters, frits, or plastic housing?
- Will interferences leak from plastic housings, filters, or frits into the injection matrix?
- Is the filtration membrane type compatible with measurand(s) hydrophilicity/hydrophobicity?
- Is pre-rinsing of the filter recommended to reduce potential leaching of contaminants?

Factors that may affect reproducibility include filter break-through, pre-analytical handling (fresh versus frozen biofluids, sample pH), and ULF centrifugation conditions (e.g., time, temperature, relative centrifugal force) [54–56]. As with any sample prep method that minimally depletes the sample matrix, robust testing for ion suppression is key. A longer-term issue is whether matrix residue remaining after ULF sample prep will shorten LC column lifetimes or necessitate more frequent cleaning of the MS.

Modifying Measurands—Hydrolysis and Derivatization

Hydrolysis is used to remove conjugates, such as glucuronides and sulfates, which have been added to measurands during phase II metabolism. It can also simplify (fewer total measurands) a method by detecting only parent measurands in lieu of detecting parent compounds plus one or more conjugated metabolites. Conversion of all conjugated metabolites to the parent drug may also improve sensitivity for total drug exposure when there are multiple, low concentration conjugated metabolites. However, hydrolysis adds complexity to sample prep and requires additional quality control materials to assess hydrolysis efficiency. Hydrolysis can be accomplished through pH manipulation or by using a glucuronidase enzyme. For any hydrolysis procedure, temperature, pH, incubation time, and reaction buffer composition must be optimized.

Hydrolysis through pH manipulation can be accomplished under both acidic and basic conditions. An acidic solution combined with high temperatures efficiently cleaves acetalic and acylalic glucuronides and sulfuric esters [57], but it may degrade measurands and cause conversion into other metabolites (e.g., oxycodone to oxymorphone and hydrocodone to hydromorphone) [58]. Basic hydrolysis is less common. It is usually performed at room temperature or slightly elevated temperatures, but is generally less effective than acid hydrolysis.

Enzymatic hydrolysis via glucuronidase enzymes is a popular alternative. Some enzymes require long incubation times and high temperatures, but more recently developed recombinant enzymes hydrolyze efficiently at room temperature in under 15 min (e.g., IMCS, Integrated Micro-Chromatography Systems; Irmo, SC). Each enzyme has varying rates of efficiency for different compounds/functional groups, so it is best practice to optimize for all of the measurand-conjugates in a method instead of using a single compound as a proxy for others [59]. Vendors can guide in enzyme selection, but several options should be tried. Most vendors will offer free samples for this purpose.

Ideal hydrolysis conditions should be determined by optimizing parameters one at a time. For example, using the same enzyme concentration for the same amount of time (e.g., 60 min) but at varying temperatures (45 °C, 55 °C, 65 °C). Once the optimal temperature is determined, the experiment can be repeated for incubation time, pH, or enzyme concentration. Note that most enzymes do not function optimally in solutions with high percentages of organic solvents or under extreme pH conditions.

Derivatization is less commonly used for medical LC-MSMS than for GC–MS. LC-MSMS derivatization is most often done to achieve sufficient LLOQs for hormone and drug testing by enhancing MSMS detection [60]. Measurands may also be derivatized to improve stability or LC performance [60]. There can be notable drawbacks to derivatization workflows. A common limitation is MSMS fragmentation that yields a derivative moiety as the most abundant product ion, instead of a fragment specific to the measurand [60]. Isobaric interferences that react with the derivatization reagent will produce the same product ion as the measurand, and a major selectivity advantage is lost [60]. Other potential problems include loss of distinction between stereoisomers and creation of multiple species from a single measurand [61]. Use cases where extremely high concentrations of target measurands may occur (e.g., newborn screening) require validation with appropriate patient samples to confirm that derivatization reagent concentrations/conditions are sufficient for the very wide concentration range that may be encountered [62].

Common derivatization use cases in medical laboratories include dansylation for serum estradiol and 4-phenyl-1,2,4- triazole-3,5-dione (PTAD) derivatization for 1,25 dihydroxy Vitamin D [63, 64]. Alternate derivatization protocols include MPPZ for estradiol [65] and Amplifex-Diene for 1,25 dihydroxy Vitamin D [66]. Direct-matrix (pre-extraction) derivatization with propionic anhydride followed by online SPE of plasma metanephrines and catecholamines has been described [67]. Derivatization has been used routinely in newborn screening, e.g., butyl esterification of amino acids and acylcarnitines with DBS [68]. New derivatization options and solutions proposed to avoid derivatization altogether continue to be reported. A comprehensive literature review may be warranted before accepting previously described derivatization methods for medical LC-MSMS by default. Reviews of LC-MSMS derivatization for a wide range of use cases, categorized by measurand functional groups, include [69, 70].

Selecting a Small Molecule Sample Prep Method

Summary: Navigating the sample prep selection process for small molecule measurands should be guided by multiple factors (see Tables 4.1 and 4.2 and Fig. 4.2). Discussion of the tables and figure content follows. See section "Protein and Peptide Sample Prep" for the advantages and disadvantages of protein/peptide sample prep methods.

Table 4.1 Summary of characteristics for small molecule sample preparation methods

Sample prep method	Sample type	Cost	Can concentrate measurands?	Matrix depletion capability	Protocol complexity	Automation development complexity
D&S	[a]U, O-LP	$	No	Minimal	Simple	Simple
PPT	[a]S/P, WB, O-HP	$	No	Protein, variable	Simple	Simple[b]
LLE	[a]S/P, WB, U, O	$	Yes	Extensive	Complex	Complex[b]
SLE	[a]S/P, WB, U, O	$$$	Yes, moderate	Extensive	Moderately complex	Moderate[b]
SPE	[a]S/P, WB, U, O	$$$	Yes	Sorbent and protocol dependent	Complex	Moderate[b]
Online SPE	[a]S/P, WB, U, O	$$$	Yes	Trap column and protocol dependent	Manual steps are simple	Complex[c]
PLD	[a]S/P, WB	$$$	No	[a]PL and protein	Simple	Simple[b]
DME	[a]U, O	$$$	No	See note[d]	Simple	Simple[b]
IP	[a]S/P, U, CSF	$$$	Yes	Extensive	Complex	Moderate
MMP	[a]S/P, U, WB	$$$	[e]	[e]	[e]	[e]
QuEChERS	[a]S/P, WB, U, O	$$	Yes	Moderate	Simple	Moderate[f]
ACP	[a]S/P, U, O	$$$	Yes, moderate	Moderate	Simple	Simple
ULF	[a]S/P, O-HP	$$	No	Protein	Simple	Simple

[a]Cerebrospinal fluid (CSF), other(O), other high/low protein matrices [O-HP, O-LP]), phospholipid (PL), serum/plasma(S/P), urine(U), whole blood (WB)
[b]Ancillary equipment maybe necessary, e.g., positive pressure or vacuum module(s), evaporator
[c]An ALH may be required for sample barcode scanning, adding, and mixing of sample with I.S. to plates or vials as preliminary steps before automated online SPE
[d]Vendor states removal of urine pigments, salts, urea, creatinine, and residual hydrolysis enzyme; no description of sorbent type(s) is available
[e]MMP-SPE and MMP-PPT characteristics differ—see section
[f]May require dedicated automation, check for updates/modifications for use with standard ALH

Table 4.2 Sample prep selection and evaluation criteria for small molecule measurands

#	Category	Criteria	Notes
1	Measurand chemistry	Charged vs neutral, functional groups, pKa, Log P, Log D, MW.	Log P & Log D = polarity indicators.
2	LLOQ target	Default goal of ≤20% CV at the LLOQ.	See Rappold [62] on S:N limitations related to LLOQ
3	Sample type, extent of biological matrix depletion (serum, plasma, urine, whole blood, etc.)	Matrix = everything in the sample except the measurands. See also section "Introduction" on blood phospholipids & ion suppression and Table 4.1.	More extensive and/or selective matrix depletion can reduce MS ion suppression [71, 72]
4	Staff competence	LC-MSMS experience, programming capability, attention to detail & tolerance for high failure rates.	See also section "Automating Sample Prep" on automation; method complexity.
7	Time factors	Reporting deadlines, hands-on time, true extraction TAT start to finish, instrument time.	Total extraction TAT is often underestimated.
8	96 well format	Most productive but best with ALH.	Accurate manual pipetting into 96-well format is challenging.
9	Automation options	ALH; on-ALH-deck vacuum/positive pressure/evaporation/mixing/magnetic modules for cartridge/96 well format; online extraction.	In-house programming capability is key for both faster ALH development & custom optimization.
10	LC quality and tracking	Baseline; Rs of critical peak pairs; peak widths; LC back pressure; Rts.	
11	MSMS signal quality and tracking	SST mean peak area each day of use (at least 3 replicates); between day %CV at LLOQ; low concentration quality control materials.	

Sample prep and instrument performance: New users of LC-MSMS for patient care often want to keep sample prep simple—e.g., dilution (D&S) for urine and protein precipitation (PPT) for serum/whole blood (see Fig. 4.2). D&S and PPT can work well for drugs and metabolites at ng/mL to ug/mL concentrations but may lead to more frequent cleaning of the MSMS due to insufficient matrix depletion. The extent of matrix depletion by sample prep is related to the natural history of performance loss over time for LC columns and MSMS hardware [72]. Residual matrix components adhere to the LC column stationary phase, compromising flow and measurand to stationary phase interactions. LC pressure can rise, and leaks may occur. Eventually, LC peak height, shape, width, retention time, and Rs degrade. As matrix residue deposits on the MSMS source, ion guide, and eventually, the quadrupole rail, ion transmission is debased and the MSMS will deliver less signal. When a new column is installed or after the MSMS is cleaned, performance can be restored [62]. Then the cycle repeats (see Fig. 4.3).

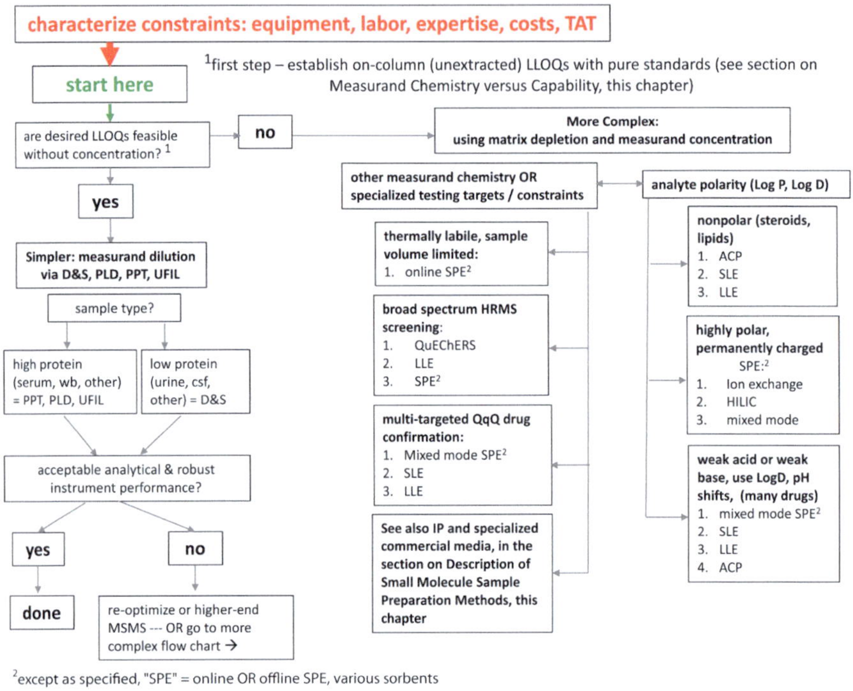

Fig. 4.2 A flow chart to navigate initial selection of small molecule sample prep—see Table 4.1 for a summary of method characteristics

Fig. 4.3 Simulated tracking of SST peak areas over time, decreasing instrument performance is followed by recovered signal after MSMS interface cleaning or LC column replacement [73]

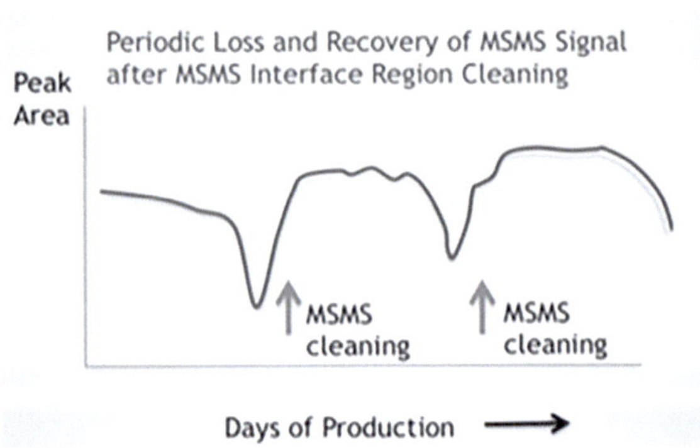

Recognizing this sample prep related effect on instruments is difficult because any protocol may work well initially. Only as matrix residue from extracted samples slowly accumulates on the instrument will performance loss be observed. This lag phase complicates assigning inadequate matrix depletion as the primary source of instrument problems. Tracking of SST parameters can detect worsening instrument trends before quality failures occur (unacceptable peak areas and precision at the LLOQ, decreased linearity, inaccuracy for closely eluting measurand pairs) [62].

Conversely, with no tracking, or no/inappropriate tracking thresholds, instruments may appear to fail suddenly. Of course, if this degradation of instrument performance occurs after an acceptable interval—the method is, by definition, robust. Other useful metrics of sample prep robustness include frequency of MSMS cleaning, LC column replacements, and maximum injections before failure, frequency of TAT exceptions, batch/sample repeats, LC leaks, and over-pressure shutdowns [62]. The question becomes, what extent of sample cleanup is needed?

Fit for Purpose and Selection Criteria: A fit-for-purpose approach is recommended for selecting sample prep protocols. Minimal sample prep may be appropriate for a given instrument and set of performance and operational expectations [61]. Under other circumstances, extensive sample clean-up may be necessary for longer instrument maintenance-free intervals and to meet more demanding performance criteria [72]. Although sample prep protocols are widely available from LC-MSMS/extraction media vendors and the scientific literature, longer-term effects of many protocols on instrument performance in a production environment are often unknown or not stated. Protocols with documented robustness, recommended by medical laboratory colleagues, are therefore particularly valuable. Tables 4.1 and 4.2 above summarize initial factors to consider when selecting sample prep protocols [3, 61, 72]. Detailed characteristics of the common small molecule techniques are described in section "Description of Small Molecule Sample Preparation Methods". It is useful to remember that LC-MSMS is a powerful measurement technique in part because so many options exist to adjust LC conditions, MSMS parameters, or sample prep details to compensate for limitations in other phases of the analysis. Thus, choices and optimization of sample prep should be highly interactive with and informed by the features and settings of the LC and MSMS systems.

Measurand Chemistry Versus Capability: Limitations of personnel, expertise, and budget are common to medical laboratories implementing LC-MSMS. This means choosing a sample prep method may be heavily influenced by practical workflow considerations as well as by measurand chemistry and method goals [61, 72]. For example, deciding if the simple, cheaper sample prep options (D&S and PPT) will suffice (Fig. 4.2). The sensitivity of the MSMS is a first consideration. Purchasing the most sensitive MSMS the laboratory can afford has many advantages. Sample prep protocols such as D&S, PPT, and PLD that do not concentrate measurands are more likely to achieve the desired LLOQ with a higher end MSMS. The performance of a more sensitive MSMS may take longer to degrade, because less matrix is introduced with each injection. To evaluate if a simpler sample prep is likely to succeed, first assess the nature of the measurand(s), sample type, and required LLOQ (Fig. 4.2) [72]. With exceptions, sample prep for endogenous measurands such as serum steroid hormones with picomolar quantitation limits requires more complex protocols, e.g., LLE, ACP, or SLE that concentrate measurands and deplete matrix. In contrast, drugs and metabolites at higher concentrations are often amenable to D&S, PPT, or PLD, even with a less sensitive MSMS. First, define the required LLOQ and then measure on-column detection limits with pure standard (no biomatrix). This is the first step to determine if concentration versus dilution of measurands with sample prep will be needed [61].

If the desired LLOQ can be met with dilution, the sample type is the next parameter to consider [72]. D&S is appropriate for low protein matrices such as urine or CSF, whereas PPT or PLD are needed for high protein matrices such as serum/plasma/whole blood [72]. PPT is the protocol with the most risk for ion suppression and matrix residue contamination of the LC-MSMS. Details of the PPT protocol can make a difference in the extent of matrix depletion [27]. Modifying the LC gradient may ameliorate the ion suppression seen with D&S and PPT but stay aware to the reduction in throughput that occurs with any increase in min/injection [61]. PLD is probably the simplest technique to accomplish major matrix depletion (protein, phospholipids) [72].

Beyond simple sample prep: If a technique with greater selectivity, concentrating capability or matrix depletion is needed, evaluate measurand(s) chemistry—charged vs neutral, acid/base status (pKa), polarity (Log P, Log D), and thermostability (Fig. 4.2). Neutral, non-polar compounds tend to have good recovery and matrix depletion when there is partitioning in and out of a nonpolar phase, as in LLE, ACP and SLE [74]. Although reversed-phase SPE has good retention of neutral, non-polar measurands such as steroids, depletion of blood phospholipids can be difficult. Solvent washes that remove matrix may also wash neutral measurands to waste [74]. But mixed-mode ion exchange SPE for weakly acidic/basic measurands can be highly selective. Wash solutions can be pH-tuned to retain charged measurands with ion exchange while depleting lipophilic matrix from the reversed phase. Then, a pH shift converts the measurands to their uncharged form for elution with organic solvent [72]. Thermally labile or highly volatile measurands may not tolerate heating during the evaporation step needed with LLE, SLE or offline SPE. Alternatives include online SPE (no evaporation step) and ACP or µElution SPE (also SPME, other newer micro-formats), as the smaller elution volumes used may not need evaporation [75]. When the decision is between LLE and other concentrating techniques (e.g., SLE, ACP, SPE, SPME)—lower materials costs favor LLE, whereas SLE et al. require less labor and have higher throughput. SPE and LLE have the greatest ability to concentrate measurands. Manual LLE is easy to launch for small batch sizes (e.g., <10), but the manual labor and ergonomic burden of scaling up to larger batches (e.g., >20) can be problematic. LLE, ACP, and SLE do not have good recovery for highly polar or permanently charged measurands.

Using commercial media: A wide range of innovative commercial media have been developed and applied over the last 5–10 years in non-medical use cases (pharma, environmental, food and forensic testing) but they are likely underutilized by medical laboratories [18, 72, 75, 76]. The trend has been towards miniaturization and "greener" chemistry—decreasing volumes of solvents and plastic used [75]. Commercial sample prep media (ACP, PLD, SLE, SPE, DME, newer options) used with automation can vastly improve productivity and throughput. Vendors may be interested in collaboration with medical laboratory partners to optimize and validate applications for recent-generation media and small automation platforms for sample prep. If more than one complex technique appears to be an option, vendor demonstrations and trials at your laboratory using in-house patient samples can provide comparison data as well as a hands-on evaluation of workflow.

Scaling up: Medical laboratories implementing LC-MSMS for the first time often launch with a single method, few samples, manual pipetting, and D&S or PPT sample prep. As test volumes and menus expand, a need develops for automation and more sophisticated sample prep [61, 72]. Introducing more complex sample prep protocols for small batch sizes can be done incrementally, without a major investment. Relatively low-cost (sometimes below capital equipment thresholds) evaporators and vacuum or positive pressure manifolds can enable a laboratory to perform high-quality manual LLE, and cartridge-based SPE or SLE. Scaling up for sample prep of larger sample numbers involves capital investment, with key decisions being the switch from tubes/vials/sample prep cartridges to 96-well plate format and purchasing of an ALH, and/or implementing online extraction [61]. Except for LLE and QuEChERS, the techniques described in this chapter can be done in 96-well format, which will deliver the single, most significant improvement in sample prep productivity that can be implemented. ALH is not required for use of 96-well format, but (from personal experience) manually pipetting small volumes into plate wells is highly vulnerable to sample misidentification (wrong well) and false <LLOQ results (no sample added). The difficulty of thoroughly mixing immiscible liquids in 96-well plates and the risk of cross-contamination between wells means that automating LLE can be challenging and requires extensive validation.

Cost analysis and conclusions: Materials cost/sample is low and relatively easy to calculate for D&S, PPT, and LLE. But cost/reportable may be higher than anticipated for these techniques if accurate labor expenses are included. Painstaking cost analysis of automation via online SPE or use of commercial media with ALH may yield favorable cost/reportable test ratios compared to manual D&S, PPT, or LLE because of reduced labor/sample. Finally, the best sample prep choice is whatever protocol matches optimally with the capability and finances of your laboratory while delivering consistent, good assay quality and reliable instrument operations (robustness)—in short, fit for purpose.

Special considerations for general unknown screening (GUS—also broad spectrum drug screening): GUS has been problematic at US medical laboratories due to technical complexity (use of chromatography/MS) and debatable value for patient care [77]. Untargeted LC–high resolution mass spectrometry (HRMS) has broader detection capability than targeted unit resolution LC-MSMS (QqQ), but the clinical utility needs further study [77, 78]. A primary challenge of LC-HRMS GUS sample prep is balancing sensitivity (maximum measurand recovery across a broad range of Log D) versus selectivity (greater matrix depletion to decrease ion suppression).

Drug metabolites are often present in urine at higher concentrations than the parent drug, thus of interest for GUS [79]. Urine GUS sample prep may include hydrolysis to convert polar conjugated metabolites into more non-polar moieties for improved extraction recovery [79]. Arguments against hydrolysis include the potential for modifying measurand structure such that both false negatives and positives may occur [80] and reports that a more abundant ESI signal may be seen for glucuronides than for the matching aglycones [81, 82]. In comparisons of simple vs complex sample prep, the selective, concentrating options detected more compounds in some studies with better precision and less matrix effect (LLE, QuEChERS, HLB or online SPE) [79, 81, 83]. However, such techniques also missed hydrophilic compounds that were detected by less selective, dilutional D&S and PPT [79, 81]. Better serum GUS results using PLD (less matrix effect) versus PPT have been described [84, 85]. Two highly automated methods, TurboFlow®, [79] and Shimadzu CLAM-2040, [86] needed minimal expertise/time for GUS sample prep. To develop a fit-for-purpose GUS sample prep, consider measurand menu with limit of detection, sample type(s), TAT, ease of use, cost, concentrating capability, hydrolysis, and use of evaporation, flow through, and magnetic modules. The wider the polarity range/diversity of functional groups there are in a measurand menu, the less likely it is that a single GUS sample prep will have acceptable recovery/matrix effect for all measurands [87, 88]. Common solutions are multiple sample types and extractions (e.g., acidic for blood/basic for urine), reporting disclaimers, and test panels for GUS (e.g., including immunoassays, quantification of serum salicylates, and acetaminophen) [77].

Automating Sample Prep

Options for automated sample prep, such as ALH can improve throughput and minimize human error during sample prep. ALHs come with various pipetting arms or "channel" options from 1 to 96. The most flexible system for medical LC-MSMS use would be a 4- or 8-channel system that can pipette from primary sample tubes and in and out of various reagent and extraction containers. There are many options available, so lab requirements and ALH capability should be fully understood prior to purchase [89]. It should be noted that programming the software typically requires training from the vendor, the software is very different between vendors, and although vendors have custom programming services, care should be taken when implementing vendor-provided methods [90].

ALH can accommodate a wide range of labware including various sizes of tubes, 96 well plates and reagent troughs. Standard and custom racks are available from manufacturers as well as third-party vendors (i.e., www.konnis.com). Institutions with clinical engineering groups may be able to have in-house custom rack solutions 3D printed, e.g., see Fig. 4.4.

Vials vs 96 well plates Ideally, to minimize the amount of user intervention required in a sample prep process, all extraction steps would be performed in a 96 well plate. However, there are limitations to using 96-well plates, including sample

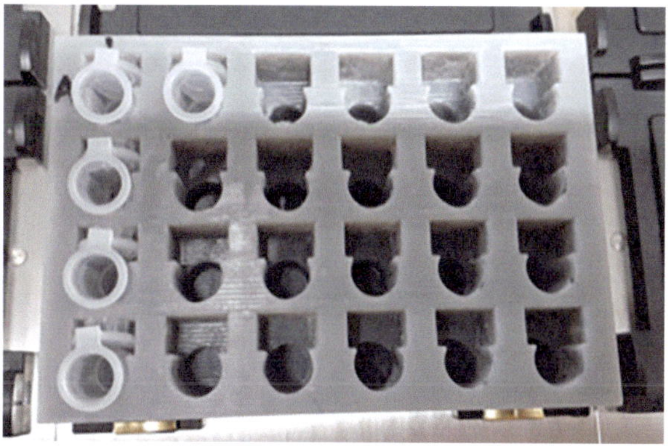

Fig. 4.4 3D printed rack to hold 1.5 mL snap cap tubes with caps secured

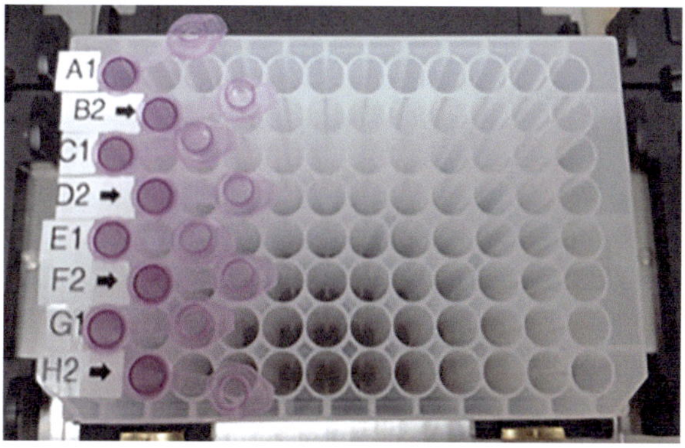

Fig. 4.5 Use of a 2 mL deep 96-well plate to hold calibrators and QCs stored in 0.5 mL microcentrifuge tubes

and extraction solvent maximum volumes, solvent compatibility with cap mats, and the ability to properly mix the sample with solvent in the narrow wells of plates. Additionally, absorption (an issue with many peptides) to certain plastics may play a role in the selection of vials over plates.

There are challenges to using vials in an ALH. Many labs use vials with snap cap lids. The ALH vendor may have specific racks that accommodate vials with snap cap lids, but labs are often in the position where they do not have the budget for additional racks and components other than what came with the ALH. Creative solutions may be required, as shown in Fig. 4.5.

Manual user intervention is a significant downside of using vials. Each vial needs to be labeled, capped following removal from the ALH, and mixing and centrifugation steps need to be handled off-deck. Subsequent ALH steps require replacing the tubes in the correct order in the appropriate rack, followed by uncapping prior to re-loading. Opportunities for human error when using vials can be mitigated by using 96 well format plates and extraction media (Table 4.3).

Best practices for partial plate use may be needed at small volume labs, where it may not be feasible to consume an entire 96 well plate in a single run. In that instance, used wells can be marked and the unused wells saved for the next run. A

Table 4.3 Example method adaptations from the authors' labs

Measurand	Original sample prep method summary	Changes to improve process
25-hydroxyvitamin D	LLE in 1.5 mL snap-cap tubes *Manual intervention required:* *Tube labeling* *Capping* *Transfer to rack for off-deck mixing* *Transfer to centrifuge rack and centrifuging* *Sorting for reloading to ALH rack* *Uncapping*	PPT in 2 mL 96 DWP *Reduced amount of user intervention* *No labeling, uncapping, or sorting required.*
Aldosterone	LLE in 5 mL snap cap tubes *Manual intervention required:* *Tube labeling* *Capping* *Transfer to rack for off-deck mixing* *Transfer to the centrifuge rack and centrifuging* *Sorting for reloading to ALH rack* *Uncapping*	SLE in Biotage SLE+ plate [91] *Reduced the amount of user intervention* *All SLE steps done on ALH deck* *Less MTBE solvent used* *Increased measurand extraction recovery with SLE* vs *LLE*

common way to do this is to cover the used wells with lab tape. This is easiest when an entire row can be taped off because it minimizes the opportunity for contamination from a neighboring well and makes partial plate use more ALH-friendly by allowing the next batch to start in row A. However, this practice will lead to wasted wells, adding cost to the assay. If starting from the next available position instead of a new row, the correct starting position must be included in the ALH programming.

Alternatively, since 96 format well plates and sample prep media are typically the same dimensions at the top left and bottom right, the partially used plate can be flipped so that position H12 becomes position A1. Care must be taken to ensure the number of wells needed for a run do not exceed the available wells remaining in a partial plate. Labs should consider the usability versus cost savings when deciding whether to block off individual wells versus entire rows.

Avoiding cross-contamination: ALH software comes pre-programmed with liquid classes which have set parameters for various liquids. Settings include parameters controlling how quickly a liquid is aspirated and dispensed, if air gaps are used, air gap volumes, and the pressure used to hold the volume of aspirated liquid in the pipette tip, depending on the viscosity of the liquid. However, (a) the pre-programmed vendor list is often limited to common solvents, and user-defined liquid classes may need to be defined, and (b) special pipetting programming may be needed for most solvents, as even with the appropriate liquid class, the solvent may

Table 4.4 Recommended precautions for minimizing the risk of cross-contamination during ALH pipetting steps

Process step	Recommended precaution
Aspirating volatile solvents	Pre-wetting step to prevent dripping
Dispensing steps	Adjust dispense speed and/or depth of tip into receiving container to minimize splashing
Travel across deck	1. Assign tubes/plates/vials positions on ALH deck to minimize the tips traveling above sample tubes and extraction containers, as well as reagent troughs 2. Only add solvents, I.S.s, and reagents to the ALH deck as needed, or keep covered when not in use (avoid any dripping into reagent trough)

still drip from the pipette tip. Dripping can be dealt with by programming pipet tip pre-wetting steps for the solvent in question to equilibrate solvent vapor pressure in the pipette channel ("conditioning") prior to the pipetting step. Cross-contamination from ALH tips could happen if dripping or bubbles are formed at the tip of the tip, and subsequently released over the deck as the tips are moved after aspirating or dispensing, and travel over other sample tubes, reagent containers, and/or the extraction containers. Splashing of liquids if the dispense speed is too high could also cause cross contamination (Table 4.4).

Protein and Peptide Sample Prep

Basic principles (see Table 4.6): Sample prep of biological samples for the analysis of peptides and proteins by LC-MSMS is complex. Due to the limited range of triple quadrupoles, proteins above a certain mass cannot be directly measured by LC-MSMS. Quantitative clinical protein LC-MSMS applications use bottom-up analysis which requires digestion of the protein and measurement of proteolytic peptides as a surrogate for the protein of interest. Pre and/or post-digestion extraction steps, such as SPE or IP, may be required to improve the sensitivity of the assay for low-level proteins and peptides, and to remove matrix and reagents used in the digestion procedure.

Internal Standard Selection and Digestion Variance: Proteins are present in biological matrices spanning 10 orders of magnitude. To achieve adequate peptide signal from low-abundance proteins, the plasma volume required may mean that 1 mg or more of protein is being digested. This poses a challenge for digestion completion and can contribute to digestion variability between samples [92]. Ideally, to control for this variability, a stable isotope labeled (SIL) protein should be used [92–94]. SIL proteins remain difficult to obtain and are expensive. SIL peptides—easier to synthesize and can be custom-made at a reasonable cost—are more frequently used as I.S.s in quantitative LC-MSMS protein assays. SIL peptides will not normalize for digestion variability, and thus it is important that the digestion protocol be strictly controlled to minimize variability and ensure accuracy.

Table 4.5 Protein/peptide sample prep characteristics

Sample type	Cost	Can concentrate?	Matrix removal	Complex or Simple	Automation?
S/P, U, CSF*	$ – $$$	Yes	+ to +++	Varying complexity	Yes

*Serum/plasma (S/P), urine (U), cerebral Spinal Fluid (CSF)

Table 4.6 General bottom up protein digestion protocol steps

Step	Purpose	Details	Selected references
Pre digestion sample prep	Purify and/or concentrate the protein measurand (i.e., remove matrix components)	IP SPE PPT Size exclusion filtration LLE	Kilpatrick and Bunk [95]; Rauh [96]; Ackermann [31]; Neubert et al. [97]; Al-Amrani et al. [98]; Asicioglu et al. [99]
Denatu-ration	Unfold the protein to allow access for trypsin to the needed areas of the protein for efficient digestion.	Denaturing chemicals include: Chaotropes[a] Surfactants Solvents These can be used in the presence of heat or in addition to heat.	Proc et al. [100]; Zheng and DeMarco [101]
Reduction	Breaking of cysteine disulfide bridges	Commonly used reagents are dithiothreitol (DTT) and tris(2- carboxyethyl) phosphine (TCEP). DTT is more commonly used as its neutral pH is more compatible with trypsin digestion	Proc et al. [100]; Al-Amrani et al. [98]
Alkylation	Prevents the reformation of cysteine disulfide bridges by blocking cysteine thiol groups	The most common reagent used is iodoacetamide	Proc et al. [100]
Digestion	Enzymatically break the protein into proteolytic peptides	Various trypsin grades are available and may be important depending on the measurand. Buffer selection may impact digestion effectiveness. Digestion is often stopped by adding acid, but anti-trypsin reagents can be used if, for example, IP will follow digestion	Van Den Broek et al. [102]; Shuford et al. [94]; Zheng and DeMarco [101]

(continued)

Table 4.6 (continued)

Step	Purpose	Details	Selected references
Post digestion cleanup	Peptide purification and/or concentration	IP SPE	Kuhn et al. [103]; Dufield and Radabaugh [104]; Ackermann [31]; Hoofnagle and Roth [105]; Neubert et al. [97]; Van Der Gugten et al. [106]; Shi et al. [107])

[a]Chaotropes inhibit trypsin, so they must be diluted to appropriate concentrations if used

Selecting an appropriate calibrant for endogenous proteins can also be challenging, as endogenous proteins and synthetic proteins may behave differently during the digestion process [94]. Efforts have been made to standardize and harmonize medical LC-MSMS protein assays as well as produce reference materials for thyroglobulin [107, 108], apolipoproteins [109], lipoprotein(a) [110], and C-Reactive Protein (CRP) [95].

Standard digestion protocols involve multiple steps including denaturation, reduction, alkylation, and digestion. Structural variations between proteins affect how accessible cleavage sites are to the enzyme used for digestion [100]. Modifications of the generic digestion workflow are common, including buffer selection and concentration, trypsin selection, incubation times, and temperatures [96, 101, 111–113]. For example, proteins that do not contain cysteines may not require reduction and alkylation, steps that help unfold the protein to facilitate cleavage [114, 115].

IP is a widely used technique in protein analysis, and can be used at the protein level, before digestion, and/or at the peptide level, after digestion [31, 95, 116, 117]. IP can improve specificity and sensitivity by concentrating and isolating the protein and/or proteolytic peptides [31]. Thyroglobulin (Tg) is present at orders of magnitude lower than abundant proteins like albumin, and a large sample volume is required to achieve the necessary lower limits of quantitation. The interferences present following a standard digest protocol would not allow for adequate detection of Tg peptides. Stable isotope standards and capture by anti-peptide antibodies (SISCAPA), where digested peptides undergo IP, is a commonly used technique for LC-MSMS Tg measurement [97, 105–107, 118, 119].

A digestion time course experiment should be done for any protein LC-MSMS assay (see Fig. 4.6). All peptides that may be used in the assay should be monitored to determine the optimal digestion time. Digestion times have traditionally been overnight, but many clinically relevant protein targets require a much shorter digestion time to reach complete digestion for the peptides of interest [100]. Ideally, complete digestion of the protein will occur with a steady state following the maximum observable peptide signal, so that slight changes in digestion time would not impact digestion reproducibility [100].

Clinically relevant in-use protein LC-MSMS assays (see Fig. 4.7): While protein LC-MSMS assays are prevalent in the proteomics literature, methods in use in

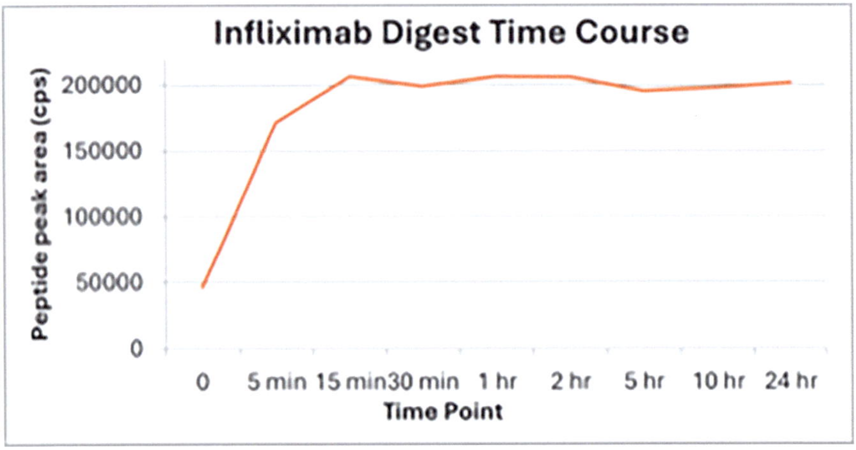

Fig. 4.6 Example digestion time course result for infliximab. Each experiment was performed in triplicate (original data generated by G. van der Gugten). For this peptide, digestion is complete in 1 h

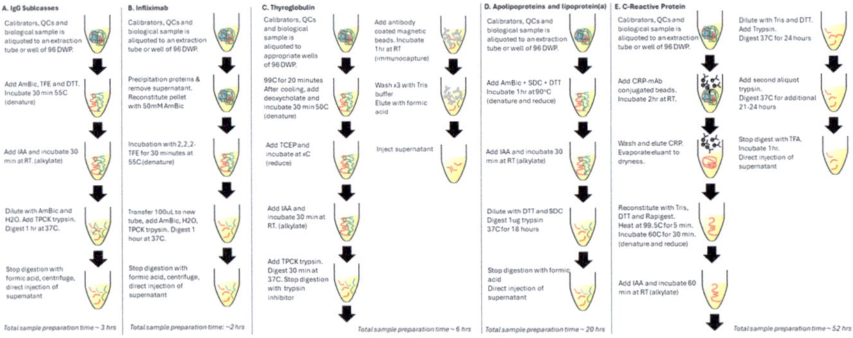

Fig. 4.7 Graphical representation of example clinically relevant protein assays performed by medical LC-MSMS. Each protein is different, requiring different sample prep approaches

medical LC-MSMS laboratories are few including thyroglobulin [105–107, 117–119], infliximab [120, 121], IgG Subclasses [122, 123], apolipoproteins and lipoprotein [70, 114, 124], and CRP [95].

Endogenous peptide analysis (see Table 4.7): Clinically relevant endogenous peptides such as angiotensin I, amyloid beta, hepcidin and insulin do not require digestion prior to LC-MSMS analysis. Special care in assessing non-specific binding of the peptides to labware, as well as to LC components, should be taken. The use of specially treated plastics such as Eppendorf LoBind, Waters QuanRecovery, and Axygen Maxymum Recovery products, pre-treatment of labware, or addition of carrier proteins may be required. It should be noted that not all plastics are the same and may perform differently even between container formats within a brand (i.e., tube vs 96-well plate).

Table 4.7 Example peptide targets and procedures

Peptide measurand & matrix	Example extraction method	Special considerations	Reference(s)
Angiotensin I from plasma	SPE of incubated plasma samples using reversed-phase sorbent	Endogenous renin cleaves angiotensinogen to angiotensin I at 37 °C. Samples are collected cold, in EDTA tubes, centrifuged cold, and plasma frozen immediately to inhibit renin activity during sample collection and storage	Van Der Gugten and Holmes [125]
Amyloid beta peptides in CSF	1. SPE using µSPE and mixed-mode sorbent 2. IP	Non-specific binding of Ab peptides requires special handling	Ford et al. [126]; Lame et al. [127]; Lin et al. [128]; DeMarco et al. [129]; Korecka and Shaw [130]; Oztug et al. [131]
Hepcidin in plasma	1. Protein precipitation 2. SPE 3. IP	Non-specific binding should be assessed	Enko et al. [132]; Chen et al. [133]; Punt et al. [134]
Endogenous insulins/ insulin analogues	1. Precipitation and reduction of disulfide bonds 2. SPE 3. IP	Insulin is not stable at room temperature in plasma or in solution. Non-specific binding should be assessed	Chen et al. [135]; Chambers et al. [136]; Van Der Gugten et al. [137]; Shen et al. [138]
ACTH	IP	ACTH is not stable at RT, and samples should be collected in pre-chilled tubes, and plasma immediately frozen following centrifugation. Excessive freeze-thaw cycles should be avoided	Shi et al. [139]

Dried Blood Spots (DBS) Sample Prep

DBS cards have been in use as a sample collection technique since the 1960s when Robert Guthrie introduced them for use in newborn screening for phenylketonuria (PKU). Sampling is typically done by collecting drops of blood from the heel for newborn screening (finger for other patients) and allowing the blood spots to dry on a filter paper card. A wide range of LC-MSMS applications using DBS cards have been reported in the literature. DBS are primarily used in newborn screening but have potential to be used in many areas of the clinical laboratory, including toxicology, therapeutic drug monitoring, endocrinology, proteomics, metabolomics, and lipidomics [140–143]. Measurand extraction from DBS requires special considerations:

Pre-analytical Considerations

Filter paper and blood distribution The type of paper used for DBS sampling will affect adsorption and dispersion of the blood and can cause variation in sample attributes that could impact measurand stability, volume per area, as well as analytical effects [143]. Whatman 903 (W903) and Ahlstrom 226 (A226) filter papers are recommended by the Clinical and Laboratory Standards Institute (CLSI) and approved by the Food and Drug Administration (FDA) and the Centers for Disease Control (CDC) [144, 145]. The whole blood drop should be spotted in the middle of the pre-printed circular collection area of the blood spot card to allow for radial dispersion of the blood to the edge of the spot. Chromatographic effects of the filter paper can cause the distribution of blood to be uneven throughout the spot [143, 144]. This can be assessed by analyzing punches at various positions in the DBS to determine if the measurand concentration varies due to this effect.

Hematocrit effect (see Fig. 4.8): Variation in hematocrit (Hct) is viewed as a significant factor in DBS analysis [145]. Hct is the proportion of blood volume taken up by red blood cells. Directly proportional to viscosity—it affects the distribution of the blood across the filter paper [144, 146]. A higher Hct causes less distribution of blood through the spot, and subsequently, a punch will contain more blood volume than from a DBS with a lower Hct value [142–145]. Hct also affects the percentage of plasma in punches made in different areas of the DBS and is an important variable to assess, particularly for measurands found mainly in the serum or plasma portion of blood [143]. Hct may also affect extraction recovery [147].

Hct effect can be assessed by spiking measurand(s) into a blank blood matrix prepared at varying Hct levels for spotting and analysis. If varying Hct levels cause variation in measurand concentrations, the Hct value may be required to normalize the results, but this may not be practical—rather, calibrators and controls can be prepared at Hct levels corresponding to the study samples. Hct levels can be assessed visually, and pictorial guidelines can be referred to in routine analysis for what is acceptable [145].

Blood volume: The volume of blood spotted onto the DBS card may result in variation in the measured measurand concentration for a fixed punch, depending on the compound being measured. This can be assessed by spotting various volumes of blood samples on the DBS cards and determining if the resulting measurand

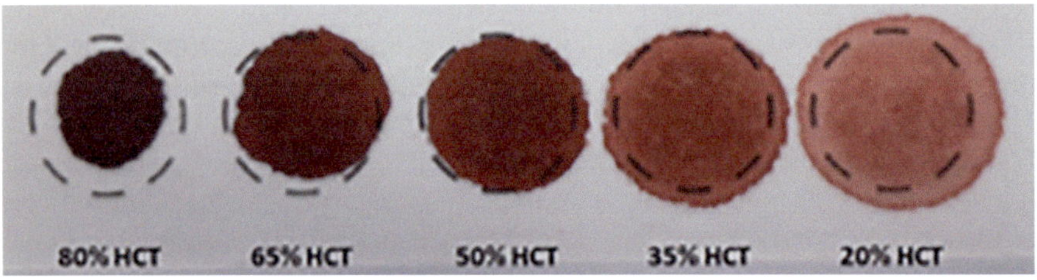

Fig. 4.8 Effect of hematocrit on blood distribution on filter paper

concentrations from various punch locations (i.e., center, peripheral) are within acceptance criteria. Based on the results of this assessment, recommendations regarding both acceptable spot size and where sub punches should be made from the DBS to ensure the most accurate result should be included in the method procedures [144, 145].

Alternative microsampling techniques have been developed in an attempt to overcome the challenges associated with the inaccuracy of exact volume measurement of a DBS punch. There are a number of commercial products available that make use of microfluidics, polymer-assisted volumetric sampling, and capillary flow to enable precise volumes of blood to be collected and dried [148]. These sampling approaches may be more feasible in a controlled clinical study, rather than in programs such as newborn screening where filter card DBS is globally well established.

Sample Prep Considerations

Punch equivalent volume: A typical DBS spot contains 50–100 μL of blood volume. In most cases, a 3.2 mm or 6.4 mm punch will be used for extraction of the measurands of interest. Equivalent blood volumes in a 3.2 mm punch are between approximately 2.7 μL and 3.4 μL for Hct levels between 40 and 65% [149, 150]. This Hct-dependent variation in blood volume may affect assay accuracy. The small equivalent blood volume, and equivalent serum volume (approximately 1.54 μL [151]) contained in a single 3.2 mm DBS punch can pose challenges for achieving a desired LLOQ, depending on the measurand and the sensitivity of the mass spectrometer being used. Larger sample sizes are feasible by using a larger punch size (i.e., 6.4 mm, approx. 11.2 uL) [149] or by analyzing multiple punches, although there are limits on the number of available punches that can be made from a single DBS.

Internal standard (I.S.) addition: I.S. mixing and equilibration as is employed in biological fluid sample prep, is not possible with DBS, as the I.S. is most often added as part of the extraction or elution reagent. Because of this, the I.S. may not thoroughly compensate for the measurands of interest during the sample prep process [152].

Preparation of calibrators and controls: Blank matrix for DBS can be prepared in-house using washed blood cells which are mixed at an appropriate Hct concentration (i.e., 55%) with a charcoal-stripped serum or buffer. This surrogate matrix is then spiked with the measurands of interest and spotted onto the DBS filter paper. The same type of DBS filter paper should be used for sample collection and calibrators, and controls [144–146]. The techniques used to prepare calibrators and controls—including the type of blood cells used, the Hct content, and the volume of blood applied to filter paper—can affect the measured concentration of the measurand(s) [145, 146]. Gentle mixing or rocking of the calibrators and controls for 30 min up to 24 h may be required to allow for equilibration of the spiked measurand(s) to the blank matrix before spotting to the filter paper.

It can be challenging to accurately add a whole blood blank matrix to the fill line of a volumetric flask. Alternative approaches include (a) preparing calibrators gravimetrically by weighing the equivalent amount of whole blood blank matrix, (b) preparing calibrators volumetrically in charcoal stripped serum (or alternative buffer) followed by mixing with washed blood cells to obtain the appropriate Hct level, or (c) purchasing commercially available serum or plasma calibrators, and mixing with washed blood cells to the appropriate Hct level. Proficiency testing agencies such as the CDC NSQAP, ERNDiM, and UKNEQAS have DBS quality controls and proficiency testing materials that can assist laboratories in ensuring in-house prepared calibrators are accurate, but these are limited to compounds specific to newborn screening programs. Commercially available DBS calibrators and controls are specific to newborn screening applications, so laboratories may be in the position where they must prepare DBS calibrators and controls in house.

Carryover concerns specific to DBS are twofold: (1) Physical contact of the DBS between cards, and (2) carryover from the puncher. Physical contact between cards during transport and storage can be easily dealt with by ensuring a physical barrier is present between exposed blood spots to protect from card-to-card carryover. Puncher carryover should be tested thoroughly, and if it is determined that there is carryover from a high sample to a subsequent punch, procedures to clean the puncher between samples should be implemented [143, 152].

Assessment of matrix effects and recovery: Matrix effects assessments should be performed for DBS as for any other sample type [153]. Because the I.S. may not give appropriate analytical compensation for the recovery of the measurand from the DBS and/or filter paper, evaluation of recovery may need a more thorough assessment, including assessment of impacts of the age of the DBS [152].

General Sample Extraction Procedures for DBS (See Table 4.8)

DBS sample prep requires a sub punch or the entire DBS to be removed from the filter paper to enable extraction and quantitation of the measurand [145]. This can be done manually, with handheld punches, or with semi-automated punching instruments which integrate barcode reading, have cameras indicating sub punch location, and distribute the tracked samples to 96-well plates [145]. Punch location should be assessed based on the pre-analytical variables that can cause inaccuracy as described above, since the punch location, depending on size and quality of the DBS, can impact the accuracy of the results obtained [145].

Typically, one or more DBS punches are taken and transferred into tubes or appropriate wells of a 96 well plate, followed by addition of the extraction solvent mixture containing the I.S. Binding of the measurand to the protein in the matrix, or to the filter paper material, as well as measurand solubility must be taken into consideration when choosing the extraction solvent [141, 144]. The extraction process often includes incubation with or without shaking, sonication, or microwave extraction [144]. Optimal extraction time should be determined empirically and is often longer than what is typically employed for liquid biological specimen protein

Table 4.8 Example DBS sample prep methods

Measurands tested	Example extraction	Considerations	References
Amino acids and acylcarnitines for NBS—FIA-MSMS	1 × 3.2 mm punch 100 μL extraction solution containing I.S. Shake 650 rpm, 45 °C, 45 min Transfer supernatant to new well plate	Some measurands (e.g., leucine and isoleucine) cannot be differentiated using the example method. An alternative method is to use butylation.	De Jesús et al. [68]
CAH steroid panel: cortisol, 17OHP, 11Deoxycortisol, 21Deoxycortisol, androstenedione—LC-MSMS	1 × 3.2 mm punch in a filter plate seated on top of collection plate 200 μL of methanol containing I.S. Let sit at RT for 30 min Centrifuge to collect supernatant in collection plate Evaporate to dryness Reconstitute with 40 μL	MSMS must be sufficiently sensitive to reach the LLOQ using only one 3.2 mm punch. Alternatively, multiple or larger diameter punches can be used	Example from author's current lab
Second Tier NBS—LC-MSMS	1 × 3.2 mm punch in a 96 well plate 100 μL of extraction solution containing I.S.s 12 μL of DTT Shake 45 min at RT Evaporate extract to dryness Reconstitute, shake 5 min.	Example procedure from Kilgore 2023. There are many approaches to second tier testing including small disease specific panels [154] to large universal panels [155].	Dubland et al. [154]; Kilgore et al. [155]

precipitation procedures. Measurand recovery can be optimized by examining the various extraction parameters such as extraction solvent composition, temperature, time and if using additional solvation energy such as sonication or microwaves. A centrifugation step may be employed to help remove any DBS or filter paper particulates, and the supernatant transferred or filtered to a new vial or 96-well plate. Further processing may include evaporation, reconstitution, derivatization, dilution, or direct injection to the MS/MS system [144].

More extensive sample prep can be performed, depending on the measurands of interest: The DBS punch can be incubated in a buffer or water to rehydrate the blood, followed by the standard biological fluid extraction techniques such as PPT, LLE, SLE, or SPE.

References

1. Williams ML, Olomukoro AA, Emmons RV, et al. Matrix effects demystified: strategies for resolving challenges in analytical separations of complex samples. J Sep Sci. 2023;46:2300571. https://doi.org/10.1002/jssc.202300571.
2. Zhou W, Yang S, Wang PG. Matrix effects and application of matrix effect factor. Bioanalysis. 2017;9:1839–44. https://doi.org/10.4155/bio-2017-0214.
3. Stone J. A practical guide to sample preparation for liquid chromatography-tandem mass spectrometry in clinical research and toxicology. Spectrosc Eur. 2018;30:15–8, 21
4. Vogeser M, Seger C. A decade of HPLC–MS/MS in the routine clinical laboratory—goals for further developments. Clin Biochem. 2008;41:649–62. https://doi.org/10.1016/j.clinbiochem.2008.02.017.
5. Ferslew KE. Specimen preparation/extraction. In: Levine BS, Kerrigan S, editors. Principles of forensic toxicology. Cham: Springer; 2020. p. 109–25.
6. Jackson TC, Zhang YV, Sime PJ, et al. Development of an accurate and sensitive method for lactate analysis in exhaled breath condensate by LC MS/MS. J Chromatogr B Analyt Technol Biomed Life Sci. 2017;1061–1062:468–73. https://doi.org/10.1016/j.jchromb.2017.07.041.
7. Hasan M, Schumacher G, Seekamp A, et al. LC–MS/MS method for the determination of clodronate in human plasma. J Pharm Biomed Anal. 2014;100:341–7. https://doi.org/10.1016/j.jpba.2014.08.022.
8. Margaryan T, Sargsyan M, Gevorgyan A, et al. High-throughput protein precipitation method with 96-well plate for determination of doxepin and nordoxepin in human plasma using LC–MS/MS. Biomed Chromatogr. 2020;34:e4844. https://doi.org/10.1002/bmc.4844.
9. Marney LC, Laha TJ, Baird GS, et al. Isopropanol protein precipitation for the analysis of plasma free metanephrines by liquid chromatography-tandem mass spectrometry. Clin Chem. 2008;54:1729–32. https://doi.org/10.1373/clinchem.2008.104083.
10. Mikayelyan A, Aleksanyan A, Sargsyan M, et al. Protein precipitation method for determination of clobazam and N-desmethylclobazam in human plasma by LC–MS/MS. Biomed Chromatogr. 2020;34:e4710. https://doi.org/10.1002/bmc.4710.
11. Polson C, Sarkar P, Incledon B, et al. Optimization of protein precipitation based upon effectiveness of protein removal and ionization effect in liquid chromatography–tandem mass spectrometry. J Chromatogr B. 2003;785:263–75. https://doi.org/10.1016/S1570-0232(02)00914-5.
12. Wohlfarth A, Roth N, Auwärter V. LC–MS/MS analysis of Δ9-tetrahydrocannabinolic acid A in serum after protein precipitation using an in-house synthesized deuterated internal standard. J Mass Spectrom. 2012;47:778–85. https://doi.org/10.1002/jms.3021.
13. French D. Advances in clinical mass spectrometry. Adv Clin Chem. 2017;79:153–98. https://doi.org/10.1016/bs.acc.2016.09.003.
14. Carmical J, Brown S. The impact of phospholipids and phospholipid removal on bioanalytical method performance. Biomed Chromatogr. 2016;30:710–20. https://doi.org/10.1002/bmc.3686.
15. Badawy MEI, El-Nouby MAM, Kimani PK, et al. A review of the modern principles and applications of solid-phase extraction techniques in chromatographic analysis. Anal Sci. 2022;38:1457–87. https://doi.org/10.1007/s44211-022-00190-8.
16. Restek. The fundamentals of solid phase extraction.

17. Turoňová D, Kujovská Krčmová L, Švec F. Application of microextraction in pipette tips in clinical and forensic toxicology. TrAC Trends Anal Chem. 2021;143:116404. https://doi.org/10.1016/j.trac.2021.116404.
18. Mahdavijalal M, Petio C, Staffilano G, et al. Innovative solid-phase extraction strategies for improving the advanced chromatographic determination of drugs in challenging biological samples. Molecules. 2024;29:2278. https://doi.org/10.3390/molecules29102278.
19. MacNeill R. Hydrophilic-phase extraction: a new avenue of solid-phase extraction for oligonucleotide bioanalysis. LCGC Eur. 2022:46–51. https://doi.org/10.56530/lcgc.eu.kt3381t8.
20. Wang J, Kong S, Yan J, et al. Hydrophilic interaction liquid chromatography-solid phase extraction directly combined with protein precipitation for the determination of triptorelin in plasma. J Chromatogr B. 2014;960:214–21. https://doi.org/10.1016/j.jchromb.2014.04.036.
21. Zheng N. Automated and high-throughput extraction approaches. In: Solid-phase extraction. Elsevier; 2020. p. 573–88.
22. Kuklenyik Z, Calafat AM, Barr JR, Pirkle JL. Design of online solid phase extraction-liquid chromatography-tandem mass spectrometry (SPE-LC–MS/MS) hyphenated systems for quantitative analysis of small organic compounds in biological matrices. J Sep Sci. 2011;34:3606–18. https://doi.org/10.1002/jssc.201100562.
23. Gaudio FD, Cucina A, Indelicato S, et al. Turbulent flow chromatography: a unique two-dimensional liquid chromatography. In: High performance liquid chromatography – recent advances and applications. IntechOpen; 2023.
24. Cortese M, Gigliobianco MR, Magnoni F, et al. Compensate for or minimize matrix effects? Strategies for overcoming matrix effects in liquid chromatography-mass spectrometry technique: a tutorial review. Molecules. 2020;25:3047. https://doi.org/10.3390/molecules25133047.
25. Brown S, Carmichael J. Phospholipid depletion techniques in LC–MS bioanalysis. In: Sample preparation in LC–MS bioanalysis. Wiley; 2019. p. 52–67.
26. Pucci V, Di Palma S, Alfieri A, et al. A novel strategy for reducing phospholipids-based matrix effect in LC–ESI-MS bioanalysis by means of HybridSPE. J Pharm Biomed Anal. 2009;50:867–71. https://doi.org/10.1016/j.jpba.2009.05.037.
27. Stone J. High-throughput serum 25-hydroxy vitamin D testing with automated sample preparation. Methods Mol Biol. 2016;1378:301–20. https://doi.org/10.1007/978-1-4939-3182-8_32.
28. Biotage A note (2018) ISOLUTE®HYDRO DME+Dual Mode Extraction Columns.
29. Biotage A note (2019) Extraction of Illicit and Prescribed Drugs from Enzyme-Hydrolyzed Urine Using ISOLUTE® HYDRO DME+ Prior to UPLC–MS/MS Analysis.
30. Biotage A note (2020) Sample Preparation Techniques for Synthetic Benzodiazepines.
31. Ackermann BL. Understanding the role of immunoaffinity-based mass spectrometry methods for clinical applications. Clin Chem. 2012;58:1620–2. https://doi.org/10.1373/clinchem.2012.193714.
32. Delaunay N, Pichon V, Hennion M-C. Immunoaffinity solid-phase extraction for the trace-analysis of low-molecular-mass analytes in complex sample matrices. J Chromatogr B Biomed Sci Appl. 2000;745:15–37. https://doi.org/10.1016/S0378-4347(00)00116-X.
33. Laha TJ, Strathmann FG, Wang Z, et al. Characterizing antibody ross-reactivity for immunoaffinity purification of analytes prior to multiplexed liquid chromatography–tandem mass spectrometry. Clin Chem. 2012;58:1711–6. https://doi.org/10.1373/clinchem.2012.185827.
34. Stanley B, Dai J, Xu A, et al. A sensitive and cost-effective LC–MS-MS method for determination of 1α,25-dihydroxyvitamin D3 in human plasma. LC GC N Am. 2015;13
35. Vogeser M, Geiger A, Herrmann R, Kobold U. Preparation of plasma samples for chromatographic analyses using functionalized ferromagnetic micro-particles manipulated in a high pressure liquid system. Clin Biochem. 2009;42:915–8. https://doi.org/10.1016/j.clinbiochem.2009.01.018.
36. Ma X, Zou Y, Wang D, et al. Novel magnetic-bead-assisted sequential extraction method for liquid chromatography-mass spectrometry (MS)/MS of components with diverse properties:

gastrin determination as a case study. Anal Chem. 2023;95:802–10. https://doi.org/10.1021/acs.analchem.2c02970.
37. Yu S, Zhou W, Yu J, et al. An automated magnetic bead extraction method for measuring plasma metanephrines and 3-methoxytyramine using liquid chromatography tandem mass spectrometry. Anal Bioanal Chem. 2022;414:3541–9. https://doi.org/10.1007/s00216-022-03984-x.
38. König K, Goethel SF, Rusu VM, Vogeser M. Deproteination of serum samples for LC–MS/MS analyses by applying magnetic micro-particles. Clin Biochem. 2013;46:652–5. https://doi.org/10.1016/j.clinbiochem.2013.01.003.
39. Wiesen MHJ, Blaich C, Streichert T, et al. Paramagnetic micro-particles as a tool for rapid quantification of apixaban, dabigatran, edoxaban and rivaroxaban in human plasma by UHPLC–MS/MS. Clin Chem Lab Med. 2017;55 https://doi.org/10.1515/cclm-2016-0888.
40. Anastassiades M, Lehotay SJ, Štajnbaher D, Schenck FJ. Fast and easy multiresidue method employing acetonitrile extraction/partitioning and "dispersive solid-phase extraction" for the determination of pesticide residues in produce. J AOAC Int. 2003;86:412–31. https://doi.org/10.1093/jaoac/86.2.412.
41. Lehotay S. The QuEChERSER Mega-Method. LC GC N Am. 2022;40:13–9.
42. Socas-Rodríguez B, González-Sálamo J, Herrera-Herrera A, et al. Recent advances and developments in the QuEChERS method. In: Comprehensive analytical chemistry; 2017.
43. Rejczak T, Tuzimski T. A review of recent developments and trends in the QuEChERS sample preparation approach. Open Chem. 2015;13 https://doi.org/10.1515/chem-2015-0109.
44. Pouliopoulos A, Tsakelidou E, Krokos A, et al. Quantification of 15 psychotropic drugs in serum and postmortem blood samples after a modified mini-QuEChERS by UHPLC–MS-MS. J Anal Toxicol. 2018;42:337–45. https://doi.org/10.1093/jat/bky006.
45. Alves V, Conceição C, Gonçalves J, et al. Improved analytical approach based on QuECHERS/UHPLC–PDA for quantification of fluoxetine, clomipramine and their active metabolites in human urine samples. J Anal Toxicol. 2017;41:45–53. https://doi.org/10.1093/jat/bkw077.
46. Dulaurent S, El Balkhi S, Poncelet L, et al. QuEChERS sample preparation prior to LC–MS/MS determination of opiates, amphetamines, and cocaine metabolites in whole blood. Anal Bioanal Chem. 2016;408:1467–74. https://doi.org/10.1007/s00216-015-9248-3.
47. Rodrigues TB, Morais DR, Gianvecchio VAP, et al. Development and validation of a method for quantification of 28 psychotropic drugs in postmortem blood samples by modified micro-QuEChERS and LC–MS-MS. J Anal Toxicol. 2021;45:644–56. https://doi.org/10.1093/jat/bkaa138.
48. Settle V, Foster F, Roberts P, et al. Automated QuEChERS extraction for the confirmation of pesticide residues in foods using LC/MS/MS.
49. Trent J. Pesticide analysis using the AutoMate-Q40: an automated solution to QuEChERS extractions application note pesticide analysis; 3-Apr-13. LC GC N AM. 2013.
50. Tecan. Tecan AC extraction plate; 2017.
51. Baecher S, Geyer R, Lehmann C, Vogeser M. Absorptive chemistry based extraction for LC–MS/MS analysis of small molecule analytes from biological fluids—an application for 25-hydroxyvitamin D. Clin Chem Lab Med. 2014;52:363–71. https://doi.org/10.1515/cclm-2013-0534.
52. Couchman L, Subramaniam K, Fisher DS, et al. Automated analysis of clozapine and norclozapine in human plasma using novel extraction plate technology and flow-injection tandem mass spectrometry. Ther Drug Monit. 2016;38:42–9. https://doi.org/10.1097/FTD.0000000000000231.
53. Stone JA, van Staveren DR, Fitzerald RL. Automated sample preparation enables LC–MS/MS as a routine diagnostic analysis for serum testosterone. J Appl Lab Med. 2017;2:33–46. https://doi.org/10.1373/jalm.2016.022772.
54. Johnsen E, Brandtzaeg OK, Vehus T, et al. A critical evaluation of Amicon Ultra centrifugal filters for separating proteins, drugs and nanoparticles in biosamples. J Pharm Biomed Anal. 2016;120:106–11. https://doi.org/10.1016/j.jpba.2015.12.010.

55. Nilsson LB. The bioanalytical challenge of determining unbound concentration and protein binding for drugs. Bioanalysis. 2013;5:3033–50. https://doi.org/10.4155/bio.13.274.
56. Toma C-M, Imre S, Vari C-E, et al. Ultrafiltration method for plasma protein binding studies and its limitations. PRO. 2021;9:382. https://doi.org/10.3390/pr9020382.
57. Wang L, Yuan W, Reuschel S, Meng M. Hydrolysis of phase II conjugates for LC–MS bioanalysis of total parent drugs. In: Handbook of LC–MS bioanalysis. Wiley; 2013. p. 471–7.
58. Sitasuwan P, Melendez C, Marinova M, et al. Degradation of opioids and opiates during acid hydrolysis leads to reduced recovery compared to enzymatic hydrolysis. J Anal Toxicol. 2016;40:601–7. https://doi.org/10.1093/jat/bkw085.
59. Yang HS, Wu AHB, Lynch KL. Development and validation of a novel LC–MS/MS opioid confirmation assay: evaluation of β-glucuronidase enzymes and sample cleanup methods. J Anal Toxicol. 2016;40:323–9. https://doi.org/10.1093/jat/bkw026.
60. Higashi T. Derivatization to generate a product ion containing analyte-specific moiety in ESI–MS/MS. Anal Sci. 2024;40:973–4. https://doi.org/10.1007/s44211-024-00567-x.
61. Rappold BA. Review of the use of liquid chromatography-tandem mass spectrometry in clinical laboratories: part I-development. Ann Lab Med. 2022a;42:121–40. https://doi.org/10.3343/alm.2022.42.2.121.
62. Rappold BA. Review of the use of liquid chromatography-tandem mass spectrometry in clinical laboratories: part II–operations. Ann Lab Med. 2022b;42:531–57. https://doi.org/10.3343/alm.2022.42.5.531.
63. Aronov PA, Hall LM, Dettmer K, et al. Metabolic profiling of major vitamin D metabolites using Diels–Alder derivatization and ultra-performance liquid chromatography–tandem mass spectrometry. Anal Bioanal Chem. 2008;391:1917–30. https://doi.org/10.1007/s00216-008-2095-8.
64. Tai SS-C, Welch MJ. Development and evaluation of a reference measurement procedure for the determination of estradiol-17β in human serum using isotope-dilution liquid chromatography−tandem mass spectrometry. Anal Chem. 2005;77:6359–63. https://doi.org/10.1021/ac050837i.
65. Denver N, Khan S, Stasinopoulos I, et al. Derivatization enhances analysis of estrogens and their bioactive metabolites in human plasma by liquid chromatography tandem mass spectrometry. Anal Chim Acta. 2019;1054:84–94. https://doi.org/10.1016/j.aca.2018.12.023.
66. Chan N, Kaleta EJ. Quantitation of 1α,25-dihydroxyvitamin D by LC–MS/MS using solid-phase extraction and fixed-charge derivitization in comparison to immunoextraction. Clin Chem Lab Med. 2015;53 https://doi.org/10.1515/cclm-2014-0884.
67. Van Faassen M, Bischoff R, Eijkelenkamp K, et al. In matrix Derivatization combined with LC–MS/MS results in ultrasensitive quantification of plasma free metanephrines and catecholamines. Anal Chem. 2020;92:9072–8. https://doi.org/10.1021/acs.analchem.0c01263.
68. De Jesús VR, Chace DH, Lim TH, et al. Comparison of amino acids and acylcarnitines assay methods used in newborn screening assays by tandem mass spectrometry. Clin Chim Acta. 2010;411:684–9. https://doi.org/10.1016/j.cca.2010.01.034.
69. Baghdady YZ, Schug KA. Review of in situ derivatization techniques for enhanced bioanalysis using liquid chromatography with mass spectrometry. J Sep Sci. 2016;39:102–14. https://doi.org/10.1002/jssc.201501003.
70. Zhang Y, Ren X, Zhou Z, et al. Simultaneous quantitative LC–MS/MS analysis of 13 apolipoproteins and lipoprotein (a) in human plasma. Analyst. 2024;149:3444–55. https://doi.org/10.1039/D4AN00221K.
71. Guo X, Lankmayr E. Phospholipid-based matrix effects in LC–MS bioanalysis. Bioanalysis. 2011;3:349–52. https://doi.org/10.4155/bio.10.213.
72. Marin S, Smith J, Neifeld J, Gairloch E. Bioanalytical analysis of small-molecule drugs and metabolites in physiological samples by LC–MS, part 2: sample preparation. LC GC N Am. 2021;39:372–83.

73. Stone JA, van der Gugten JG. Quantitative tandem mass spectrometry in the clinical laboratory: regulation and opportunity for validation of laboratory developed tests. J Mass Spectrom Adv Clin Lab. 2023;28:82–90. https://doi.org/10.1016/j.jmsacl.2023.03.001.
74. Stone J. Chapter 3 – Sample preparation techniques for mass spectrometry in the clinical laboratory. In: Nair H, Clarke W, editors. Mass spectrometry for the clinical laboratory. San Diego: Academic Press; 2017. p. 37–62.
75. Dugheri S, Marrubini G, Mucci N, et al. A review of micro-solid-phase extraction techniques and devices applied in sample pretreatment coupled with chromatographic analysis. Acta Chromatogr. 2021;33:99–111. https://doi.org/10.1556/1326.2020.00790.
76. Kanu AB. Recent developments in sample preparation techniques combined with high-performance liquid chromatography: a critical review. J Chromatogr A. 2021;1654:462444. https://doi.org/10.1016/j.chroma.2021.462444.
77. Van Wijk XMR, Goodnough R, Colby JM. Mass spectrometry in emergency toxicology: current state and future applications. Crit Rev Clin Lab Sci. 2019;56:225–38. https://doi.org/10.1080/10408363.2019.1585415.
78. Partridge E, Trobbiani S, Stockham P, et al. A validated method for the screening of 320 forensically significant compounds in blood by LC/QTOF, with simultaneous quantification of selected compounds. J Anal Toxicol. 2018;42:220–31. https://doi.org/10.1093/jat/bkx108.
79. Helfer AG, Michely JA, Weber AA, et al. LC–HR-MS/MS standard urine screening approach: pros and cons of automated on-line extraction by turbulent flow chromatography versus dilute-and-shoot and comparison with established urine precipitation. J Chromatogr B. 2017;1043:138–49. https://doi.org/10.1016/j.jchromb.2016.06.036.
80. Maurer HH. Pitfalls in drug testing by hyphenated low- and high-resolution mass spectrometry. Drug Test Anal. 2020;12:172–9. https://doi.org/10.1002/dta.2744.
81. Musatadi M, Andrés-Maguregi A, De Angelis F, et al. The role of sample preparation in suspect and non-target screening for exposome analysis using human urine. Chemosphere. 2023;339:139690. https://doi.org/10.1016/j.chemosphere.2023.139690.
82. Pourchet M, Debrauwer L, Klanova J, et al. Suspect and non-targeted screening of chemicals of emerging concern for human biomonitoring, environmental health studies and support to risk assessment: from promises to challenges and harmonisation issues. Environ Int. 2020;139:105545. https://doi.org/10.1016/j.envint.2020.105545.
83. Guo Z, Huang S, Wang J, Feng Y-L. Recent advances in non-targeted screening analysis using liquid chromatography—high resolution mass spectrometry to explore new biomarkers for human exposure. Talanta. 2020;219:121339. https://doi.org/10.1016/j.talanta.2020.121339.
84. Ogawa T, Kondo F, Iwai M, et al. Novel extraction method using an ISOLUTE PLD+ protein and phospholipid removal column for liquid chromatography-tandem mass spectrometry analysis of 20 psychoactive drugs in postmortem whole blood samples. Forensic Sci Int. 2022;331:111130. https://doi.org/10.1016/j.forsciint.2021.111130.
85. Valero AMR, Jorge OQ, Serrano BB, Tejedor SA. Optimization of a rapid method for screening drugs in blood by liquid chromatography tandem mass spectrometry. Adv Lab Med. 2023;4:365. https://doi.org/10.1515/almed-2023-0154.
86. Robin T, El Balkhi S, Dulaurent S, et al. First-line toxicological screening with fully automated extraction. J Anal Toxicol. 2021;45:252–68. https://doi.org/10.1093/jat/bkaa075.
87. Abushareeda W, Vonaparti A, Saad KA, et al. High resolution full scan liquid chromatography mass spectrometry comprehensive screening in sports antidoping urine analysis. J Pharm Biomed Anal. 2018;151:10–24. https://doi.org/10.1016/j.jpba.2017.12.025.
88. Chaker J, Kristensen DM, Halldorsson TI, et al. Comprehensive evaluation of blood plasma and serum sample preparations for HRMS-based chemical exposomics: overlaps and specificities. Anal Chem. 2022;94:866–74. https://doi.org/10.1021/acs.analchem.1c03638.
89. Torres-Acosta MA, Lye GJ, Dikicioglu D. Automated liquid-handling operations for robust, resilient, and efficient bio-based laboratory practices. Biochem Eng J. 2022;188:108713. https://doi.org/10.1016/j.bej.2022.108713.

90. Britt-Rodriquez K, Daniel J, Hayden J. Surreptitious pipetting errors on a vendor-programmed liquid handler. J Mass Spectrom Adv Clin Lab. 2024;33:1–3. https://doi.org/10.1016/j.jmsacl.2024.05.001.
91. Van Der Gugten JG, Crawford M, Grant RP, Holmes DT (2012) Supported liquid extraction offers improved sample preparation for aldosterone analysis by liquid chromatography tandem mass spectrometry. J Clin Pathol 65:1045–48. https://doi.org/10.1136/jclinpath-2012-200990.
92. Hoofnagle AN, Wener MH. The fundamental flaws of immunoassays and potential solutions using tandem mass spectrometry. J Immunol Methods. 2009;347:3–11. https://doi.org/10.1016/j.jim.2009.06.003.
93. Faria M, Halquist MS, Yuan M, et al. Comparison of a stable isotope labeled (SIL) peptide and an extended SIL peptide as internal standards to track digestion variability of an unstable signature peptide during quantification of a cancer biomarker, human osteopontin, from plasma using capillary microflow LC–MS/MS. J Chromatogr B. 2015;1001:156–68. https://doi.org/10.1016/j.jchromb.2015.05.040.
94. Shuford CM, Walters JJ, Holland PM, et al. Absolute protein quantification by mass spectrometry: not as simple as advertised. Anal Chem. 2017;89:7406–15. https://doi.org/10.1021/acs.analchem.7b00858.
95. Kilpatrick EL, Bunk DM. Reference measurement procedure development for C-reactive protein in human serum. Anal Chem. 2009;81:8610–6. https://doi.org/10.1021/ac901597h.
96. Rauh M. LC–MS/MS for protein and peptide quantification in clinical chemistry. J Chromatogr B. 2012;883–884:59–67. https://doi.org/10.1016/j.jchromb.2011.09.030.
97. Neubert H, Shuford CM, Olah TV, et al. Protein biomarker quantification by immunoaffinity liquid chromatography–tandem mass spectrometry: current state and future vision. Clin Chem. 2020;66:282–301. https://doi.org/10.1093/clinchem/hvz022.
98. Al-Amrani S, Al-Jabri Z, Al-Zaabi A, et al. Proteomics: concepts and applications in human medicine. WJBC. 2021;12:57–69. https://doi.org/10.4331/wjbc.v12.i5.57.
99. Asicioglu M, Oztug M, Karaguler NG. Development of an ID-LC–MS/MS method using targeted proteomics for quantifying cardiac troponin I in human serum. Clin Proteomics. 2023;20:40. https://doi.org/10.1186/s12014-023-09430-z.
100. Proc JL, Kuzyk MA, Hardie DB, et al. A quantitative study of the effects of chaotropic agents, surfactants, and solvents on the digestion efficiency of human plasma proteins by trypsin. J Proteome Res. 2010;9:5422–37. https://doi.org/10.1021/pr100656u.
101. Zheng YZ, DeMarco ML. Manipulating trypsin digestion conditions to accelerate proteolysis and simplify digestion workflows in development of protein mass spectrometric assays for the clinical laboratory. Clin Mass Spectrom. 2017;6:1–12. https://doi.org/10.1016/j.clinms.2017.10.001.
102. Van Den Broek I, Niessen WMA, Van Dongen WD. Bioanalytical LC–MS/MS of protein-based biopharmaceuticals. J Chromatogr B. 2013;929:161–79. https://doi.org/10.1016/j.jchromb.2013.04.030.
103. Kuhn E, Addona T, Keshishian H, et al. Developing multiplexed assays for troponin I and interleukin-33 in plasma by peptide immunoaffinity enrichment and targeted mass spectrometry. Clin Chem. 2009;55:1108–17. https://doi.org/10.1373/clinchem.2009.123935.
104. Dufield DR, Radabaugh MR. Online immunoaffinity LC/MS/MS. A general method to increase sensitivity and specificity: how do you do it and what do you need? Methods. 2012;56:236–45. https://doi.org/10.1016/j.ymeth.2011.08.012.
105. Hoofnagle AN, Roth MY. Improving the measurement of serum thyroglobulin with mass spectrometry. J Clin Endocrinol Metabol. 2013;98:1343–52. https://doi.org/10.1210/jc.2012-4172.
106. Van Der Gugten JG, Razavi M, Holmes DT. Quantitation of thyroglobulin in serum using SISCAPA and liquid chromatography-tandem mass spectrometry (LC–MS/MS). In: Garg U, editor. Clinical applications of mass spectrometry in biomolecular analysis. New York, NY: Springer; 2022. p. 473–83.

107. Shi J, Phipps WS, Owusu BY, et al. A distributable LC–MS/MS method for the measurement of serum thyroglobulin. J Mass Spectrom Adv Clin Lab. 2022;26:28–33. https://doi.org/10.1016/j.jmsacl.2022.09.005.
108. Netzel BC, Grant RP, Hoofnagle AN, et al. First steps toward harmonization of LC–MS/MS thyroglobulin assays. Clin Chem. 2016;62:297–9. https://doi.org/10.1373/clinchem.2015.245266.
109. Cobbaert CM, Althaus H, Begcevic Brkovic I, et al. Towards an SI-traceable reference measurement system for seven serum apolipoproteins using bottom-up quantitative proteomics: conceptual approach enabled by cross-disciplinary/cross-sector collaboration. Clin Chem. 2021;67:478–89. https://doi.org/10.1093/clinchem/hvaa239.
110. Marcovina SM, Clouet-Foraison N, Koschinsky ML, et al. Development of an LC–MS/MS proposed candidate reference method for the standardization of analytical methods to measure lipoprotein(a). Clin Chem. 2021;67:490–9. https://doi.org/10.1093/clinchem/hvaa324.
111. Li F, Schmerberg CM, Ji QC. Accelerated tryptic digestion of proteins in plasma for absolute quantitation using a protein internal standard by liquid chromatography/tandem mass spectrometry. Rapid Comm Mass Spectrometry. 2009;23:729–32. https://doi.org/10.1002/rcm.3926.
112. Lowenthal MS, Liang Y, Phinney KW, Stein SE. Quantitative bottom-up proteomics depends on digestion conditions. Anal Chem. 2014;86:551–8. https://doi.org/10.1021/ac4027274.
113. Shuford CM, Grant RP. Cheaper, faster, simpler trypsin digestion for high-throughput targeted protein quantification. J Mass Spectrom Adv Clin Lab. 2023;30:74–82. https://doi.org/10.1016/j.jmsacl.2023.11.002.
114. Shi J, Zheng YZ, Sin DD, DeMarco ML. A streamlined method for quantification of apolipoprotein A1 in human plasma by LC–MS/MS. Clin Chem. 2018;64:1782–4. https://doi.org/10.1373/clinchem.2018.293530.
115. Wojtkiewicz M, Berg Luecke L, Kelly MI, Gundry RL. Facile preparation of peptides for mass spectrometry analysis in bottom-up proteomics workflows. Curr Protoc. 2021;1:e85. https://doi.org/10.1002/cpz1.85.
116. Anderson NL, Anderson NG, Haines LR, et al. Mass spectrometric quantitation of peptides and proteins using stable isotope standards and capture by anti-peptide antibodies (SISCAPA). J Proteome Res. 2004;3:235–44. https://doi.org/10.1021/pr034086h.
117. Hoofnagle AN, Becker JO, Wener MH, Heinecke JW. Quantification of thyroglobulin, a low-abundance serum protein, by immunoaffinity peptide enrichment and tandem mass spectrometry. Clin Chem. 2008;54:1796–804. https://doi.org/10.1373/clinchem.2008.109652.
118. Clarke NJ, Zhang Y, Reitz RE. A novel mass spectrometry–based assay for the accurate measurement of thyroglobulin from patient samples containing antithyroglobulin autoantibodies. J Investig Med. 2012;60:1157–63. https://doi.org/10.2310/JIM.0b013e318276deb4.
119. Kushnir MM, Rockwood AL, Roberts WL, et al. Measurement of thyroglobulin by liquid chromatography–tandem mass spectrometry in serum and plasma in the presence of antithyroglobulin autoantibodies. Clin Chem. 2013;59:982–90. https://doi.org/10.1373/clinchem.2012.195594.
120. Van Der Gugten JG, Bressler B, DeMarco ML. An automated mass spectrometric blood test for therapeutic drug monitoring of infliximab. Clin Mass Spectrom. 2019;12:16–22. https://doi.org/10.1016/j.clinms.2019.01.003.
121. Willrich MAV, Murray DL, Barnidge DR, et al. Quantitation of infliximab using clonotypic peptides and selective reaction monitoring by LC–MS/MS. Int Immunopharmacol. 2015;28:513–20. https://doi.org/10.1016/j.intimp.2015.07.007.
122. Ladwig PM, Barnidge DR, Snyder MR, et al. Quantification of serum IgG subclasses by use of subclass-specific tryptic peptides and liquid chromatography–tandem mass spectrometry. Clin Chem. 2014;60:1080–8. https://doi.org/10.1373/clinchem.2014.222208.
123. Van Der Gugten G, DeMarco ML, Chen LYC, et al. Resolution of spurious immunonephelometric IgG subclass measurement discrepancies by LC–MS/MS. Clin Chem. 2018;64:735–42. https://doi.org/10.1373/clinchem.2017.282319.

124. Van Den Broek I, Romijn FPHTM, Nouta J, et al. Automated multiplex LC–MS/MS assay for quantifying serum apolipoproteins A-I, B, C-I, C-II, C-III, and E with qualitative apolipoprotein E phenotyping. Clin Chem. 2016;62:188–97. https://doi.org/10.1373/clinchem.2015.246702.
125. Van Der Gugten JG, Holmes DT. Quantitation of plasma renin activity in plasma using liquid chromatography–tandem mass spectrometry (LC–MS/MS). In: Garg U, editor. Clinical applications of mass spectrometry in biomolecular analysis. New York, NY: Springer; 2016. p. 243–53.
126. Ford MJ, Cantone JL, Polson C, et al. Qualitative and quantitative characterization of the amyloid β peptide (Aβ) population in biological matrices using an immunoprecipitation–LC/MS assay. J Neurosci Methods. 2008;168:465–74. https://doi.org/10.1016/j.jneumeth.2007.11.019.
127. Lame ME, Chambers EE, Blatnik M. Quantitation of amyloid beta peptides Aβ1–38, Aβ1–40, and Aβ1–42 in human cerebrospinal fluid by ultra-performance liquid chromatography–tandem mass spectrometry. Anal Biochem. 2011;419:133–9. https://doi.org/10.1016/j.ab.2011.08.010.
128. Lin P, Chen W, Yuan F, et al. An UHPLC–MS/MS method for simultaneous quantification of human amyloid beta peptides Aβ1-38, Aβ1-40 and Aβ1-42 in cerebrospinal fluid using micro-elution solid phase extraction. J Chromatogr B. 2017;1070:82–91. https://doi.org/10.1016/j.jchromb.2017.10.047.
129. DeMarco ML, Nguyen Q, Fok A, et al. An automated clinical mass spectrometric method for identification and quantification of variant and wild-type amyloid-β 1-40 and 1-42 peptides in CSF. Alzheimers Dementi. 2020;12 https://doi.org/10.1002/dad2.12036.
130. Korecka M, Shaw LM. Mass spectrometry-based methods for robust measurement of Alzheimer's disease biomarkers in biological fluids. J Neurochem. 2021;159:211–33. https://doi.org/10.1111/jnc.15465.
131. Oztug M, Vatansever B, Altin G, et al. An LC–MS/MS-based platform for the quantification of multiple amyloid beta peptides in surrogate cerebrospinal fluid. J Mass Spectrom Adv Clin Lab. 2024;31:40–8. https://doi.org/10.1016/j.jmsacl.2024.01.002.
132. Enko D, Zelzer S, Fauler G, Herrmann M. Evaluation of a commercial liquid-chromatography high-resolution mass-spectrometry method for the determination of hepcidin-25. Biochem Med. 2019;29:292–301. https://doi.org/10.11613/BM.2019.020701.
133. Chen M, Liu J, Wright B. A sensitive and cost-effective high-performance liquid chromatography/tandem mass spectrometry (multiple reaction monitoring) method for the clinical measurement of serum hepcidin. Rapid Comm Mass Spectrometry. 2020;34:e8644. https://doi.org/10.1002/rcm.8644.
134. Punt Arjen M, Wieman JC, Van Der Elst KC, et al. An easy, fast, and efficient assay for the quantification of peptide Hepcidin-25 in serum and plasma with LC–MS/MS. Ann Clin Biochem. 2022;59:330–7. https://doi.org/10.1177/00045632221095490.
135. Chen Z, Caulfield MP, McPhaul MJ, et al. Quantitative insulin analysis using liquid chromatography–tandem mass spectrometry in a high-throughput clinical laboratory. Clin Chem. 2013;59:1349–56. https://doi.org/10.1373/clinchem.2012.199794.
136. Chambers EE, Fountain KJ, Smith N, et al. Multidimensional LC–MS/MS enables simultaneous quantification of intact human insulin and five recombinant analogs in human plasma. Anal Chem. 2014;86:694–702. https://doi.org/10.1021/ac403055d.
137. Van Der Gugten JG, Wong S, Holmes DT. Quantitation of insulin analogues in serum using Immunoaffinity extraction, liquid chromatography, and tandem mass spectrometry. In: Garg U, editor. Clinical applications of mass spectrometry in biomolecular analysis. New York, NY: Springer; 2016. p. 119–30.
138. Shen Y, Prinyawiwatkul W, Xu Z. Insulin: a review of analytical methods. Analyst. 2019;144:4139–48. https://doi.org/10.1039/C9AN00112C.
139. Shi J, Dhaliwal P, Zi Zheng Y, et al. An intact ACTH LC–MS/MS assay as an arbiter of clinically discordant immunoassay results. Clin Chem. 2019;65:1397–404. https://doi.org/10.1373/clinchem.2019.306365.

140. Malsagova K, Kopylov A, Stepanov A, et al. Dried blood spot in laboratory: directions and prospects. Diagnostics. 2020;10:248. https://doi.org/10.3390/diagnostics10040248.
141. Sharma A, Jaiswal S, Shukla M, Lal J. Dried blood spots: concepts, present status, and future perspectives in bioanalysis. Drug Test Anal. 2014;6:399–414. https://doi.org/10.1002/dta.1646.
142. Skogvold HB, Rootwelt H, Reubsaet L, et al. Dried blood spot analysis with liquid chromatography and mass spectrometry: trends in clinical chemistry. J Sep Sci. 2023;46:2300210. https://doi.org/10.1002/jssc.202300210.
143. Zakaria R, Allen KJ, Koplin JJ, et al. Advantages and challenges of dried blood spot analysis by mass spectrometry across the total testing process. EJIFCC. 2016;27:288–317.
144. Li W, Tse FLS. Dried blood spot sampling in combination with LC-MS/MS for quantitative analysis of small molecules. Biomed Chromatogr. 2010;24:49–65. https://doi.org/10.1002/bmc.1367.
145. Moat SJ, George RS, Carling RS. Use of dried blood spot specimens to monitor patients with inherited metabolic disorders. IJNS. 2020;6:26. https://doi.org/10.3390/ijns6020026.
146. Keevil BG. The analysis of dried blood spot samples using liquid chromatography tandem mass spectrometry. Clin Biochem. 2011;44:110–8. https://doi.org/10.1016/j.clinbiochem.2010.06.014.
147. Deprez S, Stove C. Application of a fully automated dried blood spot method for therapeutic drug monitoring of immunosuppressants: another step toward implementation of dried blood spot analysis. Arch Pathol Lab Med. 2023;147:786–96. https://doi.org/10.5858/arpa.2021-0533-OA.
148. Thangavelu MU, Wouters B, Kindt A, et al. Blood microsampling technologies: innovations and applications in 2022. Anal Sci Adv. 2023;4:154–80. https://doi.org/10.1002/ansa.202300011.
149. Baruteau J, Khalil Y, Grunewald S, et al. Urea cycle related amino acids measured in dried bloodspots enable long-term in vivo monitoring and therapeutic adjustment. Meta. 2019;9:275. https://doi.org/10.3390/metabo9110275.
150. Hall E, Flores S, De Jesús V. Influence of hematocrit and total-spot volume on performance characteristics of dried blood spots for newborn screening. IJNS. 2015;1:69–78. https://doi.org/10.3390/ijns1020069.
151. Hannon WH, Therrell BL. Overview of the history and applications of dried blood samples. In: Li W, Lee MS, editors. Dried blood spots. 1st ed. Wiley; 2014. p. 1–15.
152. Timmerman P, White S, Globig S, et al. EBF recommendation on the validation of bioanalytical methods for dried blood spots. Bioanalysis. 2011;3:1567–75. https://doi.org/10.4155/bio.11.132.
153. Matuszewski BK, Constanzer ML, Chavez-Eng CM. Strategies for the assessment of matrix effect in quantitative bioanalytical methods based on HPLC−MS/MS. Anal Chem. 2003;75:3019–30. https://doi.org/10.1021/ac020361s.
154. Dubland JA, Rakić B, Vallance H, Sinclair G. Analysis of 2-methylcitric acid, methylmalonic acid, and total homocysteine in dried blood spots by LC–MS/MS for application in the newborn screening laboratory: a dual derivatization approach. J Mass Spectrom Adv Clin Lab. 2021;20:1–10. https://doi.org/10.1016/j.jmsacl.2021.03.001.
155. Kilgore MB, Platis D, Lim T, et al. Development of a universal second-tier newborn screening LC–MS/MS method for amino acids, lysophosphatidylcholines, and organic acids. Anal Chem. 2023;95:3187–94. https://doi.org/10.1021/acs.analchem.2c03098.

Specific Lab Techniques for LC-MS/MS Analysis

5

Brittany K. Casey, Heidi R. Schimmelbusch,
Daniel T. Holmes, Rong Yi, and Robert A. Middleberg

Introduction

Clinical laboratories rely on advanced analytical techniques to detect compounds quickly, reliably, and often at very low concentrations in complex biological matrices. LC-MS/MS has seen widespread use in clinical applications such as drug monitoring, biomarker quantification, toxicology, and endocrinology for this reason due to its sensitivity, specificity, and multiplexing capabilities. For laboratories with little or no prior experience with LC-MS/MS, practical guidance for its proper implementation and operation is useful. This includes understanding and control of environmental conditions to ensure adequate site preparation, thorough vendor evaluation, selection, and verification of equipment and reagents to ensure they are fit for use, and familiarity with associated laboratory techniques. This chapter provides detailed considerations for implementing LC-MS/MS in a clinical laboratory setting.

Equipment Qualification

Several qualification steps are designed to assess the LC-MS/MS system on the way to analyzing patient samples. Design qualification outlines the functional and performance specifications before equipment is purchased. This assures the equipment

B. K. Casey · H. R. Schimmelbusch · R. A. Middleberg (✉)
NMS Labs, Horsham, PA, USA
e-mail: robert.middleberg@nmslabs.com

D. T. Holmes · R. Yi
University of British Columbia Department of Pathology and Laboratory Medicine,
Vancouver, BC, Canada

Y. V. Zhang, U. Garg (eds.), *Practical Guide to Implementing Liquid Chromatography Mass Spectrometry in Clinical Laboratories*,
https://doi.org/10.1007/978-3-032-03852-4_5

will be suitable for the intended applications and includes vendor qualification. Installation qualification is a documented collection of activities required to install equipment into the user's environment. This includes site preparation before installation. After installation, the vendor will perform a series of performance checks before releasing the equipment to the user. Operational qualification is ultimately performed by the end user. This process demonstrates that the equipment functions according to operational specifications in the selected environment. Both hardware and software are assessed and documented during this qualification step. Lastly, performance qualification is performed on a periodic basis to ensure continued suitable performance.

Site Preparation

The first step in implementation typically involves site preparation to ensure successful and reliable operation of the equipment necessary to perform testing. The most stringent operating conditions are applied to instrumentation, and adequate site preparation is a vendor requirement before installation is initiated (Table 5.1). Requirements are very similar between LC-MS/MS manufacturers.

Table 5.1 Typical site preparation guidelines for LC–MS/MS instrumentation

Power	Voltage fluctuation allowances by vendor Uninterrupted power supply Power outlet compatibility with power cords supplied by the vendor Individual power requirements per instrument component Length of cords supplied and accessibility
Gas	Dry, oil-free nitrogen, 95% purity or higher Nitrogen must be regulated to specified setting using a two-stage gas regulator with an appropriate outlet range Copper gas tubing must be chemically cleaned Stainless steel gas tubing must be medical grade Joints should be compression fittings to avoid contamination from soldered or brazed joints Tubing size specified by vendor Nitrogen consumption is large, recommend using a liquid nitrogen dewar for heavy usage Dry, oil-free Argon, 99.997% purity If an alternate gas is allowed by the vendor, verify purity requirements Argon must be regulated to a specified setting using a two-stage gas regulator with an appropriate outlet range Medical-grade stainless steel is recommended for the collision gas supply Joints should be compression fittings to avoid contamination from soldered or brazed joints Tubing size specified by vendor Consumption is minimal so a tank is appropriate for this purpose

(continued)

Table 5.1 (continued)

Extraction and waste collection	Exhaust venting must comply with all local safety and environmental regulations. The ANSI/AIHA Z9.2-2012 standard "fundamentals governing the design and operation of local exhaust ventilation systems" provides guidance Systems can be vented to a fume hood or laboratory exhaust system Liquid waste container should be sized based on usage Degasser outlet requires ambient ventilation Source and rough pump exhaust require proper negative pressure ventilation to ensure a safe working environment for both personnel and the equipment. Negative pressure ensures contaminants and gas vapors are drawn out of the work area Exhaust speed generally must maintain a minimum of 100 fpm to prevent backflow
Shipping container handling	Temperature and humidity requirements vary by vendor Keep boxes unopened and on pallets ahead of installation
Space and load	Flat surface and level within +/−1° Table should support the weight of components, not subject to vibrations, and have adequate clearance on all sides of the system for service access clearances may be stated by the vendor for service requirements Rough pump will be on the floor under the system. Allow adequate air flow to maintain temperature and venting Data system allowances should be evaluated and have proper cord lengths
Environmental[a]	Temperature requirements for operating temperature variation need to be carefully planned to ensure compliance To calculate the overall heat dissipation into the room, add together the applicable power consumption values given in the electrical specification section. You may need to install or upgrade air conditioning systems to accommodate additional heat load in the room when installing these systems, particularly from nitrogen generators Humidity needs to be monitored to avoid condensation and to meet requirements for operating Due to exhaust and fluidic systems, leaks are a potential risk for consideration Instrument performance may be impacted by altitude Systems cannot be used within magnetic or radio frequency fields above a certain level
Customer-supplied items	Check the vendor site preparation guide for items required for installation not provided by the vendor This may include solvents, glassware and gas fittings, and regulators

[a]Equipment such as balances will also have vibration and static electricity requirements or considerations

Vendor Qualification

Thorough vendor evaluation prior to material selection is critical to ensuring quality, traceability, and compliance with regulatory standards. Instrument manufacturers are generally well-established entities, and the selection of instrumentation is influenced by factors such as existing purchasing agreements, familiarity with the manufacturer, and documented performance through demonstrations and technical notes. Due to the high degree of individualization involved, this chapter will not cover the evaluation of instrument manufacturers but will focus on evaluating vendors of other types of equipment, services, reagents, or consumables.

This evaluation is especially vital for reference materials and calibration vendors, as these directly affect the accuracy and reliability of laboratory results. Rigorously evaluating vendors mitigates the risk of compromised results, regulatory non-compliance, and operational inefficiencies. Laboratories should prioritize vendors with established quality credentials or recognized accreditations, such as ISO 9001 for quality management systems, ISO/IEC 17025 for testing and calibration laboratories, or ISO 17034 for reference material producers. These qualifications demonstrate adherence to quality standards and provide confidence in the vendor's reliability.

In addition to verifying accreditation status, laboratories may request and review certificates of analysis (CoA) for reagents or calibration certificates for equipment or vendors. These documents should detail critical parameters, such as purity, concentration, and traceability to national or international standards. A thorough review ensures the products or services meet the laboratory's specifications and are fit for purpose [1].

Reagent Selection

Solvent Grades

Choosing the appropriate grade of solvent is important to the performance of the chromatographic system and the quality of the results generated (Table 5.2). Solvents and water may contain dissolved inorganic and organic compounds, gases, microorganisms, and particulates.

Although the most expensive of the options, "LC/MS" grade solvent is recommended by most vendors for optimal results and care of the system [2].

Water for sample preparation and instrument use must be Type I water. To meet the requirements for Type I water, it must have resistivity greater than 18 MΩ-cm, conductivity less than 0.056 μS/cm, and total organic carbons less than 50 ppb. Deionization is the only process that can produce water with the required resistivity. The quality of the deionized water is impacted by storage and age. Opening containers frequently will lead to contamination of the water from the laboratory environment. While bottled water may start with the same level of purity as water from a deionized water system, as the bottled water is opened multiple times, the purity

Table 5.2 Laboratory solvent grades

Grade	Purity	Use	Other specifications	Recommendations
Spectrophotometric	97–99%	Spectrophotometric analysis, HPLC, trace compound, metal and contaminant detection	Multiply distilled, ultra-fine borosilicate glass, UV impurities removed	Not recommended for LC-MS/MS
HPLC	≥99%	HPLC	Filtered through 4.0 μm or less polycarbonate filters. Low residue and solid count	Suitable for HPLC. Not recommended for MS/MS detectors.
LC/MS	≥99%	LC–MS LC–MSMS TOF	Typically same grade as HPLC but filtered through 0.2 μm or less polycarbonate membranes to remove residual particles	Use for analysis by LC-MS/MS

will degrade. Water stored in open or non-airtight containers is susceptible to bacterial growth and environmental contamination. If deionized water will be generated and stored in large volumes from a purification system, a UV treatment option is recommended to reduce bacterial growth. Ideally, laboratories with high water consumption should produce ultrapure water daily from a water purification system. Bottles for daily use should be cleaned with each refill and can be stored in amber glass to reduce bacterial growth [3].

Reserpine, an antihypertensive drug, is commonly used to demonstrate the performance of a mass spectrometry system. Signal-to-noise ratio can be measured using this compound as a reference point. LC/MS grade water specifications dictate that no peak in the mass spectrum may be higher than the reserpine peak $[M + H] +$ ($m/z = 609$). Although the LC/MS grade water of many vendors may consistently pass control quality tests, the reserpine signals obtained using water obtained from different vendors can differ. For example, an evaluation of a solution of 50 ppb reserpine prepared using LC/MS grade bottled water from three different vendors and freshly produced Milli-Q® water was performed. Prior to the evaluation, all bottled waters were opened three times a day for 28 days to expose the solvent to the laboratory atmosphere. Direct injection of these samples into the MS revealed the signal suppression of the $[M + H] +$ peak for all bottled waters except the Milli-Q® water. This demonstrates that the storage and handling of laboratory water will impact the quality, which directly impacts the analytical results [3].

Table 5.3 Laboratory reagent grades

Grade	Purity	Use	Recommendation
ACS	≥95%	Food, drug, and medicinal	Use for sample preparation for LC-MS/MS
Reagent	≥95%	Food, drug, and medicinal	Use for sample preparation for LC-MS/MS
USP	Meets or exceeds USP requirements	Food, drug, and medicinal	Meets or exceeds LC-MS/MS analytical requirements
NF	Meets or exceeds National Formulary requirements	Chemical and biological drug substances, dosage forms, and compounded preparations	Meets or exceeds LC-MS/MS analytical requirements
Laboratory	Unknown	Educational	Not recommended for LC-MS/MS
Purified	Meets no official standard	Non-medical	Not recommended for LC-MS/MS
Technical	Meets no official standard	Commercial and industrial	Not recommended for LC-MS/MS

Reagent Grades

Reagents used to prepare samples for analysis can be different from those used during instrumental analysis. A number of different grades may be present in your laboratory already. Below are guidelines for selection (Table 5.3) [2].

Internal Standards

LC-MS/MS analysis typically utilizes an internal standard, which is added to calibrators, QC samples, and case specimens to normalize some of the potential variability in analytical methods. The amount of internal standard added is determined during method validation and may vary depending on the expected concentration of the analyte of interest. Typically, it will be added so that its concentration in the prepared sample is similar to the analyte of interest in the case samples. Once the appropriate internal standard quantity is determined, the same amount is added to every sample.

Isotopically labeled analog(s) of the analyte(s) of interest are commonly used as internal standards since the labeled analog mimics the behavior of the analyte of interest, therefore mitigating sources of variation. The most common isotopic labels are deuterium, carbon-13, and nitrogen-15. The number of isotopic labels must be sufficient to differentiate the standard from the analyte during MS detection. This is minimally 3 amu but preferably more. The position of isotopic labels within the molecule should be such that chemical exchange with protons or solvent is unlikely and interference is minimized for both parent and fragment ions. Deuterium labels should not be positioned on heteroatoms such as oxygen or nitrogen for this reason or on other positions with acidic hydrogens. Carbon-13, and nitrogen-15 labels are preferable, as they are unable to exchange, but they are also more costly than deuterium labels. Additionally, the labelled site needs to be on the analytically relevant portion of the molecule so that the internal standard fragments differ from the analyte fragments by the desired mass unit. Labels in more than one position on the molecule may be necessary to achieve this. Internal standard cost generally increases with the complexity of the synthesis as well as the number of isotopic labels, so finding a compromise between cost and differentiation is important.

The use of isotopically labeled internal standards in an analysis may be precluded due to lack of availability, cost, or the number of analytes in the panel. In such situations, one or more internal standards with chemical properties sufficiently close to those of the analytes of interest may be used instead (Fig. 5.1).

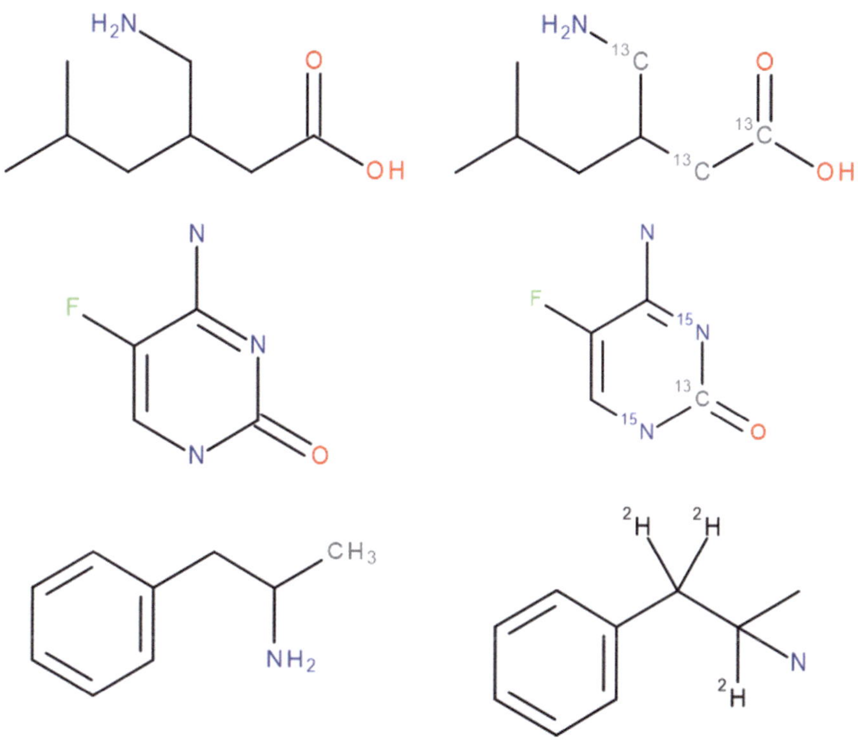

Fig. 5.1 Chemical structures of representative analytes of interest (left) and potential internal standards with different types of isotopic labels (right)

Calibrators

When selecting materials for use as calibrators, it is important to select those with the highest quality and purity, sourced from a reputable vendor with a detailed Certificate of Analysis (CoA). To maintain metrological traceability during preparation, they should be prepared using balances that have been qualified and calibrated using ISO 17025 requirements and NIST traceable weights. Verification of the solution standard involves multiple aspects, such as assessing mass balance purity (with necessary salt adjustments), examining spectral and physical data, and confirming the stability of the solution [1].

Quality Controls

An alternate vendor should be used for the control material than the one selected for the calibrator material when possible. If an alternate is not available, it is recommended to prepare material using a different lot and at a separate time from the calibrator. Staggering calibrator and control preparations will monitor degradation of materials over time, whereas preparation at the same time may lead to erroneous results due to similar degradation patterns. Prior to use, a comparison of calibrator and control material should be done by standard verification or quantitative comparison.

Typically, a minimum of two controls per analytical run is required, though it's common to use three levels along with a blank. Controls should be strategically positioned at the upper, middle and lower end of the analytical measurement range (AMR) or, alternatively for endogenous compounds, within and flanking the normal range of patient samples. Blank controls play an important role in monitoring for matrix interferences and contamination.

Controls should mimic patient samples and be handled in the same way throughout the process. The control matrix should match patient samples, and in cases where patient samples include multiple matrices, studies must be performed to ensure comparable performance across different matrices. Otherwise, calibrator, control, and patient samples must be matrix-matched.

Fortified controls are the most common, though authentic patient samples may also be used in select cases, for example when the presence of analyte metabolites is preferred or natural matrix is easier to prepare than purchase. Fortified control material should be prepared and verified before being used with patient samples and can be prepared by a commercial vendor or internally. Pooled patient samples may serve to create an authentic control. When considering free versus bound analytes in controls, it is important to match the preparation method to that used for patient samples. For instance, if patient samples are prepared using protein removal filters to analyze free drug concentrations, controls should be prepared in the same way. Hydrolysis is a process used to revert a compound to its free state from its conjugated state. If sample preparation involves hydrolysis, controls should include a hydrolysis monitoring compound to ensure the reaction reaches completeness.

Lastly, it is beneficial to include a control to monitor the effects of dilution on patient samples and the effectiveness of liquid handling devices. Dilution studies should be performed during method development to determine the maximum allowable dilution for each matrix type. While advanced techniques like LC-MS/MS are essential for achieving high sensitivity and specificity in complex analyses, their success often relies on mastering fundamental laboratory practices [1].

Equipment and Reagent Verification

After evaluating and selecting a vendor, ensuring the quality and suitability of equipment does not end with its acquisition. Verification of these items, including instrumentation, prior to use is a critical step to confirm that they meet acceptability criteria and perform as expected prior to use with patient samples. After installation, the vendor will evaluate the system against their internal qualification criteria. The end user should perform a similar evaluation using criteria based on the intended use of the equipment. The validation or verification of one or more representative methods or processes should be performed and documented. Once the equipment is deemed acceptable post-installation, day of use verification is recommended. The frequency of checks for certain equipment is based on use and impact on results [4].

Performance qualification can be fulfilled by incorporating day of use verification in the form of a system suitability test (SST). An SST is a neat solution (SST mix) containing analytes of interest, which is analyzed to ensure the chromatographic and MS components of the system are performing properly. The SST mix typically comprises a mix of analytes that have different retention times, polarities, and molecular weights. The ideal SST composition spans the range of the LC program and is chemically similar to the analytes included in the analysis. In the event of a failure of a reagent or piece of equipment to pass the day of use check, remediation is performed, and the system is re-checked. Chapter 8 provides additional detail on troubleshooting for LC-MS/MS. Day of use verification for reagents prepared by the laboratory such as calibrator and QC solutions comprises a comparison of the newly prepared lot against the previously used/verified lot to ensure the performance of the new lot is comparable or improved relative to the previously used lot. Day of use verification for other laboratory equipment will be covered in the subsection specific to that equipment.

Basic Laboratory Equipment and Techniques

Basic lab techniques, such as accurately measuring and transferring liquids or precisely weighing standards or samples, provide the foundation for reliable and reproducible analytical results. Equipment considered to have a potential impact on the analytical result will be covered (e.g., volumetric flasks and balances), while general laboratory equipment (e.g., centrifuges) will not.

Volumetric Glassware

Volumetric glassware is commonly used for achieving precise and accurate volume measurements in a laboratory. When using volumetric glassware, solvent is added to the glassware until the meniscus, the liquid curve seen in the glassware, is even with the graduation line. The meniscus may be concave or convex depending on the solvent used. Volumetric glassware is typically mixed by inversion; however, the mixing technique depends on the nature of the solute and the desired level of homogeneity in the solution. Solute should be added to the solvent slowly to promote dissolution. When mixing by inversion, care should be taken to not overly agitate the liquid and avoid creating air bubbles. Viscous liquids can be mixed using a magnetic stir bar. Some solutes may require heat to encourage dissolution in solvent. If solvents being mixed can be predicted to generate gases, care should be taken when removing the vessel stopper [5].

Type A glassware is preferred for quantitative analyses, as it has a tighter tolerance/specification than non-type A glassware. Day of use verification for glassware typically involves a visual inspection of the equipment for damage, confirming its cleanliness, and conducting volume checks when necessary. Laboratories should follow manufacturer guidelines or established protocols for periodic recalibration to ensure the glassware continues to deliver reliable measurements over time. In certain applications, such as working with hydrofluoric acid or other corrosive chemicals, plastic volumetric glassware made of materials like polypropylene is necessary due to its chemical resistance and durability. The accuracy of plastic glassware may differ from traditional glassware, however, so its use should be carefully evaluated based on the specific requirements of the analysis.

Proper glassware storage and care is vital to prevent warping or etching that can compromise accuracy and/or integrity. Additionally, as glassware is commonly shared across multiple procedures in the clinical laboratory, effort should be made to prevent cross-contamination. This is generally accomplished through thorough cleaning of the glassware between uses. A variety of glass washing methods are available from hand washing to automated glassware washers. Once the cleaning procedure has been selected and detailed in policy, validation of the procedure is necessary regardless of the method used to ensure removal of any cleaning agent residue and previous analyte(s). This is accomplished through the spiking of a representative drug into test solutions. The glassware used is then cleaned according to policy and rinsed iteratively with a suitable solvent. The rinse solutions are ultimately analyzed for the presence of the representative drug. Glassware can also be rinsed with purified water to check whether any residue from cleaning agents remains. This can be accomplished by a comparison of the UV spectrum and/or pH of the purified water before and after rinsing. If comparing the pH, a pH meter or a colorimetric indicator such as Bromothymol Blue may be used. An analysis of total organic carbon (TOC) may also be performed [6].

Liquid Handling Devices

Liquid handling devices are used to accurately, precisely, and efficiently transfer specific volumes of liquids. Choosing the appropriate device for your application is crucial. Air displacement and positive displacement devices can be manual piston-stroke pipettes or multifunction dispensers. Piston-stroke devices have the flexibility to dispense fixed or adjustable volumes across a wide range. Single and multichannel devices cater to different lab techniques, with multichannel devices operating on the air displacement principle.

Dispensers can significantly reduce the number of individual pipetting processes by repeatedly dispensing a certain volume from a previously aspirated one. Using a handheld dispenser to dispense a single volume into several destination (e.g., 8 channel) containers can be an effective alternative to full automation.

The pipette tip is a major component of the dispensing system, with its shape, material, and fit impacting measurement accuracy. It is recommended to match the manufacturer's tips with their devices. Wide orifice tips are available for use with viscous or fragile liquids. The fit of the tip also affects the measurement; tips with a large air gap require more pre-wetting than those with minimal air gap due to the air above the liquid needing conditioning.

Air displacement devices are ideal for measuring aqueous liquids. The accuracy and precision of these devices depend on environmental conditions such as temperature and humidity, as well as the user's proper operation. Pre-wetting the tip helps equilibrate the air above the sample, accounting for evaporation due to room conditions and sample volatility. The depth of the tip in the liquid impacts the aspirated volume due to the surrounding liquid pressure. However, air displacement devices are not recommended for very volatile liquids because they can increase air pressure above the sample, forcing liquid to drip out of the tip and lowering the measured volume. Positive displacement devices, which can be used for both aqueous and organic liquids, are recommended for measuring volatile liquids as they mitigate environmental conditions by measuring within a closed system. The properties of the liquid, such as temperature, viscosity, and volatility, become less impactful within the tip of the dispenser. Positive displacement devices can be manual or electronic and may utilize disposable tips. Syringes are also used for volatile liquid measuring but require specific techniques for accuracy and precision.

For air displacement devices, choosing between fixed or adjustable volume devices should be based on the frequency of the required volume and the task's performance criteria. Adjustable pipettes vary in accuracy and precision from their low to high end, with the low end having a wider range based on the manufacturer's performance specifications for new devices. Fixed volume devices generally offer tighter performance specifications than adjustable ones. Single-channel devices are effective for non-repetitive dispensing using disposable tips, while multichannel devices enhance efficiency for well-plate applications by dispensing the same volume across multiple samples.

Evaluating accuracy and precision, considering systematic and random errors, depends on the application. The volume measurement and device used will impact the result, so determining an acceptable error amount for the application and choosing an appropriate device is crucial. Criteria can be established using performance testing data or ISO 8655 criteria and should be stringent enough to detect performance issues before they affect measurement results. Equipment like pipettes is typically evaluated with a quick check to ensure accuracy and precision, a process often performed by the laboratory rather than a calibration vendor. The frequency of performance verification should reflect the regularity of use and the potential impact of a failure on results. However, incorrect measurements are most frequently attributed to operator technique or improper use.

The successful use of liquid handling devices largely depends on the operator, making training a critical component of performance. Developing a training system that includes initial and periodic assessments of the operator is essential. Control, calibrator preparation and proficiency testing are all ways to assess proper technique [7].

Type of Pipettes

Air displacement pipettes are the preferred choice for working with aqueous solutions. The piston moves to the appropriate position when the volume is set. When the operating button is pressed to the first stop, the piston expels the same volume of air as indicated on the volume setting. After immersing the tip into the liquid, the operating button is released. This creates a partial vacuum, and the specified volume of liquid is aspirated into the tip. As the volume depends on the air displacement, many factors may affect the performance of air displacement pipettes, including the volatility, viscosity and specific gravity of the solution. Therefore, air displacement pipettes are most commonly used for aqueous solutions and biological samples which are non-volatile and have a specific gravity near 1.0S (Fig. 5.2).

Air displacement pipettes come with fixed or adjustable volume and can have mechanical or electronic controls. If the volume is adjustable, there is a fixed range of operation. Selection between manual or electronic pipettes should be based on the requirements for precision, lab task throughput, and ergonomics consideration. Manual pipettes are easy and quick to operate and allow the operator to control the speed of aspiration and dispensing. In contrast, the electronic pipettes will aspirate and dispense at a set, adjustable speed to deliver maximum repeatability. They also prevent repetitive motion injuries.

Positive displacement pipettes are the best choice for organic solutions and piston components come into direct contact with the liquid. In this case, pipette tips contain both the cylinder and the piston. When the operating button is pressed, the piston migrates to the end of the tip to contact the sample. Releasing the button, the piston moves up, drawing the sample into the tip. In the absence of an air cushion, positive displacement pipettes are less affected by temperature and barometric pressure changes. By way of benefit over air displacement pipettes, positive displacement pipettes (1) minimize liquid dripping due to volatile solvent evaporating to the top space; (2) avoids liquids with higher viscosity clinging to the pipette tip (3)

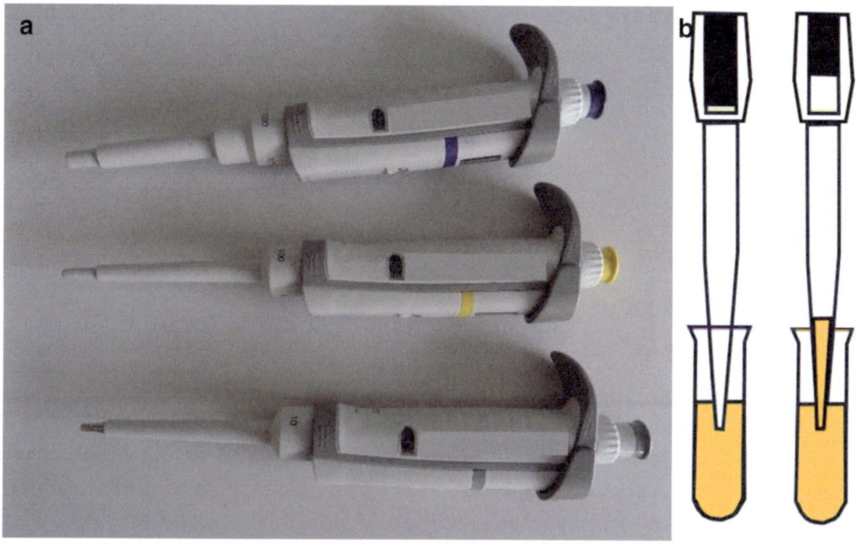

Fig. 5.2 (**a**) Typical commercial air displacement pipettes used in clinical laboratories. Devices are shown without disposable tips attached. (**b**) Pipetting action of an air displacement pipette

Fig. 5.3 A: Typical commercial positive displacement pipette. B: Pipetting action of a positive displacement pipette showing the plunger contacting the sample

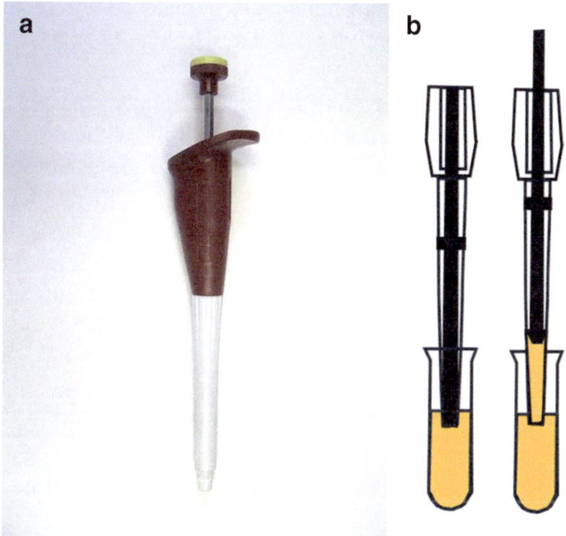

protect inside of the pipette from cross-contamination. Therefore, the positive displacement pipettes are the best choice when working with highly volatile organic solvent, high-density solutions, and samples with high viscosity, such as resin and oil (Fig. 5.3).

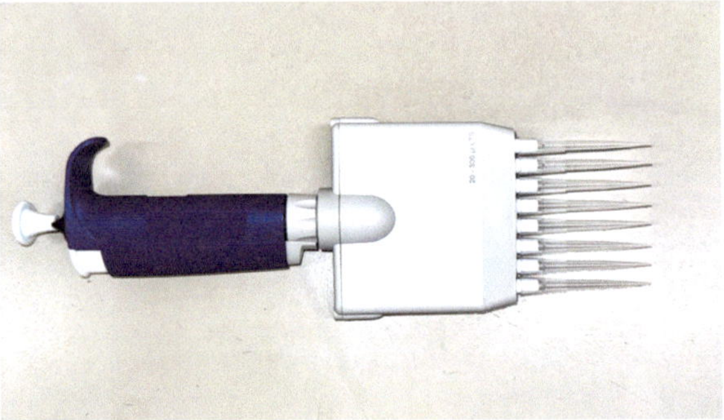

Fig. 5.4 A commercial multichannel pipette with disposable tips attached

Multi-channel Pipettes Multi-channel pipettes come with 4, 6, 9, 12 or 96 channels and can hold multiple tips for pipetting multiple samples at once (Fig. 5.4). They are very convenient when transferring samples from a 96-well plate to another or adding reagent to a well plate. Using an 8- or 12-channel pipette to transfer from a 96-well plate can expedite the operation yet reduce human error of miscounting or misreading the position. However, caution should be taken when pipetting critical volumes, such as transferring samples or adding an internal standard into samples, as it may not be obvious if one channel is not pipetting properly due to a clog, air bubble, or loose fit of a pipette tip. Some multi-channel pipettes have adjustable channels that can fit sample racks or plates of different sizes. Most have fixed channels that fit standard 96-well plates.

Repeater Pipettes Repeater pipettes allow repeated dispensing of the same volume of liquid into multiple tubes or wells without the need to aspirate more liquid between each step. Wide volume ranges are achievable on a repeater pipette, via attaching different-sized cartridges (0.1 mL to 50 mL), allowing dispensed volume ranging from 1uL to 10 mL. The cartridges are positive-displacement tips in nature and therefore carry all the related benefits. They provide superb accuracy and repeatability when used for volatile organic solvents such as methanol, acetonitrile, and methyl-tertbutyl ether.

Bottle Top Dispensers Bottle-top dispensers are liquid measuring devices that attach to the top of the bottles to allow safe and reproducible liquid distribution without contamination. Bottle-top dispensers should be selected based on top diameter, material to be dispensed (to ensure chemical compatibility), and dispensing volume range.

Pipette Techniques

The forward mode is widely used for most air displacement devices, requiring the user to pre-wet the tip and not needing more volume than intended to dispense. To successfully use the forward mode technique, several steps should be followed.

Table 5.4 Immersion depth by volume for pipette tips

Volume, μL	Immersion Depth, mm
<1	1–2
1–100	2–3
101–1000	2–4
1.1–10 mL	3–6

First, using a tip type created by the manufacturer ensures the best fit to the pipette nosecone. Minimally handling the pipette helps ensure the air inside does not increase in temperature from the operator's hand, as increased internal air temperature will expand and force liquid out of the pipette tip, lowering the dispensed volume. Room temperature can also have an impact on this process.

When aspirating, hold the pipette straight and parallel with the container, and immerse the tip to the proper depth (see Table 5.4). Deeper immersion may cause droplets to cling to the outside of the tip or force more liquid inside the tip. Consistent plunger button pressure and speed are essential. Each time a new tip is applied, pre-wet the pipette tip to condition the inside and humidify the air within the pipette. Pre-wetting requires multiple full aspiration and dispense cycles, depending on the air gap above the liquid. Aspirate to the first stop and dispense to the second stop at least three times to pre-wet. Allow the plunger to return to its top stop before beginning the next cycle.

Pause for 1 s after aspiration to allow the liquid to fully travel into the pipette tip. After dispensing, examine the tip and employ a tip-touch by touching the tip and dragging it along the wall on the way out of the container. This technique helps ensure accurate and consistent liquid handling [7].

Forward Mode Pipetting

To ensure accurate pipetting, begin by installing the appropriate tip and pre-wetting it at least three times. When aspirating, hold the pipette parallel to the container and aspirate from the first stop. For dispensing, position the pipette at an angle, push through to the second stop, and touch the tip to the side of the container. Drag the tip along the wall on the way out before releasing the plunger and discarding the tip.

In cases where a positive displacement device is not available, you can use reverse mode and wide-bore tips with an air displacement device to handle very viscous liquids effectively [7].

Reverse Mode Pipetting

Begin by installing the appropriate tip onto the pipette. When performing aspiration, ensure you hold the pipette parallel to the container. Depress the plunger all the way to the second stop and aspirate the liquid. For dispensing, gently depress the plunger to the first stop while positioning the pipette at an angle. Touch the tip to the side of the container to ensure all liquid is expelled [7].

Balances

The principles discussed for volumetric measurements and the operation of liquid handling devices extend equally/analogously to the use of balances in the laboratory. Accurate weighing is foundational to preparing solutions, calibrators, and samples, ensuring correct proportions and concentrations for downstream analyses. Day-of-use verification of balances, such as ensuring they are level, clean, and performing a quick check with certified reference weights, is essential to confirm proper balance function before use. The selection of a balance should be based on the sensitivity or resolution required for the specific application, with microbalances or analytical balances being ideal for tasks demanding increased accuracy and precision. Certified Type 1 weights, which meet the strictest metrological standards, are indispensable for calibration and verification of balances, ensuring traceability and regulatory compliance. By combining proper balance selection with regular verification and appropriate use of high-quality weights, laboratories can achieve consistent and reliable results across a wide range of measurements and time. At least annual balance calibration should be performed by an ISO 17025 vendor.

There are generally three types of balances used in the lab: top-loading balances, analytical balances, and micro balances.

The top-loading balance (Fig. 5.5a) is the least delicate and with a higher weight capacity (up to 5 kg), making it a good choice for routine weighing of large amounts of chemicals and/or their containers. It is also handy to keep a top-loading balance near a lab centrifuge to conveniently verify that the weights of two centrifuge racks or plates are within a desired tolerance.

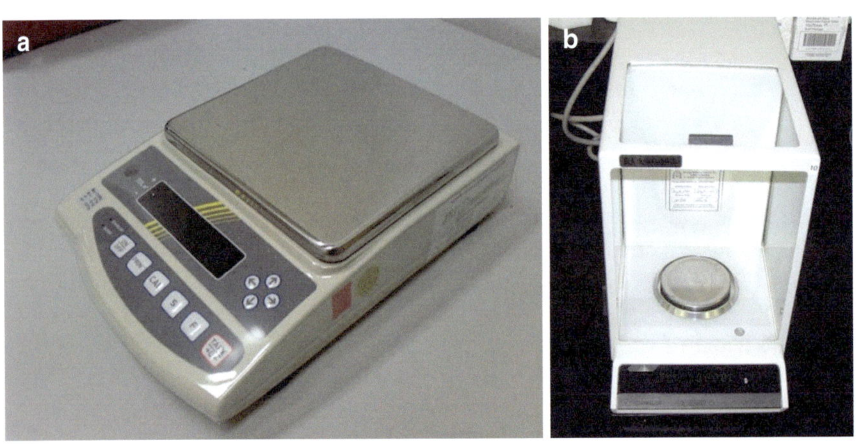

Fig. 5.5 (**a**) a top loading balance (**b**) an analytical balance

The analytical balance (Fig. 5.5b) is designed to provide high-precision measurements where the weights are crucial, such as when weighing standards to prepare calibrators. Analytical balances are capable of measuring mass with a higher level of accuracy. They typically have a readability (i.e., a minimum increment) of 0.01 mg or 0.1 mg. Analytical balances are enclosed in a glass chamber to protect them from air currents, dust, and other environmental variables that can affect their accuracy. The maximum weighing capacity is usually 200 g to 300 g for analytical balances.

When high accuracy is required (i.e., sub milligram) micro balances or ultra-micro balances should be used. By incorporating a non-magnetic weight pan, air draft protection and separating the electronic box from the weighing module, micro and ultra-micro balances can reach a readability of 0.0001 mg to 0.001 mg. The maximum weighing capacity is usually 2–10 g. Extreme care should be taken when operating micro balances, as force or heavy weight can easily damage them.

Balances should be placed on a stable, vibration-free surface away from drafts, direct sunlight, and temperature fluctuations. They should be calibrated regularly using certified weights, following the manufacturer's or laboratory guidelines for calibration frequency and procedures. Certified weights need to be handled using tools (e.g., tweezers) to prevent oil or moisture transfer from hands, which will alter the mass of the calibrator.

When weighing chemical powders, use clean, dry containers or weighing paper to avoid contamination. Close the balance doors before reading to prevent air currents from affecting the measurement. Hygroscopic compounds must be weighed inside a dry box.

Specific Laboratory Techniques for LC-MS/MS

Impact of Extract Quality

Extract quality has a direct impact on the performance of the LC-MS/MS system. Extraction should be sufficient to remove large particles, proteins, and other non-target substances from samples. Unwanted components from sample matrices will shorten the lifespan of the analytical column, instrument plumbing, and detector. Clean-up steps in preparation can include filtering, protein precipitation and centrifugation, dilution, liquid-liquid and solid phase type extractions, or any combination of these techniques. Final extracts should be free of particulates and oils.

Impact of Mobile Phase Preparation

The components and conditions of the mobile phase will also impact the performance of the detector over time. Mobile phase modifiers (e.g., buffers) and mixing of different mobile phases in the system can create salt buildup within the liquid pump system, as well as forming deposits on the detector. Deposits on the detector can create active sites, which reduce sensitivity. Contaminants in the mobile phase from age and improper storage can lead to high background and ion suppression. High background will suppress the signal of lower masses to a higher degree, but it depends on where the background is highest. Modifiers in the mobile phase aid in the ionization of target compounds as well as in adjusting the pH of the eluent. Choose modifiers that are volatile, like adducts of ammonium such as acetate, carbonate, formate, and hydroxide, to avoid salt buildup on the MS source. In addition to these buffers, formic, or acetic acid or trimethylamine will work to adjust the eluent pH.

Conditioning, Equilibration, and Column Storage

If the LC-MS/MS system will be idle for long periods of time, the LC system should be purged with organic solvent. Leaving aqueous solution in the system will encourage bacterial growth, which leads to clogs in the small inner-diameter tubing of LC systems. A periodic flush of the injection path can be incorporated with preventative maintenance to extend the life of the solvent delivery system. The flush solution should be comprised of a larger percentage of organic solvent to water, using similar components as the mobile phases. Mobile phase lines should have a filter end of the bottle and will pass through a degasser as part of the LC system. Analytical columns should be conditioned prior to the first use. The conditioning varies based on the stationary phase of the column and the manufacturer's storage solvent. New columns are packaged with a certificate of analysis indicating the storage solvent. Most columns are stored with a solution >50% organic solvent. Flush the column with 10 column volumes of a 10–20% less organic solvent than the storage solvent. Then switch over to the desired mobile phase for another 10 column volumes. Column volume can be calculated with the eq. $V = \pi r^2 L$, where V = volume, r = radius and L = column length. After initial column conditioning, equilibrate the column for each use with the mobile phase for analysis. Equilibration allows the mobile phase to saturate the stationary phase. This will stabilize retention times and allow detection of leaks before analysis begins. Equilibration encourages the sample to travel through the pores and interact with the functional groups of the stationary phase.

Tube Cutting, Fitting, and Connection

Specific techniques, including tube cutting, fitting and connecting tubing, and fitting guard columns, are everyday techniques to maintain optimum LC-MS/MS performance.

Tube Cutting

Two types of tubing are commonly used for HPLC application: stainless steel tubing and PEEK (polyether ether ketone) tubing (Fig. 5.6). For stainless steel tubing, it is best to purchase pre-cut tubing. For PEEK tubing, a guillotine-style

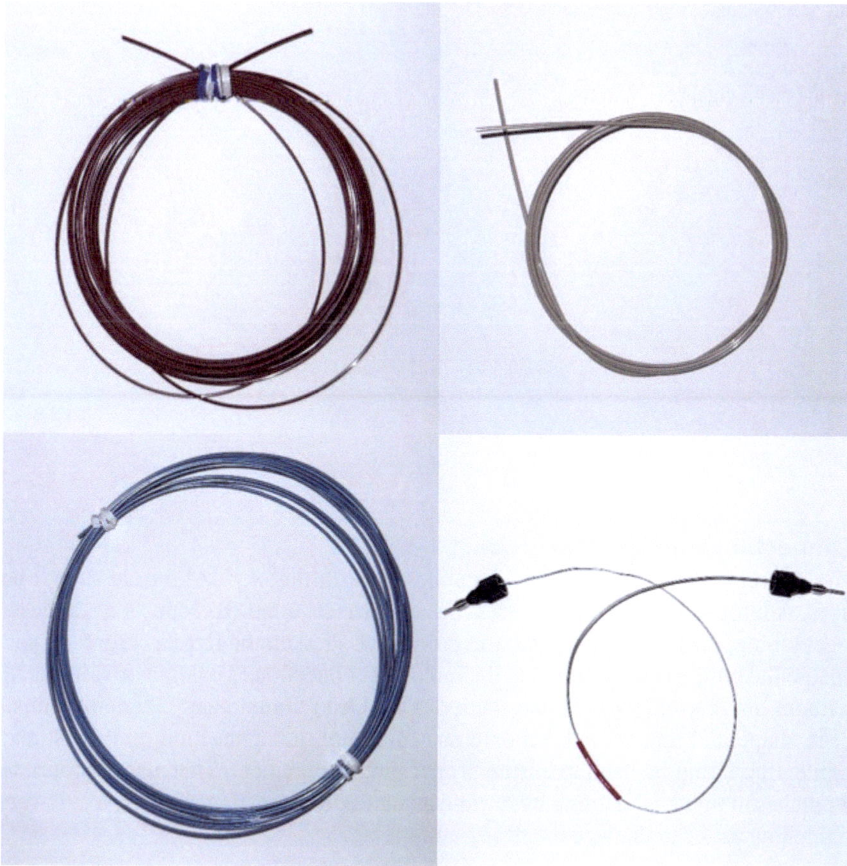

Fig. 5.6 PEEK tubing and stainless steel tubing with color coding

Fig. 5.7 Razor cutter for PEEK tubing

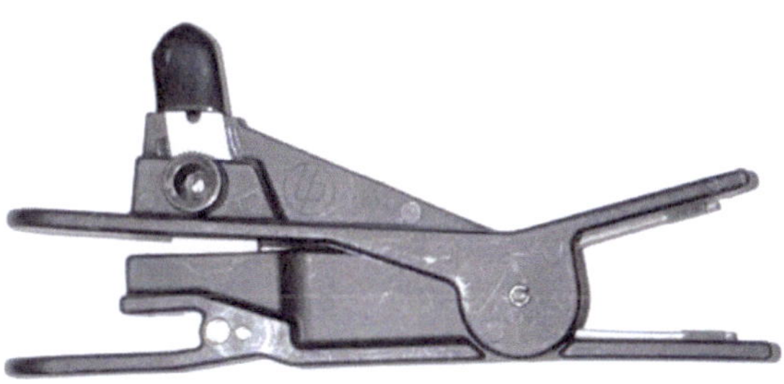

tubing cutter should be used (Fig. 5.7). Never use a razor blade, knife, or scissors to cut PEEK tubing, as these will crimp the tubing and restrict the flow, causing high pressure or a leak. A guillotine-style tubing cutter ensures a smooth cut that does not affect tubing calibre. It is sometimes recommended to rotate the cutter around the tubing 5–6 times to make a flat and even cut.

Fig. 5.8 Stainless steel HPLC fittingss. The nut is shown on the left and the ferrule on the right

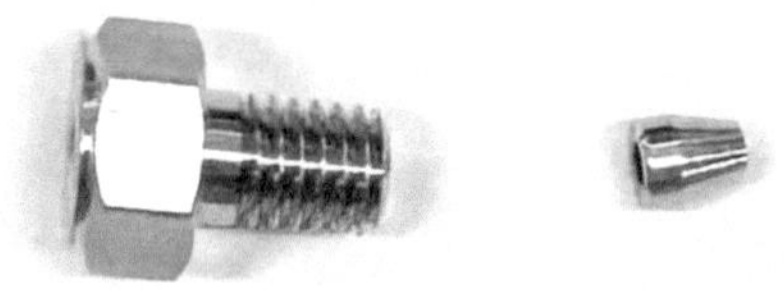

Connecting Stainless Steel Tubing

To connect stainless steel tubing, a stainless steel fitting nut and ferrule should be used. Appropriate tools such as wrenches are also required. To connect a stainless-steel tubing, insert the tubing into the fitting nut, slide on the ferrule (Fig. 5.8), and ensure the tubing is fully seated at the inlet of a connection (a column or valve, etc.) without any gap. Leaving a gap increases the dead volume and can compromise peak shape and separation on a column. To secure the connection, first twist and tighten the fitting by hand to ensure proper thread alignment. Then use appropriate wrenches to tighten the fitting by turning a quarter turn past finger-tight. Avoid over-tightening as it can damage the fitting and tubing.

Connecting PEEK Tubing

PEEK tubing requires the use of a PEEK fitting (Fig. 5.9). Some PEEK fittings have a built-in ferrule, and some need a separate ferrule (Fig. 5.8). Insert the PEEK tubing into the PEEK fitting, ensuring the tubing is fully seated at the inlet of the connection, without any gap. Tighten the fitting by hand until it is snug. PEEK fittings are designed to be tightened by hand only; over-tightening can lead to high pressure or damage.

Guard Columns

A guard column is a column-based protection system designed to prevent HPLC columns from being contaminated and thereby intended to maintain chromatographic performance and lengthen the lifespan of the column. They are available in different designs, but all have a similar function (Fig. 5.10). The inlet end of the guard column usually fits both PEEK tubing and metal tubing. The outlet end has a floating fitting, adaptable to different columns with various inlet depths.

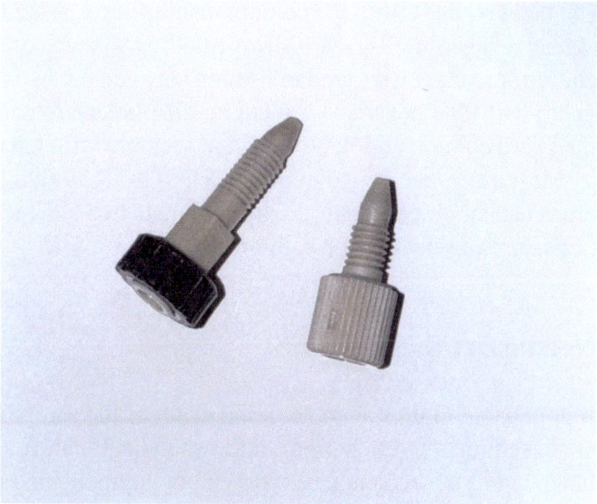

Fig. 5.9 Plastic peak tubing HPLC fittings

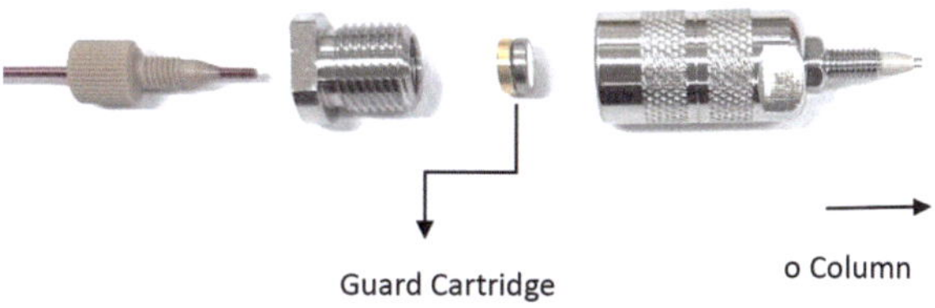

Fig. 5.10 An illustration of proper guard cartridge installation

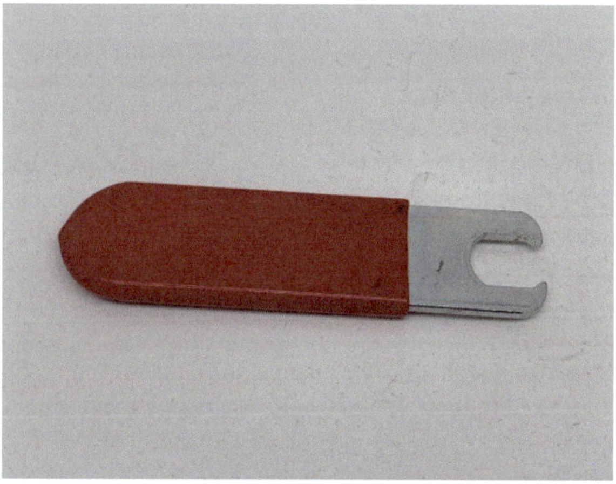

Fig. 5.11 A guard cartridge wrench

When installing a cartridge into the guard column, follow the manufacturer's instructions provided carefully as the cartridge has directionality. Connect the two parts of the guard column, first by finger tightening, then by a wrench for a secure connection. This connection needs to be very tight to withstand the same pressure as on the analytical column. Specialized wrenches (Fig. 5.11) are usually required and can be purchased from the column manufacturer. After the guard column is securely connected, run the LC-MS/MS method on a blank or system suitability sample to check for leaks. Leaks tend to form in between the two component metal parts of the guard-cartridge housing—the nut and the holder. When a leak is observed, remove the guard column and tighten it more securely with the appropriate tools.

Mastering specific techniques such as tube cutting, fitting, and fitting guard columns can significantly improve continuous LC-MS/MS operation without interruption caused by leaking or high pressure.

Needle Depth Selection

If applicable to the LC system, the depth of the sampling needle can be adjusted to avoid sediment at the bottom of the analytical vial. If sample clean-up is not possible to avoid the presence of sediment or components falling out of solution, needle adjustment can be a preventative measure to avoid clogs in the path of the sample.

Lab Safety

Universal precautions observed for general laboratory settings will apply for LC-MS/MS analysis as well. Personal protective equipment (PPE), engineering controls, waste disposal and air handling considerations are detailed below. PPE that fits well and is comfortable to wear will encourage compliance with laboratory safety guidelines.

Glove Selection

Gloves should be selected based on the hazards presented in the application. Clinical LC-MS/MS presents both chemical and biological hazards. The type of chemical, nature of the contact, duration of contact, grip requirements, thermal protection, size, and comfort are some variables when choosing a glove type. While latex is a popular general-purpose glove material, allergic reactions are a risk factor. Nitrile gloves have become a more common alternative and provide extended use to prolonged exposure to some chemicals that would cause other materials to break down. Known limitations to nitrile gloves are oxidizing agents, aromatic solvents, ketones, and acetates. Butyl and neoprene gloves are also available [8].

Eye Protection

Eye protection should protect against specific hazards, which in this application are chemical and biological. Eyewear should fit properly and comfortably, not restrict vision, be durable and cleanable, and not interfere with other PPE. Safety spectacles and face shields are appropriate for this application. Goggles are an alternative to full eye protection and pair well with corrective lenses. Ordinary prescriptive lenses are not suitable protection against the hazards presented [8].

Laboratory Coats

While in the laboratory, appropriate laboratory attire should be worn at all times to mitigate potential hazardous material contact with the skin. This includes long pants, closed-toe shoes, and a task-appropriate laboratory coat. The determination of what constitutes a task-appropriate laboratory coat depends on the task being performed. The standards applicable to the different types of laboratory hazards that may be encountered are shown below (Table 5.5).

Routine cleaning of laboratory coats is necessary to remove potential contaminants and hazardous materials and maintain a safe working environment. Laboratory coats may be laundered in-house or sent out for cleaning. If laundering is outsourced, it is important to select a vendor with knowledge of and experience in decontamination processes. Heavily contaminated lab coats should be disposed of properly through the applicable waste stream rather than attempting to clean them [9].

Air Turnover

Maintaining proper air turnover in clinical laboratories is essential for ensuring a safe and healthy environment. Air Changes Per Hour (ACH) is a critical metric that defines how frequently the air within a space is replaced with fresh air. High ACH rates help to rapidly remove hazardous fumes and contaminants and reduce deposition of liquids or condensable solids in exhaust systems, thereby enhancing air quality and minimizing exposure to potentially harmful substances. The previous NFPA 45 recommendation for air turnover rate for laboratories using chemicals was greater than 8 ACH when occupied, and a minimum of 4 ACH when unoccupied; the most recent recommendation is for continuous turnover but doesn't specify a minimum number of ACH. Adhering to these standards ensures that laboratories maintain optimal air quality while balancing energy efficiency [10].

Table 5.5 Types of laboratory hazards and the applicable standards for laboratory coats

Type of laboratory hazard	Applicable test standard
Biological (bloodborne pathogens)	ASTM F1670[a] (penetration by synthetic blood) and ASTM F1671[a] (bloodborne pathogen exposure)
Chemical (carcinogens, flammable or corrosive materials)	AATCC Method 42 (resistance to the penetration of water by impact) and ASTM F903 (liquid chemical barrier)

[a]Of the two standards, F1671 is more stringent in its resistance requirements and is the more conservative option when it is unclear which standard is more suitable

Mixed Waste Disposal

LC-MS/MS systems generate mixed organic waste. Mobile phases are typically weak acids or bases and a mixture of aqueous and organic chemicals. Waste disposal is dependent on location. EPA guideline Part 261 (Identification and Listing of Hazardous Waste) should be reviewed. Hazardous waste disposal records need to be retained and abatement actions recorded. Abatement means action by an employer to comply with a cited standard or regulation or to eliminate a recognized hazard identified by OSHA during an inspection.

Conclusions

The information provided in this chapter, while fairly comprehensive, is meant to reflect minimal considerations for LC-MS/MS utilization in the clinical laboratory setting. Many such considerations have locally-prescribed mandates and each laboratory should become familiar with such standards before undertaking the steps outlined in this section. By following these steps, clinical laboratories will be well on their way to implementation of LC-MS/MS for routine testing purposes.

References

1. Moffat AC, Clarke EGC. Clarke's analysis of drugs and poisons: in pharmaceuticals, body fluids, and postmortem material. 4th ed. London: Pharmaceutical Press; 2011.
2. Nelson ML, P.D.V.o.B.a.S.D. A guide to solvent grades. CP Lab Chemicals; 2022.
3. Corporation EM. Solutions for Mass Spec. 2014: p. 48.
4. Chan CC. Practical approaches to method validation and essential instrument qualification. Wiley; 2010.
5. Team, C.P.B., How to use a volumetric flask. 2018.
6. Detergent Residue Testing. 3.
7. Best Practices for the Use of Micropipettes. 2015.
8. Labor, U.S.D.o. and O.S.a.H. Administration Personal Protective Equipment. 2023. OSHA 3151-02R 2023.
9. Committee, O.S.a.H., National Institutes of Health Guidance for the Selection of Laboratory Coats. 2016: p. 9.
10. NFPA, NFPA 45: Standard on fire protection for laboratories using chemicals. 2024, NFPA.

Method Development and Validation

6

Mark M. Kushnir and Erik Kish-Trier

Introduction

Development and validation of a liquid chromatography-tandem mass spectrometry (LC-MS/MS) method should start with definition of the intended clinical use, which informs both the performance characteristic requirements and regulatory considerations. Development of a clinical LC-MS/MS method is a complex process in which every aspect of pre-analytics, sample preparation, LC separation, MS detection, data processing, and interpretation should be optimized and thoroughly evaluated to produce a complete diagnostic testing system. Steps involved in the development and validation of LC-MS/MS methods are broadly similar (Fig. 6.1), however, analyte-specific considerations influence each step of the process [1–4].

Starting in the planning stage, project feasibility should be continually evaluated to mitigate the considerable investment needed for development, validation, and implementation of a successful assay. All aspects of the assay, including the target analyte(s), sample type(s), required analytical performance characteristics, and logistical constraints, should be assessed at this stage. In addition to the above considerations, it is important to assess the availability of certified reference materials (CRMs), reference measurement procedures (RMPs), and proficiency testing programs for the analyte(s) of interest. Peer-reviewed publications on previously developed methods can provide valuable guidance; however, it is essential to verify all

M. M. Kushnir (✉)
ARUP Institute for Clinical and Experimental Pathology, Salt Lake City, UT, USA

Department of Pathology, University of Utah, Salt Lake City, UT, USA
e-mail: kushnmm@aruplabs.com

E. Kish-Trier
ARUP Institute for Research and Innovation, Salt Lake City, UT, USA

Y. V. Zhang, U. Garg (eds.), *Practical Guide to Implementing Liquid Chromatography Mass Spectrometry in Clinical Laboratories*,
https://doi.org/10.1007/978-3-032-03852-4_6

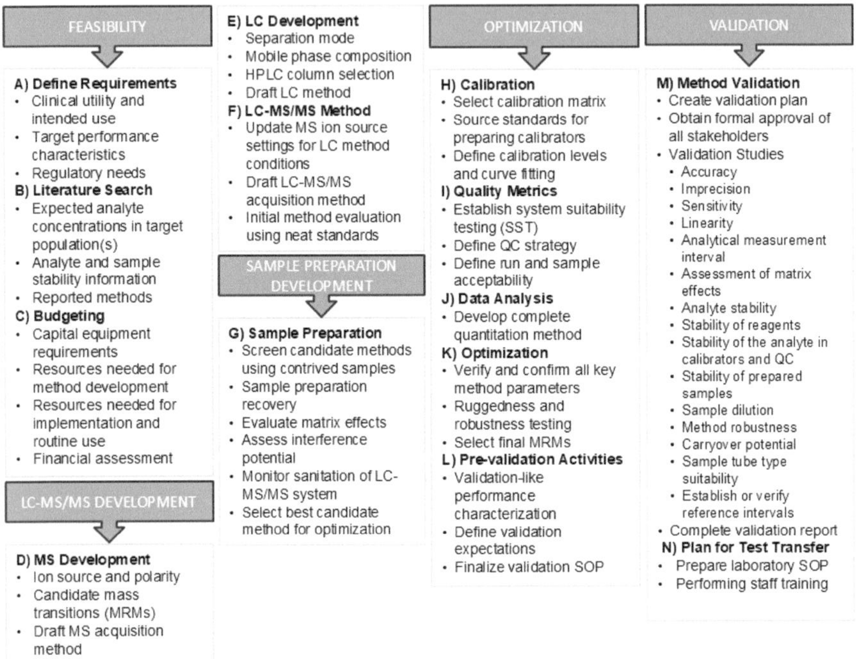

Fig. 6.1 Key steps in development and validation of clinical LC-MS/MS methods

the details, as methodological nuances and the details in the publications may differ significantly from the application under consideration.

It should be noted that MS instruments from different vendors, different models from the same vendor, and even alternate units of the same model, differ in performance from each other. Instrument settings are not transferable between individual instruments; therefore, it is important to optimize MS settings on each specific LC-MS/MS instrument that is used for the method.

Method development should start with creating an instrument method for the detection of the analyte(s) of interest, followed by the development of all other aspects of the method. For example, MS parameters for analyte monitoring are established first, followed by LC parameters for analyte separation, and lastly, development of the method for preparing samples in the matrix intended for the assay. Bracketing these efforts are pre-analytic considerations, and the data analysis informatics tools required for results interpretation and reporting.

Frequent evaluation of performance characteristics (e.g., accuracy, precision, analytical sensitivity, analytical specificity, analytical measurement interval (AMI), etc.) should be made to confirm adequacy for the intended clinical application. Good laboratory notebook practices should be utilized throughout the project, including design control, experimental plans, detailed reagent and consumable information (e.g., vendor, catalog, and lot numbers), and experimental results.

For novel methods that lack a predicate, extensive clinical validation of the method is required. Access to patient samples, corresponding to the healthy and disease states, can pose a significant challenge and should be carefully considered during the planning stages. If clinical evaluation of the method or establishing reference intervals or medical decision points is required, Institution Review Board (IRB) approval must be obtained before any research using samples from human subjects is conducted.

Once a method has been developed and optimized, pre-validation performance evaluation of the assay should be conducted to determine if the targeted performance characteristics can be achieved and to mitigate failure in validation. Only when the performance of the developed method has been fully assessed, and a locked-down analytical protocol and validation plan, are in place, should the project be advanced to the validation stage. All validation experiments should be conducted as the method is intended to be run in the clinical laboratory, including pre-analytical considerations and clinical laboratory staff and instrumentation. The validation experiments should evaluate the method as a complete test system, ideally from sample collection to result reporting. Together, these efforts will yield a robust, clinically informative LC-MS/MS method that is fully characterized and suitable for the clinical laboratory environment [5, 6].

MS Method Development

Brief Introduction of Triple Quadruple Mass Spectrometers

See chapter "Mass Spectrometry" for details on this topic. Triple quadrupole mass spectrometers (QQQ) are one of the most common types of mass spectrometers used in clinical laboratories and will be the focus of this section [7, 8]. Triple quadrupole MS consists of two mass analyzers (MS1 and MS2), arranged sequentially, with a collision cell positioned between them. Ions separated in MS1 undergo fragmentation in the collision cell via collision-induced dissociation (CID). In this process, molecular ions collide with inert gas molecules, leading to the formation of molecular fragment ions. The collision energy, type of collision gas (e.g., nitrogen, argon), and the collision gas pressure determine the efficiency of the fragmentation process.

Triple quadrupole MS can acquire data in multiple modes: product ion scan, precursor ion scan, neutral loss scan, and multiple reaction monitoring (MRM). In product ion scan mode, MS1 transmits m/z corresponding to the analyte(s), and MS2 scans through a range of m/z to acquire mass spectra of the fragment ion(s). In precursor ion scan mode, MS2 is set to transmit m/z characteristic of a specific molecular fragment ion, while MS1 scans through a range of m/z to acquire mass spectra of the precursor ion(s) that produces the selected fragment ion. In a neutral loss scan, both MS1 and MS2 are simultaneously scanned using a constant m/z offset; this mode of operation could be useful for the detection of compounds of the same class, which lose a specific neutral fragment during fragmentation (e.g., analysis of amino acid butyl ester derivatives, phosphorylated peptides).

As discussed below, there are many parameters that need to be assessed during the assay development phase. It is important to note that many of these parameters are inter-dependent, and consideration of their interactions must be made to ensure successful development.

Selection of Mass Transitions

Multiple reaction monitoring (MRM) is the most common mode of data acquisition in targeted analysis methods using QQQ instruments. In MRM mode, both, MS1 and MS2 are set to transmit ions of a specified m/z, which are characteristic of the analyte of interest. MRM acquisition is performed by isolating the precursor ion (typically the molecular ion) in MS1, fragmenting the ion in the collision cell, and then monitoring one or more fragment ions in MS2. The pairs of precursor/fragment ions are called mass transitions; typically, two mass transitions of an analyte and two mass transitions corresponding to the IS are utilized in quantitative analysis methods. Ratios of MRMs are often monitored as a means of assuring adequate specificity of analysis [13].

Development of MRM-based acquisition methods starts with optimizing the conditions for detection of the molecular ion of the analyte, followed by acquiring product ion mass spectra to identify the analyte-specific fragment ions. Precursor ions are typically protonated (in positive mode), or de-protonated (in negative ion mode) molecular ions of the analyte, though in some cases they could be fragments of the molecular ion produced by low-energy fragmentation (e.g., loss of water) in the ion source. A list of candidate mass transitions, corresponding to the most intense fragment ions, should be compiled from the product ion spectra. The choice of mass transitions for the final method depends on signal intensity and potential for interference. Fragment ions selected for use in the mass transitions should be justified based on the expected CID fragmentation of the analyte. In many cases, the chemical identity of the fragment ions could be elucidated based on the structure of the analyte, while on some occasions, fragmentation occurs through a complex, multistep mechanism via intramolecular rearrangements.

In the early stages of method development, all available analyte- and IS-specific mass transitions should be included in the acquisition method, to enable continual performance assessment. Mass transitions with the greatest signal intensity and lowest baseline noise typically provide the best sensitivity. A greater baseline noise is often observed in mass transitions using commonly encountered fragment ions [e.g., m/z 59 (methyl ester, COOCH3+), m/z 77 (aromatic ring, C6H5+), m/z 91 (tropylium ion, C7H7+), m/z 92 (McLafferty rearrangement, involving aromatic ring)]. Poor specificity could also be observed in mass transitions resulting from trivial losses [e.g., loss of water (-H2O, 18 Da), ammonia (−NH3, 17 Da), carbon dioxide (−CO2, 44 Da)], which could be produced through fragmentation of compounds isobaric to the targeted analyte. Mass transitions based on fragment ions with m/z < 50 are typically noisy and should be avoided. The best sensitivity and specificity of analysis is typically achieved using mass transitions, which are based on unique molecular fragment ions, having high signal intensity, minimal background noise, and no mass transitions in common with peaks of nearby-eluting unrelated substances.

Common methods for identifying analyte-specific mass transitions and optimizing MS settings include either infusing or serially injecting a standard of the analyte of interest. Infusion of standard, while scanning instrument parameters, permits real-time visualization of the impact of changing the settings on the MS signal, whereas serial injection is compatible with automated optimization of instrument settings. Automated optimization routines are powerful tools in the development of multi-analyte methods, though care should be taken to verify and confirm values of the settings generated by the software during the optimization process.

Identifying suitable analyte-specific fragment ions is the first step in optimizing MS parameters and building candidate MRM transitions to use during method development. Product ion scans acquired while ramping collision energy (CE) are used to generate analyte-specific fragments across a range of CE. Once individual fragments are identified, CE settings can be further refined and, generally, the voltage corresponding to the maximum signal intensity is selected for use in the method. As stated above during, the method development process, it is often useful to include as many MRM transitions as available, in order to mitigate any unforeseen issues that could be observed going forward (e.g., interference, elevated background noise).

Two mass transitions for both the analyte and the IS, which demonstrate the best analytical performance, should be selected for use in the final method. Mass transitions that provide greater sensitivity are typically used for quantification while the other selected mass transition is used to qualitatively confirm the analyte identity. The selected mass transitions should be specific to the analyte of interest, with adequate signal intensity at the lower limit of the measurement interval (LLMI) and have minimal background noise. The relative peak intensity in the secondary MRM (relative to the quantitative MRM) should be >20%. Importantly, stable-isotope labeled internal standards (SIL-IS) often track the ionization and fragmentation process of the unlabeled analyte most effectively when the corresponding MRM fragments for both, the IS and the analyte, originate from the same fragmentation pathway.

In situations where the IS has an impurity of unlabeled analyte, the addition of IS to the samples contaminates the samples with analyte, which may impact quantification. Therefore, IS purity should be assessed while selecting the IS during method development and verified for subsequent lots prior to placing them in use. Impurities impacting method performance can also be introduced by assay reagents and consumables, therefore similar precautions should be made during selection and before use of new lots of these materials. The assessment should be performed for all mass transitions used in the method, including mass transitions of the IS. A proactive screening approach to assure the quality of new lots of standards, reagents, and consumables is more effective than troubleshooting after the fact.

Optimization of Ion Source Parameters

The two most common LC-MS/MS ionization sources used in clinical laboratory methods are electrospray ionization (ESI) and atmospheric pressure chemical ionization (APCI). ESI is most suited for the ionization of polar molecules, whereas APCI is typically used in the analysis of nonpolar molecules. An advantage of APCI is that it is less impacted by competitive ionization from other sample constituents and therefore exhibits less matrix effect [9, 10]. Negative ion mode may exhibit fewer matrix effects as well, as phospholipids and other matrix constituents, which commonly cause these effects, are often not efficiently ionized in negative ion mode. When developing a new method, all available types of ion sources, as well as positive and negative polarity modes, should be evaluated.

Preliminary optimization of ion source settings can be performed by T-infusion of a standard solution into the mobile phase flow delivered by the HPLC. The ion source parameters (voltages, gas flows, and gas temperatures) are adjusted to optimize the MRM signal at the mobile phase composition expected at the retention time of the analyte peak. Importantly, it must be considered that at higher ESI voltage and APCI needle current, more matrix constituents can be ionized, which may increase the potential for matrix effects, interferences, and non-specific background noise [11, 12]. Consequently, the lowest voltage or current settings providing adequate sensitivity are typically preferred for ESI and APCI, respectively.

Ion source parameters, as well as mobile phase composition (e.g., modifiers, pH, organic solvent) and LC flow rate impact analyte ionization efficiency and stability, and consequently method performance and robustness. The optimal settings for the ion source depend on the chemical and physical properties of the molecule of interest (pKa, proton affinity, hydrophobicity, thermal stability, etc.), the mobile phase composition, and the flow rate. The selection of mobile phase modifiers and their concentration should be carefully evaluated and optimized. Often, a compromise in mobile phase composition must be made that balances optimal LC separation with optimal ionization.

If the composition or flow rate of the mobile phase is changed, the ion source settings should be reoptimized. This task could be performed by creating a method with multiple iterations of the same MRM, each using a small offset in the precursor or fragment ion m/z (e.g., 0.01 Da) to distinguish the mass transitions in the acquisition and the data analysis software. MS settings are then arrayed across these replicate MRMs, and the optimal values can be selected by comparing responses among the mass transitions. Such an approach permits the organized collection and comparison of MS parameters to select values providing the greatest sensitivity and specificity.

Determining Dwell Time

Dwell time defines how long the MS acquires signal for each data point in a method. The total time necessary for acquiring a single data point for all MRMs in a method determines the acquisition cycle time. For adequate quantitative method performance, 12–20 data points should be collected over each chromatographic peak to enable precise integration. The acquisition cycle time should be optimized to balance the collection of sufficient points across the peak with the collection of transient spectra during each data point. Collecting an insufficient number of data points over the peak will result in poor quantitative performance. Conversely, oversampling, beyond 20 points, will not improve quantitative performance and leads to increased data file size and potentially a noisier signal. During the data processing, smoothing should be performed in a manner that will provide reproducible peak integration, without distortion of peak shape, as excessive smoothing has an adverse effect on the quantitative performance of the method.

Assessment of Matrix Effects

Matrix effects occur when substances coeluting with the analyte impact its ionization [9, 10]. The mechanism can involve ion suppression, caused by coelution of less volatile compounds that alter droplet dynamics (e.g., salts, proteins, phospholipids) or due to competition in ionization with compounds that have greater proton affinity as compared to the analyte. Conversely, ion enhancement could occur due to the promotion of proton transfer to the analyte by co-eluting compounds, which results in more efficient analyte ionization.

Thorough assessment of matrix effects should be performed during method development and optimization due to the potential implications for quantitative performance. Qualitative matrix effect evaluation can be performed using post-column T-infusion of a standard solution while injecting sample extracts. In the case of endogenous compounds, where an analyte-free matrix is not available, SIL-IS may be infused instead. For complete evaluation, the sample set should include spiked reconstitution solvent, extracts of the calibrators, QC, and at least 10 patient samples. Extracted ion chromatograms (EICs) of the samples should be overlaid to assess signal suppression or enhancement in the vicinity of the analyte peak retention time. The acquired data provide a visual representation of the areas within the chromatogram that are affected by matrix effects. Evaluation of ion suppression while comparing different approaches for sample preparation may offer clues as to the source of the matrix effects and aid in mitigation.

Quantitative assessment of matrix effects can be performed by spiking identical amounts of analyte in both, the reconstitution solvent and a set of extracted samples, not containing the analyte of interest, followed by comparison of analyte peak areas. In the case of endogenous compounds, matched unspiked samples can be used to subtract background analyte levels, or alternatively, SIL-IS may be used as the spiking material. The ratio of analyte peak area in solvent to analyte peak area in spiked extracted samples is called the matrix factor, generally expressed as a percentage, and quantifies the absolute ion signal suppression or enhancement caused by the sample matrix. The matrix factor for the IS can also be calculated, and then a ratio of analyte to IS matrix factors (relative matrix factor) can be calculated. The relative matrix factor provides a useful metric to assess how effective an internal standard is at tracking analyte recovery; it is expected that for a well-developed method, the relative matrix factor should be in the vicinity of one.

Prior to locking down the method in preparation for pre-validation method evaluation, qualitative and quantitative assessment of matrix effect should be performed. Both approaches offer complementary information. For example, nearby zones of ion suppression/enhancement may be problematic in the cases of analyte-IS pairs with offset retention times. In these cases, even though the relative matrix factor may be 100%, LC performance variation may cause overlap of the ion suppression/enhancement zone with only one member of the IS-analyte pair. If only the IS or analyte is impacted, the IS would inadequately track the matrix effects, which could result in aberrant quantification. Retention time offsets between analyte-IS pairs are common with surrogate IS and are most often resolved with SIL-IS. However, in some cases, deuterated SIL-IS will exhibit RT offsets due to the 'acidic' nature of the deuterium; in such cases ^{13}C and ^{15}N would be preferred SIL-IS labels.

Matrix effects in an LC-MS/MS method can originate from various sources. Effective monitoring of matrix effects can provide valuable insights related to different aspects of method development. For example, matrix effect can vary between mobile phases prepared using solvents and modifiers acquired from different vendors and even among different lots of reagents from the same vendor. A complete method protocol should list vendors and specifications for all utilized products, which should reduce the chances for variation in performance while switching among reagent and consumable lots. In laboratories where multiple assays are performed on individual LC-MS/MS instruments, standardization of reagents can reduce supply chain related complexities and increase efficiency. Choices of plastic consumables, LC columns, sample collection tubes, etc., should be assessed in the context of their impact on matrix effect. The critical choice of calibrator matrix, especially for endogenous analytes where analyte-free biological matrices are unavailable, should also be made through evaluation of matrix effect. Overall, any substance that contacts the sample during the pre-analytical or analytical phases should be considered as a potential source of matrix effects.

Use of Internal Standards

Use of IS in LC-MS/MS methods is a key factor in achieving reliable quantitative performance, in addition it enables the quality assessment of individual sample results. Considering that the same amount of internal standard is added to every sample, the IS peak area should be comparable in all samples within a batch. During the pre-validation method evaluation, a within-batch tolerance for the IS peak area should be established. A typical target for within-batch tolerance for IS peak area is +/−50% of the mean value of the IS peak area in the calibrators of the batch. Monitoring the IS peak area across a batch permits the assessment of analyte recovery and matrix effects in the analyzed samples.

Assessment of Assay Specificity

A common approach for specificity assessment in MRM data acquisition is through monitoring peak area ratios between the qualitative and quantitative mass transitions of the analyte and the IS [13]. A target value for the within-run MRM ratio in samples is typically defined as an allowed deviation from the average value observed in the batch calibrators. Plotting concentration vs. MRM ratio is informative to understand the expected variation; the typical tolerance limits are ±20–30%. The tolerance range selected depends on the relative intensity of the peaks; a wider tolerance could be used in cases when the relative peak intensities are larger or when the required sensitivity of detection is challenging. The acceptance criteria for MRM ratio tolerance should be established prior to initiating the method validation.

Assessment of specificity should be performed in each analyzed sample as part of the sample acceptance criteria. If an interfering peak coelutes with the peak of the analyte or the IS in either the quantitative or qualitative MRM channel, the ratio of the mass transitions will deviate. Failure of the MRM ratio should be interpreted as a sign of interference. In cases when an interference is suspected, corrective actions need to be performed, and if the interference is not resolved, the quantitative results should not be reported.

One type of interference that is specific to LC-MS/MS methods is MRM crosstalk where fragment ions generated from one precursor ion interfere with the detection of fragment ions produced in an immediately following MRM. Modern collision cell design and delay time between monitoring individual MRMs have largely eliminated the issue. The presence of MRM crosstalk can be detected by adding a “mock” mass transition to the acquisition method composed of one of the product ions of interest and a spurious precursor ion (e.g., m/z lower than the product ion). Signal in this MRM at the RT of the analyte or the IS suggests the existence of a crosstalk; as a corrective action, the delay time between MRMs in the MS acquisition method should be increased.

In addition to evaluating MRM ratios, assessment of specificity should be performed by visual inspection of the chromatographic peaks in all mass transitions. The presence of split peaks or a difference in the width between the MRMs of the analyte or the IS should be interpreted as a sign of interference. For multi-analyte methods, visual inspection of all peaks is burdensome and may be alleviated by a review-by-exception workflow. It is important to properly validate all elements of an LC-MS/MS test system, this includes the data analysis workflow to be used in the assay.

Selection of Samples

Neat samples should be used for the initial instrument and sample preparation development, before introducing the additional complexity of the biological matrix. It is important to carefully define the solvent system used for preparing neat standards due to the potential impact on analyte solubility, adsorption, and stability.

Parameters to consider include the percent and identity of the organic solvent and pH. For proteins and peptides, ionic strength and the requirement for the presence of carrier protein (e.g., BSA) should also be evaluated. During assay optimization, method evaluation, and validation, it is essential to use authentic patient samples in the matrix intended for the assay.

Liquid Chromatography Development

See "Liquid Chromatography" chapter for details on this topic. The specificity and sensitivity of LC-MS/MS methods relies on an efficient LC separation. Separating target analytes into distinct chromatographic peaks enables their resolution from potential interfering substances and zones of ion suppression. In clinical laboratories, many LC-MS/MS method failures can be attributed to issues related to the chromatographic separation; thus, it is critical to develop robust and rugged LC methods. LC method development can be started when an initial MS detection method for the analyte is developed, and the MS instrument is appropriately set up (see section "MS Method Development").

Selection of LC Column

With an expansive array of LC column and mobile phases choices, it is critical to approach LC method development in an organized and informed manner. The first consideration is determining what mode of chromatographic separation is appropriate for the analyte(s) of interest. For example, a positive octanol-water partition coefficient (Log P) suggests that an analyte is nonpolar, has higher solubility in organic solvent than water, and is therefore compatible with the reversed-phase (RP) mode of separation, which is the most common, and arguably most robust, type of LC separation used in clinical LC-MS/MS methods. RP-based columns (e.g., C18, C8, phenyl) are useful for the separation of non-polar to moderately polar compounds. The alternative to RP is normal phase (NP) separation, which encompasses various techniques that use polar stationary phases (e.g., hydrophilic interaction liquid chromatography, HILIC). HILIC separations have made a resurgence in recent years, thanks to improved column chemistries, and can be useful for the analysis of polar molecules of clinical interest (e.g., basic drugs, neurotransmitters). By adding ion-pairing reagents, polar compounds can be efficiently retained under RP conditions, potentially yielding more robust methods, as compared to the methods using NP separations. Contamination of the MS and the LC flow paths with ion-pairing reagents in the mobile phase has long been a concern, especially when the same instrument is used for multiple methods. However, recently described applications using the addition of ion pairing reagents to the sample extract (instead of as a mobile phase component) may be an effective alternative [14]. This section will focus on the development of RP-based separations, while many aspects are also relevant to the development of methods using NP.

Typical LC column dimensions used in clinical LC-MS/MS methods comprise column lengths of 50 to 100 mm and internal diameters (IDs) of 2–3 mm. Longer columns can provide better separation, and smaller ID columns can be beneficial for improving sensitivity. The stationary phase packed in LC columns is typically silica or polymeric particles. Typical particle size for HPLC columns used at pressures <400 Bar is 2–3 μm, and sub-2 μm for use with ultra-HPLC (UHPLC) at pressures up to 1000 Bar. Decreased particle size increases the number of theoretical plates (N) but comes at the cost of increased backpressure. Superficially porous particles have a solid core and permeable shell, which enables UHPLC-like efficiency at HPLC pressure ranges. Stationary phase particles are highly porous, with typical pore sizes of 80–120 Å and 300–450 Å for the analysis of small molecules (<2000 Da) and proteins, respectively.

Adsorbents used as the stationary phase in RP columns are conjugated to moieties such as alkyl chains or aromatic groups (called the bonded phase), which determine the selectivity. Exposed silanol groups in the base silica in some separations contribute a secondary type interaction, which may be reduced through end-capping or conjugation of positively charged (polar-embedded) functional groups. Polar-embedded phases offer several advantages for the analysis of basic compounds at low pH, including reduced silanol interactions, improved retention and selectivity, and enhanced column longevity. Polymer-based stationary phases (vs silica based) are advantageous due to their silanol-free nature and a wide pH tolerance. The absence of silanol groups reduces the potential for unwanted ionic interactions, which facilitates improved peak shape and more efficient separations.

Overall, the initial considerations for column selection should be made based on the analyte's physical and chemical properties. Column vendors and column types that have withstood the rigors of the production environment should be considered first before bringing in new and unproven products. Knowledge of lot-to-lot variation for a given vendor and the technical support available are also prime considerations. It is important to advance several column choices through development to enable selection based on factors that may not be immediately foreseen, such as reproducibility and interference.

Selection of Mobile Phases

For RP method development, a binary solvent system of aqueous and organic solvents is typically used. The most common organic solvents for RP separations are methanol and acetonitrile. A modifier is typically added to the mobile phases to control pH and ionic strength, which are important for both LC separation and ionization of the analyte. In LC–MS methods, it is critical to use volatile mobile phase modifiers with concentrations <25 mM. A common practice is to set the mobile phase pH two units away from the analyte pKa value, so that a single microspecies is present, which enables uniform interaction of analyte molecules with column functional groups. A mix of microspecies may contribute to peak aberrations such as tailing, broadening, or splitting due to nonuniform molecular interactions. In some cases, the presence of multiple microspecies may cause retention time drift. The mobile phase pH also impacts the ionization state of silanol groups (pKa 3.5–4.5), which may lead to unwanted interactions during the LC separation. For the silanol groups to be fully neutralized, a pH within the range of 1.5–2.5 is required.

Development of an LC method is an iterative process that begins with setting up a scouting gradient where the organic solvent percentage is increased linearly over time. An LC gradient method consists of four segments, namely, sample injection/isocratic hold, the analytical gradient, column cleaning, and re-equilibration. Column volume may be estimated from the column dimensions and a typical particle porosity of ~50% or from the flow rate and retention time (RT) of an unretained compound (after subtraction of the extra column volume, consisting of the injection loop volume and volume of connecting tubing). An initial isocratic hold may be used to enable baseline signal stabilization and focusing of the analyte peak at the head of the column. In initial experiments, the gradient should transition from a low to a high percentage of organic solvent (e.g., 2–90%). Matching sample solvent conditions to the LC gradient starting conditions (or weaker) is required for consistent retention. When the desired separation is achieved, the end of the gradient may be shortened to 0.5 min past the RT of the latest eluting peak of interest, and the column cleaning and re-equilibration parts of the gradient should be optimized. The recommended mobile phase volume that needs to be delivered during the column conditioning and re-equilibration segments is 5 column volumes. Re-equilibration time may be shortened, so long as the column backpressure returns to the initial value that is observed at the time of the sample injection and reproducible performance is achieved.

Mobile phases should be prepared using LC–MS grade solvents and ultrapure water (e.g., Type I). If a mobile phase consists of a combination of solvent (e.g., water-methanol), the components should be volumetrically measured separately before pouring into the container. Mobile phase stability should be established and limited to a few days due to the volatility of the components and potential impact on analyte RT. Aqueous mobile phases should not be left at ambient conditions for prolonged periods to prevent bacterial growth and pumps should be purged with isopropyl alcohol or water: methanol (1:1) when an instrument downtime is expected. Methods for equilibrating new columns should be established per manufacturer guidelines and a shutdown method should be used to flush the system with pure solvents following completion of analytical runs. In the case of chelating compounds, such as molecules containing a phosphate group, contact with metal surfaces in the flow path should be minimized, and/or the flow path should be passivated. Guard columns with matched phase or inline filters may be used to extend HPLC column lifetime.

Other Parameters to Consider

Additional parameters that should be optimized for an efficient LC method include extra-column volume, injection volume, column oven temperature, and injection loop washing. To reduce gradient delay and maximize the separation efficiency, the extra-column volumes should be reduced by using the smallest injection loop volume and the shortest and narrowest capillaries possible upstream and downstream from the HPLC column. Capillary connections must also be made with compatible hardware; otherwise, voids may be introduced to the flow path. Injection volume in gradient LC methods is determined empirically by achieving an adequate instrument response without overloading the column, which may lead to peak broadening and abnormal peak shapes. Maximum injection volume can be estimated by plotting the volume injected vs. observed peak width and peak area. The point at which peak broadening is observed, or linearity of the response is affected, should be considered the limit. Column oven temperature has a significant impact on backpressure and accelerates mass transfer, which can improve the separation efficiency. Lastly, an effective injector washing program, including solvent choice, is critical to avoid injector carryover between sample injections. If a strong solvent is used for injector washing, a weak solvent, compatible with LC starting conditions, should be used during the last wash cycle.

Quality Metrics

The targeted assay performance metrics should guide LC method development. For example, RT should be consistent within and between runs, with a typical tolerance of +/−1% of calibrator average, enabling reproducible analytical performance. An analyte retention factor (k) of 2–10 is recommended, which permits sufficient resolution of the analyte from matrix constituents that are poorly retained or unretained, while minimizing the peak broadening and injection-to-injection time. For multiplex methods, adequate chromatographic resolution of analyte peaks ($Rs > 1.5$) is critical in cases when peaks of isobaric compounds are observed in the mass transitions. The Rs is primarily influenced by the parameter selectivity (α), which can be optimized by adjusting the gradient, mobile phase composition, pH, or the chemistry of the stationary phase. The HPLC column backpressure should be closely monitored to ensure that it returns to the baseline prior to each subsequent injection.

Sample Preparation

LC-MS/MS is a powerful analytical technique that allows the development of highly specific methods for the analysis of complex samples. However, prior to the instrumental analysis, samples must be prepared in order to assure optimal analytical performance. The aims of sample preparation are threefold: (a) separation of an analyte of interest from the biological sample matrix, (b) removal of potentially interfering sample constituents, and if necessary, (c) concentrating the analyte to enhance sensitivity. Sample preparation is specific to the chemical properties of the analyte, sample matrix type, potential matrix interferences, and the required performance characteristics of the method. Additionally, expected throughput and sample preparation complexity should inform consideration for automation of the sample preparation.

After an initial LC-MS/MS acquisition method is developed and the targeted performance characteristics are defined, development of the sample preparation method can be initiated. Though not exhaustive, the sections below provide basic information on commonly used techniques for preparing samples for LC-MS/MS analysis. Please refer to the chapter "Sample Preparation" for more details.

Liquid–Liquid Extraction

Liquid–liquid extraction (LLE) is based on leveraging the differential solubility of an analyte between two immiscible solvents. During LLE, analyte molecules are partitioned into a solvent which has comparable polarity to the analyte. For example, nonpolar steroid hormones are partitioned into organic solvent when extracted from aqueous (polar) biological matrices.

The partitioning ratio is a relative measure of the separation of an analyte between the phases when equilibrium is reached. A predicted partitioning ratio, log P, is useful to consider when deciding what sample preparation method to pursue. For example, a positive log P indicates the analyte will partition into the organic solvent, whereas a negative value indicates partitioning into the aqueous solvent. Ultimately, the selection of the extraction solvent involves empirical assessment of analyte recovery and selectivity of the analysis. Adjustment with an acidic or basic modifier can be used to neutralize ionized analytes, thereby enabling extraction into an organic solvent. For example, adjusting pH above the pKa of a weak base (e.g., nitrogen-containing biomolecules) or below the pKa of a weak acid (e.g., fatty acids) will neutralize the analyte and enable extraction into a nonpolar phase. Importantly, the sample pH should be adjusted to two or more units away from the analyte pKa to ensure that molecules of the analyte are fully neutralized.

To perform LLE, samples are aliquoted into tubes to which organic solvent (e.g., hexane, ethyl acetate, dichloromethane, methyl tert-butyl ether) is added. The tubes are tightly capped, and the solution is vigorously agitated to mix the phases, with a goal of achieving an equilibrium state for the analyte partitioning between the phases. The tubes are then centrifuged to separate the organic and the aqueous layers, followed by transfer of the layer containing the analyte into a new container (e.g., tubes, wells of a 96-well plate). The resultant organic phase is typically evaporated, and the residues reconstituted in a small volume of a solvent that is compatible with the type of HPLC separation technique used in the method. A modification of LLE, called supported liquid extraction (SLE), uses a solid, porous matrix to trap a liquid sample, enabling extraction of the analyte of interest by passing through the adsorbent an aliquot of organic solvent. An important factor to consider is that SLE offers greater compatibility with automation compared to LLE.

Solid Phase Extraction

Solid phase extraction (SPE) is one of the most effective sample preparation techniques for extracting analytes from complex biological samples. Development of an SPE method requires understanding the chemical properties of the analyte (e.g., functional groups, polarity, pKa, etc.), which enables selection of an appropriate retention mechanism. Retention by SPE can be based on such properties of the analyte as hydrophobicity, polarity, ionic interactions, or affinity. For example, molecules containing basic or acidic groups could be extracted using ion-exchange SPE adsorbents, while molecules containing hydrophobic groups could be retained using reverse-phase-based adsorbents. A wide selection of SPE adsorbents, based on different interaction mechanisms, are commercially available from multiple vendors and should be evaluated during the method development. SPE using polymeric adsorbents has advantages such as (a) a wider pH range, (b) a greater chemical stability, (c) a greater tolerance to the adsorbent drying during the extraction process, (d) the ability to provide hydrophobic and hydrophilic interactions, and (e) a greater binding capacity as compared to silica-based adsorbents.

SPE procedures typically include solvation of the adsorbent, sample pretreatment (to adjust pH, reduce ionic strength, etc.), sample loading, washing the adsorbent, drying the adsorbent, and elution of the analyte by disrupting the retention. Adequate washing of the SPE adsorbent is critical to remove substances which are non-specifically or weakly retained and may interfere with LC-MS/MS analysis. Effective elution is achieved by disrupting the interaction between the analyte and the functional groups on the surface of the adsorbent. This typically includes changing the polarity and/or adjusting the pH from the loading conditions.

In addition to the interaction of analyte molecules with functional groups on surface of the SPE adsorbent, the SPE adsorbent mass and particle size need to be considered. The required adsorbent mass depends on the content of potentially retaining compounds in the sample aliquot. Depending on the adsorbent type, the capacity of the adsorbent could range between 5% and 15%, of the dry bed weight (e.g., 30 mg of the SPE adsorbent would be expected to retain 1.5–4.5 mg of the sample constituents). If an insufficient amount of absorbent is used, a low or inconsistent recovery could be observed. Conversely, if excessive absorbent is used, incomplete recovery of the analyte during elution could be observed or a larger than desirable volume of elution solvent would be required.

The rate at which an analyte diffuses from the sample solution during loading to the porous surface of the adsorbent particles determines the extraction efficiency. By managing the flow rate, it is possible to optimize the contact time and the extraction efficiency, which is crucial for achieving reliable analytical performance. A typical flow rate, which provides adequate contact time between the sample constituents and the active sites on the surface of the adsorbent, is approximately one drop of the effluent per second. Automating the SPE processes can enhance consistency, both within and among batches. Additionally, it's important to note that smaller SPE adsorbent particle size offers larger surface area and greater diffusion rate, although they also result in higher backpressure.

Variables that need to be evaluated and optimized while developing an SPE method are (a) adsorbent type and bed mass, (b) sample aliquot volume, (c) sample pretreatment, (d) wash solvent composition and volume, (e) adsorbent drying conditions, and (f) elution solvent composition and volume. One approach for optimizing SPE steps is to systematically change the variables within the range that is planned for the evaluation. As an initial method, a generic protocol (for the class of compounds to which the analyte belongs) provided by the vendor of the SPE consumables can be used. A patient sample pool containing a measurable concentration of the analyte should be used in the optimization experiments to enable a clear interpretation of results. It is convenient to perform the experiments in a 96-well SPE plate. For example, columns 1–3, 4–6, 7–9, 10–12 of the SPE plate can be used for evaluation of different sample pretreatment methods; the first, second, and third columns in each of the four sections are used for evaluation of three compositions of SPE wash solvents; one elution solvent composition is evaluated in rows A-D of the plate, and another in rows E-H. After optimal conditions for the evaluated set of variables is determined, they can be fixed and the remaining variables optimized in the follow-up experiments, which could be performed in a similar format.

If the SPE elution solvent is compatible with the HPLC separation mode used in the method and further sample concentration is not necessary, the SPE eluate (neat or diluted) can be directly injected into the LC-MS/MS. Alternatively, the eluate can be evaporated and the residues reconstituted in a small volume of a solvent that is compatible with the HPLC separation mode used. In cases where evaporation of the SPE eluate is not desirable, for example, due to the potential for analyte degradation during evaporation or to reduce sample preparation complexity, micro-elution format SPE could enable direct injection of the extracts.

Protein Precipitation

Protein precipitation (PP) is one of the easiest approaches for sample preparation and may be effective when developing methods for analytes which are present in biological samples at high concentration, have adequate ionization efficiency and have unique mass transitions. PP involves the addition of an organic solvent (e.g., acetonitrile, methanol) or an acid (e.g., trichloroacetic acid, perchloric acid) to precipitate proteins in the sample, followed by incubation with mixing, centrifugation, and decanting the supernatant from the precipitates. The resulting supernatant can be diluted with an aqueous solution to reduce the organic content prior to HPLC separation or evaporated and reconstituted in a solvent compatible with HPLC separation used in the method. The efficiency of PP can be optimized through the use of additives (e.g., acidifying the samples, addition of salts), changing the sample-to-solvent ratio, and varying incubation time. The performance of the methods using

PP, particularly in reducing matrix effects, can be enhanced by greater dilution of the samples. Some of the drawbacks of the methods using PP include a greater potential for interference, matrix effects, and more frequent instrument downtime for LC-MS/MS instrument maintenance.

Strategies to Minimize Phospholipid Interference

Phospholipids, a significant component of blood, are one of the main classes of compounds that cause ion suppression in biological samples. In addition to causing matrix effects, phospholipids tend to accumulate in the HPLC flow path, which often leads to deterioration of separation efficiency and reduced HPLC column lifetime. To mitigate the impact of phospholipids and to improve method robustness, adequate cleaning and re-equilibration of the HPLC column at the end of every injection is required, which increases run times. Consequently, removal of phospholipids from sample extracts could enable faster chromatographic separations and more robust methods.

To minimize the harmful effects of phospholipids, it is possible to use phospholipid removal plates (PRP). PRPs are available from multiple vendors, typically in a format of 96-well plates. In addition to phospholipids, PRPs also remove proteins from biological samples. Sample pretreatment using PRP consists of protein precipitation using acidified organic solvent, followed by filtration of the supernatants through a packed bed of proprietary adsorbent packed in the wells of a 96-well plate. The obtained filtrates can be diluted (or evaporated and the residues redissolved) using a solvent compatible with HPLC separation and injected for instrumental analysis.

Derivatization

In analytical chemistry, derivatization is used to chemically modify analytes through the incorporation of a functional group into the structure of a molecule, to chemically modify the molecule and make it more amenable to analysis. In MS-based methods, derivatization can be used for modifying chromatographic behavior, enhancing ionization efficiency, and achieving more suitable fragmentation, thereby improving the sensitivity and specificity of analysis. The goals of derivatization vary, depending on the type of HPLC separation, mass analyzer, type of data acquisition and are method specific.

Internal Standards

Internal standards (IS) play an important role in quantitative analysis and monitoring assay performance. Ideally, IS should be added to the samples at the beginning of sample preparation. For an IS to effectively track an analyte during sample preparation, the IS should (a) be chemically similar to the analyte of interest, to ensure that it behaves similarly during the sample preparation, and chromatographic separation, (b) have comparable ionization and fragmentation properties to the analyte of interest, (c) be stable under conditions used during the sample preparation and the instrumental analysis, (d) not interfere with the signal of the analytes of interest, (e) provide consistent response across the calibrators, QC and unknown samples, (f) be added to the samples immediately after the sample aliquoting, and (g) be present in the samples in the same form as the analyte of interest (e.g. if an analyte is protein-bound, prior to starting sample preparation, the IS should be incubated with the samples to allow equilibration with the binding proteins).

The ideal IS in MS-based methods are structural analogs of the analyte, which contain stable isotope atoms (SIL-IS) (e.g., ^{13}C, ^{15}N, or ^{2}H). The number of incorporated isotopic atoms should be sufficient to resolve SIL-IS ions from the isotopic envelope of the analyte. For small molecules, typically three isotopic atoms (that corresponds to an increase in molecular weight by +3 Da) are sufficient, though larger molecules, or those containing an element with a higher fraction of naturally occurring isotopes (e.g., molecules containing chlorine and bromine atoms) may require larger number of isotopic ions, to separate the molecular ion of the IS from the isotopic envelope of the analyte. Isotopic distribution calculators are useful tools in evaluating IS-analyte pairs for the potential of cross-channel contribution. Chemical purity, labeling efficiency, and position of the isotopic atoms within the structure (e.g., exchangeable protons) must also be considered as potential sources of cross-channel contribution.

Complete recovery of the analyte from biological samples is typically not feasible. Internal standards (IS) are used to compensate for incomplete recovery and enable accurate quantification. As the chemical properties of the analyte and SIL-IS are nearly identical, the IS tracks recovery of the analyte during sample preparation, ionization, and the instrumental analysis, while the difference in m/z allows their separate detection. Quantification in MS-based methods is performed by normalizing analyte peak area to the IS peak area; the resulting relative response value is used for generating calibration curves and calculating analyte concentration in the unknown samples. In order for an IS to provide optimal performance, its concentration should be within 20–30% of the ULMI of the assay.

For accurate quantification, special attention should be taken to ensure that the IS peak fully coelutes with the peak of the analyte of interest. If there is an offset in retention times, quantification may be impacted adversely due to matrix effects, which are not fully compensated in regions of the analyte peak that do not overlap with the IS peak. Offset retention times in analyte-IS pairs may be observed for IS with >3 deuterium atoms, especially in the case of late eluting peaks, or when improper IS concentration is used.

Method Optimization

Development of a new LC-MS/MS method is an empirical, iterative process guided by the continual evaluation of the method's performance characteristics. Each step of the draft method procedure should be optimized, with a goal of achieving the targeted performance characteristics while ensuring the workflow is compatible with the laboratory where routine testing will be performed. Information gathered in the optimization phase of method development will enable realistic goals to be set for method performance and inform the validation acceptance criteria.

Calibration and Quality Control

Development of an approach for calibration and quality control (QC) is a critical part of method development. Certified reference materials (CRMs) are the preferred type of standards to use for preparing assay calibrators since they provide an opportunity for among-laboratory harmonization. If routine use of CRMs is cost-prohibitive, the CRM may be used to verify concentrations in laboratory-prepared calibrators, especially during bridging of manufacturing lots. If calibrators and QC samples are prepared by a laboratory, it is recommended that standards from different manufacturers or, if the standards are offered only by a single vendor, different lots of the standard be used for preparing the calibrators and the QC samples.

Analyte concentration in the calibrators should span the analytical measurement interval (AMI) of the assay and should include standards containing concentrations in the vicinity of the LLMI and ULMI of the assay. In quantitative methods, it is recommended to use at least five calibration standards. If the instrument response suggests a quadratic regression fit, or the AMI exceeds 100-fold, additional calibration levels should be considered. The ultimate number and spacing of calibration standards should be based on consideration of the AMI of the assay, the linear dynamic range of the instrument, the clinical decision points, and the type of calibration curve fitting algorithm used. In methods for qualitative analysis, it is acceptable to use a single-point calibrator prepared at the cutoff concentration of the assay. In addition to using calibration standards for generating a calibration curve, the calibrators are also used to set the target and range for the mass transition ratios for the run.

The choice of calibration matrix is paramount for the performance of a quantitative LC-MS/MS method. The matrix should be analyte-free and commutable with the patient samples to be tested (e.g., pool of negative patient samples), to act as an effective proxy. In the cases when a native analyte-free sample matrix could not be obtained or the method is intended for the measurement of an endogenous biomarker, a synthetic matrix could be used. It is important to carefully evaluate the candidate matrix for potential differences in analyte recovery and matrix effect, which would indicate non-commutability [15].

The most effective means of evaluating commutability between patient samples and a candidate calibration matrix is through "parallelism" experiments [16]. The experiment is performed as follows: two sets of calibrators are prepared, one in the candidate calibration matrix and another in a pool of patient samples containing a low concentration of the analyte of interest. If regression lines drawn through both sets of calibrators are parallel to each other, this supports the suitability of the candidate matrix for use in the assay. If the slopes of the calibration curves are significantly different, this should prompt evaluation of alternative calibration matrices or troubleshooting the assay. In addition to the use of proxy matrices for preparing calibrators, they are useful for preparing contrived samples for LLMI and AMI assessment, and in the dilution of patient samples with concentrations above the ULMI prior to sample preparation.

Once calibration levels and matrix for preparing the calibrators are selected and demonstrate acceptable performance, regression line fit type and weighting should be selected. Typically, when the AMI of the assay spans several orders of magnitude, a greater absolute variance is observed in the vicinity of the low and the upper ends of the calibration curve (generally caused by sensitivity limits, detector saturation, matrix effects, etc.). Use of weighting (e.g., 1/x or $1/x^2$), in fitting the regression line through the calibration points is often beneficial for improving the quantitative accuracy of the assay at low concentrations. Different weighting strategies could be compared retrospectively by reprocessing the acquired data.

System Suitability Testing

Prior to starting work on method validation, the targeted quality metrics for LC-MS/MS instrument performance should be established through longitudinal replicate measurements of system suitability testing (SST) standards. The SST standards should be composed of the analyte and IS in the same solvent as used for the prepared samples in the assay; the concentration of the analyte should be in the vicinity of the LLMI of the assay. Each analytical run should include replicate SST standard injections bracketed by solvent injections. SST performance assessment typically comprises evaluation of MS parameters (e.g., mass accuracy, mass resolution, signal intensity) and LC parameters (e.g., backpressure, RT, peak shape, peak height) in repeat SST injections. Reproducibility of the analyte peak area and RT in replicate injections of the SST is also informative. Data on SST analyses over the multiple runs acquired during method performance evaluation should be used for establishing SST acceptance criteria.

Longitudinal use of SST samples is important for proactively monitoring the "health" of the LC-MS/MS system. If a deviation in SST performance is observed, this could be an indication of a drift in the LC–MS system performance and should serve as a warning sign, indicating that instrument troubleshooting or maintenance is required. Importantly, SST samples should be stable, thereby enabling long-term use without concerns of the analyte degradation, which could raise false flags. Alternatively, if the SST samples are unstable, they can be prepared on the day of use, using an established procedure.

Quality Metrics and Pre-validation

Quality metrics should be established for acceptability of the runs and individual samples. The run quality metrics typically include assessment of (a) SST performance, (b) quantitative performance of the calibration standards and QC samples, (c) calibration curve metrics (e.g., R^2 and intercept), (d) boundaries for the tolerance of MRM ratios, and (e) boundaries for the tolerance of within-run IS peak area. Sample quality metrics include evaluation of (a) MRM ratios for the analyte and the IS, (b) IS peak area, and (c) assessment of chromatography in all mass transitions used in the assay (peak symmetry, peak width, presence of unresolved peaks, coeluting with the peaks of interest, etc.). The targeted quality metrics should be established prior to starting the method validation.

When method optimization efforts are deemed complete, method performance characterization should be thoroughly conducted prior to making plans for the formal assay validation. This pre-validation phase will inform on expected method performance characteristics and, importantly, minimize the risk of unexpected failures during the assay validation. Assessment of the method performance should comprise an abbreviated version of the method validation and will help to identify any potential method weaknesses.

For new methods, it is recommended to investigate analyte stability in standards, spiked samples (e.g., calibrators and QC), and patient samples. Comparison of the method to available reference measurement procedures and to validated methods of other laboratories is strongly encouraged. Analysis of external QC and proficiency testing samples (if available) is also informative in this regard and provides a foundation for monitoring the method when implemented in routine use. Any shortcomings identified in the method should be addressed prior to locking down the protocol and starting the assay validation. Addressing any inadequacies in method performance before beginning method validation is essential for achieving a successful outcome.

In addition to evaluating core performance characteristics, method robustness and ruggedness should be explored prior to starting work on the method validation. Multiple lots of critical reagents and consumables should be utilized to ensure that lot-to-lot variation does not impact the longitudinal performance of the assay. A change-of-hands experiment is also informative during this phase to determine the portability of the method from the method developer to the staff of the routine laboratory. The above-listed experiments, including pre-validation method evaluation, should ideally be conducted using the space and the equipment of the anticipated performing laboratory. If the method will be run on multiple LC-MS/MS instruments, equivalent performance needs to be confirmed.

After successful completion of the pre-validation method evaluation, a standard operating procedure (SOP) should be prepared defining all aspects of the method including the (a) purpose and principle, (b) safety requirements, (c) specimen type and pre-analytic requirements, (d) list of reagents, consumables, and equipment (e) instructions for preparing calibrators, QCs and all utilized reagents, (e) sample preparation and analysis procedure, (f) batch and samples acceptance criteria, (g) results interpretation and reporting procedure, and (h) list of supporting references. The SOP should be reviewed and approved by the Medical Director and management of the performing laboratory to ensure all method attributes are clinically appropriate and compatible with the laboratory practices. Following formal approval of the SOP by all stakeholders, no further method changes should be permitted prior to, and during the method validation.

Method Validation

Method validation is a critical part of diagnostic assay development and ensures that the method is reliable and produces accurate results, which is essential for patient care and clinical decision-making. A method should only advance to validation when sufficient data is available indicating that it meets the clinical requirements and is expected to pass performance characterization criteria. No discoveries indicating the method needs improvement should be expected to occur during the validation. Before beginning the validation studies, the SOP should be "locked-down" and formally approved by all stakeholders. All elements of the method, including reagents, consumables, instrumentation, technical procedure, data analysis, and result acceptance criteria, should be finalized.

Following pre-validation, as outlined in the above section, performance characteristic expectations should be understood and used to populate a validation plan that conforms to the appropriate regulatory environment. The validation plan should include clearly defined methods and expectations for performance characteristic evaluation and be approved by all stakeholders. Validation runs should be meticulously organized in advance of the experiments, and relevant quality metrics appropriately documented for every validation batch.

Run acceptance should be defined prior to starting method validation. Typical criteria include back-calculated calibrator concentration accuracies of ±15% (±20% at LLMI) and an $R^2 > 0.990$, with no more than one calibrator excluded (with the exception that the lowest and highest calibrators should not be excluded). The QC acceptance criteria may be based on SD limits or accuracies (if insufficient observations have been made to use SD). The QC sample sets should bracket the unknown samples of every run; no more than one control per level may fail, with a maximum of two control failures per run. The requirement for IS response criteria should be pre-established and based on the technical limitations of the assay. Additional parameters such as SST and LC peak quality parameters (RT for the analyte and IS, chromatographic peak shape, etc.) should be monitored. The acceptance of each validation batch should be documented, and only data from accepted runs should be used to determine the performance characteristics of the method.

Analytical validation of a clinical LC-MS/MS quantitative method should comprise the main performance characteristics of accuracy, precision, analytical sensitivity, analytical specificity, and reportable range. Additionally, the stability of critical reagents, the stability of the analyte in standards and patient samples, the suitability of different sample types (e.g., serum vs plasma), assessment of the effect of anticoagulants and preservatives, evaluation of potential interferences and matrix effect, and carryover should be performed. Recommended validation studies may be found in the Clinical Laboratory Standards Institute (CLSI) guideline C62A [1]. Pre-analytical parameters may also be defined during analytical validation and include sample collection and handling requirements. Depending on the availability of supporting data, clinical validation and determination or verification of reference intervals may also be required. Samples used for method performance evaluation during the validation studies should be from authentic patients (or pools of authentic patient samples); the contrived samples should be matrix-matched and have ≤5% of spiking solution volume.

Accuracy or trueness is the ability of a method to determine the accurate concentration of the analyte in a sample. Strategies for evaluating accuracy include method comparison, analysis of CRMs, and analytical recovery. Method comparison experiments should be performed, including comparison with an in-house predicate method to ensure similar or improved performance and comparison to a validated LC-MS/MS method of another laboratory to assess harmonization. Method comparison using patient samples should be performed on at least 3 different days to include inter-run variability in the analysis. Importantly, method comparison only gives an estimation of agreement unless the comparator method is a reference measurement procedure (RMP). Availability of RMPs or certified reference materials (CRMs) may be limited, so evaluation of analytical recovery in individual patient samples using high-quality standard material spiked in concentrations across the AMI may be a useful approach. Analytical recovery experiments should be evaluated by calculating percent recovery and linear regression, while data from the method comparison experiments should be assessed using Passing-Bablok or Deming regression analysis. In addition to the above-listed experiments, longitudinal performance of QC samples and calibrators should be assessed.

Performance should be evaluated in the context of the potential variation of the clinical laboratory environment to understand method repeatability and reproducibility. Accordingly, precision studies should be performed by multiple operators, including a member of the routine laboratory staff, with experiments performed on multiple days. Samples used in the evaluation of assay imprecision should comprise at least three analyte concentrations spanning the AMI, in the sample matrix intended for the assay; for example, the targeted concentrations could be 300% of the LLMI, mid-AMI, and 80% of the ULMI. When applicable, samples should also be included adjacent to medical decision points. Specific recommendations related to the assessment of assay imprecision can be found in the CLSI document EP05. A typical target for the acceptance tolerance is CVs ≤10%; alternatively, the target could be based on an available total allowable error target (TEa) for the analyte targeted in the method.

Typically, the lowest calibrator defines the LLMI and analytical sensitivity of the method. Performance of the method in the vicinity of the LLMI must be established through replicate analysis of matrix-matched samples performed on multiple days. A common target for performance at the LLMI is accuracy within 20% and imprecision ≤20%, alternatively, the target could be based on the TEa of the analyte. While not applicable to the comparison among multiple instrument platforms, signal-to-noise thresholds may be informative, with a minimum of 20:1 (in all mass transitions used in the assay), suggested as the best practice.

The linearity of the method should be confirmed over the target AMI through replicate analysis of at least six concentration levels, including the LLMI and ULMI. Use of matrix-matched calibrators, analyzed as unknowns, is appropriate. In cases when the calibrators are not matrix-matched, spiked samples or admixing low and high sample pools may be used to create the required concentration levels. If patient samples containing concentrations above the ULMI are expected, dilutional linearity of the method should be validated, as a means of extending the reportable range.

Compared to other methodologies used in clinical laboratories, LC-MS/MS provides greater specificity; however, interferences can be observed. Sample type-specific interferences such as icteric, hemolyzed, and lipemic samples, should be evaluated for compatibility with the method. Additionally, a careful survey of potentially interfering isobaric endogenous and exogenous compounds should be conducted. Special attention should be given to common over-the-counter medications and potentially co-prescribed medications for the intended patient population, since these may be present in the samples at elevated concentrations.

Establishing or verifying previously established reference intervals and medical decision points is an essential task that needs to be performed during method validation. Reference intervals are typically established using samples from healthy individuals; in order to ensure statistical significance, at least 120 participants are required. IRB approval should be obtained, and appropriate inclusion and exclusion criteria should be established prior to the enrolment of the participants. The participants should be healthy individuals, representative of the population for which the reference intervals are intended and the method utilized. The inclusion and exclusion criteria should comprise age, sex, ethnicity, health status in the context of the method's intended use, and a list of over-the-counter and prescription medications and supplements that could impact results. In addition, anthropometric characteristics, lifestyle factors such as diet, exercise, alcohol use, and smoking status should be considered. The data analysis for establishing reference intervals should be performed using appropriate statistical methods.

In cases when method comparison data demonstrate good agreement with the in-house predicate method or a validated method of another laboratory, reference interval verification may be performed to determine if adoption of the existing reference interval values is appropriate. A minimum of 40 samples should be analyzed, with a target of fewer than two of the 40 results falling outside of the targeted reference interval to support the validity of adoption. This will ensure that the existing reference interval is applicable to the targeted patient population using the new method.

Medical decision points are clinically relevant concentrations that differentiate between normal and abnormal results. These decision points are typically based on clinical studies and guidelines. Periodic review and adjustment of these decision points are necessary when new clinical evidence emerges or when the targeted patient population for the assay changes. Details on how reference intervals and medical decision points were established or verified should be included in the method validation documentation for future reference and regulatory compliance.

At the conclusion of method validation, data should be thoroughly reviewed, analyzed, and incorporated into a validation report. Each performance characteristic evaluated should be clearly marked as pass or fail. The validation report is a critical document that must be approved by all stakeholders and maintained on file in the performing clinical laboratory. The instrument data files and data analysis materials (e.g., spreadsheets) from the method validation experiments should also be on record to enable future review. If applicable, the validation report and other supporting documentation should be submitted for external regulatory review.

Successful transfer of a validated LC-MS/MS method to the routine clinical laboratory hinges on careful preparation and open communication amongst all stakeholders. Critical steps include (a) finalization of the SOP and all relevant supporting procedures (e.g., maintenance), (b) formal training of staff including method verification and proficiency studies, (c) bridging of assay specific reagent lots, as needed, (d) verification of data analysis methods, and (e) incorporation into the laboratory information management systems (LIMS), as appropriate. Careful execution of these steps will enable a smooth transfer and ensure consistent and reliable method performance.

References

1. Liquid chromatography-mass spectrometry methods, approved guideline. CLSI guidline C62-A. Clinical and Laboratory Standards Institute; 2014.
2. Rappold BA. Review of the use of liquid chromatography-tandem mass spectrometry in clinical laboratories: part II-operations. Ann Lab Med. 2022;42(5):531–57. https://doi.org/10.3343/alm.2022.42.5.531.
3. Rappold BA. Review of the use of liquid chromatography-tandem mass spectrometry in clinical laboratories: part I-development. Ann Lab Med. 2022;42(2):121–40. https://doi.org/10.3343/alm.2022.42.2.121.
4. Thomas SN, French D, Jannetto PJ, Rappold BA, Clarke WA. Liquid chromatography-tandem mass spectrometry for clinical diagnostics. Nat Rev Methods Primers. 2022;2(1):96. https://doi.org/10.1038/s43586-022-00175-x.
5. Stone JA, van der Gugten JG. Quantitative tandem mass spectrometry in the clinical laboratory: regulation and opportunity for validation of laboratory developed tests. J Mass Spectrom Adv Clin Lab. 2023;28:82–90. https://doi.org/10.1016/j.jmsacl.2023.03.001.
6. Kushnir MM, Rockwood AL, Bergquist J. Liquid chromatography-tandem mass spectrometry applications in endocrinology. Mass Spectrom Rev. 2010;29(3):480–502. https://doi.org/10.1002/mas.20264.
7. Yost RA. The triple quadrupole: innovation, serendipity and persistence. J Mass Spectrom Adv Clin Lab. 2022;24:90–9. https://doi.org/10.1016/j.jmsacl.2022.05.001.
8. Kushnir MM, Clarke NJ, Rockwood AL. Mass spectrometry. In: Rifai N, Chiu R, Young I, Wittwer C, editors. Tietz fundamentals of clinical chemistry and molecular diagnostics, vol. 2546. Philadelphia: W.B. Saunders Company; 2024. p. 211–25.
9. Annesley TM. Ion suppression in mass spectrometry. Clin Chem. 2003;49(7):1041–4. https://doi.org/10.1373/49.7.1041.

10. Bonfiglio R, King RC, Olah TV, Merkle K. The effects of sample preparation methods on the variability of the electrospray ionization response for model drug compounds. Rapid Commun Mass Spectrom. 1999;13(12):1175–85. https://doi.org/10.1002/(SICI)1097-0231(19990630)13:12<1175::AID-RCM639>3.0.CO;2-0.
11. Matuszewski BK, Constanzer ML, Chavez-Eng CM. Matrix effect in quantitative LC/MS/MS analyses of biological fluids: a method for determination of finasteride in human plasma at picogram per milliliter concentrations. Anal Chem. 1998;70(5):882–9.
12. Meikle AW, Findling J, Kushnir MM, Rockwood AL, Nelson GJ, Terry AH. Pseudo-Cushing syndrome caused by fenofibrate interference with urinary cortisol assayed by high-performance liquid chromatography. J Clin Endocrinol Metab. 2003;88(8):3521–4. https://doi.org/10.1210/jc.2003-030234.
13. Kushnir MM, Rockwood AL, Nelson GJ, Yue B, Urry FM. Assessing analytical specificity in quantitative analysis using tandem mass spectrometry. Clin Biochem. 2005;38(4):319–27. https://doi.org/10.1016/j.clinbiochem.2004.12.003.
14. Bergmann ML, Sadjadi S, Schmedes A. Analysis of catecholamines in urine by unique LC/MS suitable ion-pairing chromatography. J Chromatogr B Analyt Technol Biomed Life Sci. 2017;1057:118–23. https://doi.org/10.1016/j.jchromb.2017.04.011.
15. Miller WG, Keller T, Budd J, Johansen JV, Panteghini M, Greenberg N, Delatour V, Ceriotti F, Deprez L, Rej R, et al. Recommendations for setting a criterion for assessing commutability of secondary calibrator certified reference materials. Clin Chem. 2023;69(9):966–75. https://doi.org/10.1093/clinchem/hvad104.
16. Tu J, Bennett P. Parallelism experiments to evaluate matrix effects, selectivity and sensitivity in ligand-binding assay method development: pros and cons. Bioanalysis. 2017;9(14):1107–22. https://doi.org/10.4155/bio-2017-0084.

Instrument and Assay Maintenance for LC-MS/MS Analysis

7

Geza S. Bodor and Amanda J. Rands

Abbreviations

LC-MS/MS	liquid chromatograph–tandem mass spectrometer
LDT	laboratory-developed test
LC	liquid chromatograph
LCMS	liquid chromatography mass spectrometry (all versions)
SOP	standard operating procedure
FDA	Food and Drug Administration
LIS	laboratory information system
HPLC	high-pressure liquid chromatograph
UHPLC	ultra-high-pressure liquid chromatograph
PEEK	polyetheretherketone
SPE	solid phase extraction
ACN	acetonitrile
SST	system suitability test
RT	retention time
TAT	turnaround time
CAP	College of American Pathologists

G. S. Bodor (✉)
Department of Pathology, University of Colorado School of Medicine, Anschutz Medical Campus, Aurora, CO, USA

UCHealth University of Colorado Hospital Clinical Laboratories, Aurora, CO, USA
e-mail: Geza.Bodor@cuanschutz.edu

A. J. Rands
UCHealth University of Colorado Hospital Clinical Laboratories, Aurora, CO, USA

Y. V. Zhang, U. Garg (eds.), *Practical Guide to Implementing Liquid Chromatography Mass Spectrometry in Clinical Laboratories*,
https://doi.org/10.1007/978-3-032-03852-4_7

Introduction

Liquid chromatography–mass spectrometers (LCMS) and liquid chromatography–tandem mass spectrometers (LC-MS/MS) instruments have become more common in clinical laboratories in the past decade. In this chapter, we will use LC-MS/MS to represent both platforms, including LC-MS. These instruments are often purchased by laboratories with limited or no prior experience with LC-MS/MS. The components of the operating hardware, the liquid chromatograph, the mass spectrometer, the computer, and the software are often made by different manufacturers, and the typical application is performing laboratory developed testing (LDT). Demands on the clinical laboratory necessitate timely, accurate, uninterrupted operation, but instrument and method complexity commonly conflict with this demand due to instrument downtime, leading to frustration, and occasionally, to discontinuation of LC-MS/MS testing.

Proper maintenance of the LC-MS/MS equipment can prevent unscheduled downtime and can improve result quality, such as accuracy and precision. Although maintenance requires time and money, it keeps the instrument(s) in maximum working condition, minimizing or eliminating the need for retesting, thus saving on labor, reagent, and consumable costs. The gain in efficiency more than compensates for the time spent on maintenance. Furthermore, a properly maintained instrument is also expected to have an extended lifetime. From an economic perspective, maintenance can be considered as an investment with a significant long-term return.

LC-MS/MS maintenance must be planned, scheduled, and the required actions must be clearly defined in a standard operating procedure (SOP). Instrument manufacturers should provide instructions on the timing of maintenance and the required actions, such as inspection, cleaning, and parts replacement. Users should follow the manufacturer's instructions and use manufacturer-approved parts, but LC-MS/MS instrument wear is greatly impacted by mobile phase composition, sample type and purity, and the number of samples analyzed in a given time; therefore, each laboratory must develop its own maintenance schedule based on in-house experience. The maintenance plan or SOP must cover specific parts of the LC and MS/MS hardware, the computer and software, as well as consumables, such as the chromatography column and certain reagents. Different parts wear at different rate; therefore, separate daily, weekly, monthly, and as-needed maintenance tasks should be defined to be performed in-house. Trend monitoring by logging performance metrics either manually or electronically is an essential part of LC-MS/MS maintenance as subtle changes can precede instrument breakdown unless recognized and acted upon.

To our knowledge, no peer-reviewed literature exists that dissects LC-MS/MS instrument and method maintenance needs or that provides information on developing a maintenance plan. Instrument manufacturers supply maintenance-related information for their own hardware only, but the frequency of maintenance depends on sample and regent cleanliness, the analytical method, and the number of samples analyzed; therefore practical maintenance schedule must be developed by each laboratory based on their operating experience.

This publication is intended to aid laboratory directors and personnel who perform LC-MS/MS testing to understand the driving factors behind various aspects of maintenance delineated by instrument components and provide pointers for constructing their maintenance processes.

Instrument Maintenance

The LC-MS/MS instrument is a hybrid device. It consists of one or more liquid chromatograph (LC), a mass spectrometer with the associated ancillary instruments, such as the gas generator and the roughing pump. A desktop computer runs the chromatography program, acquires mass spectrometry data, and performs data analysis before uploading results to the laboratory information system (LIS). Each component has unique hot spots for wear or breakdown, therefore each has specific maintenance requirements according to its specific functioning. Unlike FDA-approved clinical laboratory analyzers, LC-MS/MS instruments are custom-made, often using components from different manufacturers, further increasing the complexity of maintenance that must be taken into consideration when the maintenance plan and SOP are developed.

Chromatography Maintenance

The chromatography apparatus, either high performance liquid chromatograph (HPLC) or ultra-high performance liquid chromatograph (UHPLC) consists of the autosampler, solvent pumps with inlet and outlet check valves, a column oven, and an analytical column that is often preceded by a guard column or a filter. If multiple LCs are used in multiplexed mode, multiple autosamplers, multiple pumps, and columns can be found in the hardware. The buffer flow through these parts will be directed by multiple rotary switching valves. The components of the LC instrument are connected with stainless steel or PEEK tubing using various fitting hardware. Different brands of connecting hardware exist, and they may not be compatible with each other despite similar appearance. When replacing tubing, the appropriate brand of hardware must be used for continued operation. HPLC systems typically operate between 400 and 600 bar (5000–8500 psi), while UHPLC systems may require up to 1300 bar (approximately 20,000 psi) pressure. This places the connections between the parts of LC system under significant stress that can lead to development of leaks if the connections are not made to exact specifications.

Autosampler parts, prone to wear, are the rotors, stators, needles, and the needle seats. Inadequate maintenance can lead to leaks, clogs, inconsistent injection volumes and carryover, therefore, the autosampler requires regular inspection and parts must be replaced on schedule, depending either on calendar time in service or on the number of injections. Manufacturer's recommended inspection and part replacement times are guidelines only, as sample purity has the largest impact on autosampler operation. Generally, solid phase extraction (SPE) provides cleaner sample than liquid-liquid extraction or dilute and shoot sample preparation. Particulate matter must be removed from the sample by centrifugation or filtration to prevent clogs.

LC backpressure varies between instruments and methods, but generally is consistent from run to run, with a gradual increase with increasing number of injections. The pressure also changes during the analysis of each sample in parallel with the mobile phase composition change. A sudden change of pressure can indicate clogged tubing or a leak but is not specific to one part or section of the LC. Monitoring and recording pressure changes in relation to injection numbers is a common maintenance process for detecting developing obstruction in the autosampler. Sudden large changes should initiate troubleshooting and maintenance action. Modern autosamplers contain injection counters accessible through a maintenance menu to aid in scheduling needle and seat replacement.

Rotary Valves are an integral part of the autosampler, allowing loading and injection of the sample into the solvent flow. They can also be installed in other parts than the autosampler of the liquid chromatograph to direct the flow in the chromatography system, to switch columns or to select eluents, for example. Various brands and implementations exist, each using specific parts, but their maintenance needs are similar; therefore, they can be monitored using the same parameters, such as chromatography back pressure, peak shape, and size. The parts of the rotary valves that require specific attention are the rotor, stator, and rotor seal (if applicable), and these parts are usually on a recurrent maintenance schedule, depending on time-in-service, number of injections, or turns of the rotor. If the number of injections or turns are maintenance trigger, these actions are counted by the autosampler software and can be accessed through the maintenance menu. Leaks and clogs are the common errors, requiring parts replacement that must be performed using identical hardware to the one being replaced. Use the manufacturer's part number when ordering a replacement part and follow the installation instructions carefully. Monitor the valve and tubing connections for leaks after maintenance and monitor back pressure on the system. Occasionally, small pieces of the new rotor can be dislodged during the first few hours of operation, causing clogs in downstream tubing and/or leaks in check valves or deposits on the guard column. These types of deposits can be easily cleared by applying backflow to the clogged tubing, replacing the guard column, or manually flushing the check valves.

Autosampler Needle Wash is used to clean the needle between injections. The sample must be soluble in the needle wash to prevent carryover. Fresh wash should be prepared at least weekly. Purging and priming the needle wash solution must be included in the daily maintenance before a new run is started.

Wear on autosampler needle and needle seats is proportional to the number of injections, and these parts must be replaced on condition, time in service or number of injections, according to manufacturer's recommendations.

Pumps contain moving parts, such as pistons, inlet and outlet check valves, and various seals that wear with continued use. Different HPLC manufacturers have developed different hardware; therefore intimate knowledge of the brand-specific implementation is essential for trouble-free operation. Annual inspection and replacement of pistons and seals is mandatory but may have to be done more frequently depending on usage (number of injections). Inlet and outlet check valves require closer monitoring as they frequently develop leaks from deposits of pump seal debris, leading to pressure fluctuation and retention time (RT) shift. It is good practice to purge the HPLC system with >90% water to remove salt (if used for chromatography) and acetonitrile if the instrument is used infrequently. Clogged or leaking check valves must be identified, replaced, but removed check valves can be sonicated and reinstalled. High-pressure pumps often use seal rinse, consisting of methanol, water, and isopropanol. Seal rinse must be kept fresh, replaced at least weekly. If closed-loop seal rinse is used, mark the starting volume as decreasing or increasing volume can indicate a leak around the piston seals. Purge valves are also common sources of leaks and must be kept clean for proper operation. Keep an inventory of a sufficient quantity of inlet and outlet check valves, pistons, and piston seals for continued operation, and have detailed instructions in the maintenance SOP for bench personnel to accomplish parts replacement. As before, continuous monitoring of systemic back pressure and sample retention times is essential to trigger on-condition maintenance.

HPLC Tubing replacement is a common maintenance action, most frequently demanded by extreme LC back pressure increase. HPLC tubing is made of stainless steel, polyetheretherketone (PEEK) or other material. Common internal diameters (ID) are 0.005 or 0.007 inches (0.12 or 0.17 mm, respectively). Narrower ID tubing provides lower internal volume but will increase back pressure and will be prone to clogging. Stainless steel can handle much higher back pressure than PEEK, but it is harder to cut in-house. A perfect fit between tubing and the next part is needed to eliminate dead spaces that cause peak broadening but cutting stainless steel is very difficult. Little burrs, left after cutting, will offset the fit and lead to HPLC inefficiency. It is highly recommended to purchase precut stainless-steel tubing in various lengths and replace clogged or leaking tubing with precut ones as needed. On the other hand, PEEK tubing is easy to cut to the desired length, but it may not withstand the required pressure that develops during chromatography. As a tight fit of tubing is essential, all HPLC operators must be proficient with proper tubing replacement. The distance between the ferrule and the end of the tubing must ensure a seamless fit on the first attempt, as once the ferrule is tightened, it will seat permanently on stainless steel tubing. Ferrules on PEEK tubing can be repositioned. Improperly fit stainless-steel tubing must be discarded.

Columns are considered consumables. Their efficiency changes with use, and they have a limited lifetime. Modern HPLC columns are fault tolerant but proper care can extend their useful life significantly. Particulate matter can clog the analytical column; therefore, guard columns or pre-column filters are required to retain particles that could clog the analytical column. Guard columns must be matched to the analytical column surface chemistry. Pre-column filters of 0.5–2.0 micron pore sizes are a less costly alternative to guard columns and still work well. Proteins or lipids can be deposited on analytical columns, increasing back pressure and robbing the method of efficiency. Changing system pressure, RT shift, or peak shape distortion are good indicators of column aging; therefore, monitoring of these parameters is essential. Guard columns or in-line filters must be replaced before system pressure reaches approximately 2/3 of the maximum allowed pressure. The analytical column, if removed from the HPLC, must be capped and stored according to the manufacturer's recommendations. If the columns are retained in the system, the oven must be turned off when not in use. In small laboratories, one HPLC may be used for multiple methods, using different columns that are changed as needed. In such cases, it is good practice to use quick-connect or quick-turn fittings that allow fast column exchange without the use of special tools. Some labs report good success with column regeneration, accomplished by reversing flow direction through the column, but careful method development with attention to sample preparation usually allows 10,000–15,000 injections with modern chromatography columns.

Mobile Phases can be the source of microbial, chemical, or particulate contaminants. Low-purity reagents may clog the instrument or the columns or lead to non-reproducible chromatography or ghost peaks. Always use LC-MS grade reagents, if available, or the next lower quality, such as HPLC or ACS grade, if not. Mobile phase modifiers, such as formic acid, ammonium formate, and others, can contribute contaminants even when bulk solvents are the highest grade possible. Prepared working reagents may have to be filtered after preparation using 0.5 micron filters. They must always be kept covered to prevent contamination and dust from entering. Do not exceed the reagent shelf life beyond what has been validated during method development. Keep a record of reagents purchased by lot number and date obtained. Recordkeeping is an excellent tool to trace sudden changes in method performance and to quickly identify the offending reagent(s). Observe the manufacturer's recommendation for storage temperature of chemicals.

Mobile phases made from acetonitrile (ACN) can polymerize during extended storage, which, in turn, can block fluid flow or create leakage around check valves. ACN polymerization can be prevented by preparing the mobile phase fresh before use and by rotating containers. The container that was just rotated off the HPLC must be cleaned with DI water and dried before it is refilled. If ACN polymer build up is suspected in the HPLC, the system must be washed with LCMS grade water before it is returned to service. The laboratory's LC-MS/MS maintenance SOP must specify the maximum number of days a batch of mobile phase can be used, with or without topping off the container. The date of manufacture and date of expiration must also be included on the container.

Bacterial growth may take place in mobile phases. Sodium azide, at 0.02% concentration, could be added to mobile phases if it does not interfere with the mass spectrometer, but using fresh reagents, limiting on-instrument storage time and rotating containers provide better prevention.

Even trace amounts of detergents, left behind after glassware cleaning, can adversely affect chromatography or mass spectrometry analysis; therefore, these glass containers must not be cleaned along with other laboratory ware. These require special cleaning procedures that must be described in the maintenance SOP. Multiple rinse cycles with small volumes of methanol or acetonitrile, followed by rinse with DI water and drying, is the best practice for keeping mobile phase-glassware contamination free.

The LC Column Log

The LC back pressure at the time a new column is installed depends on the hardware, the type and size of the column, the composition of the mobile phases, column oven temperature, and the flow rate of the mobile phase. The HPLC hardware contributes to the observed pressure, but each column will present a different starting pressure even when the same method is performed on the same hardware; therefore, each column must be monitored individually, in connection with the LC-MS/MS instrument it is assigned to. The initial and daily pressure readings must be performed at a set mobile phase composition, flow rate, and temperature. LC back pressure change is a non-specific sign of need for maintenance, but it is a useful parameter that can inform about the health of the LC-MS/MS system. In our laboratory, pressure reading is taken at 2 min in the equilibration, after oven temperature stabilizes at operating temperature, before any samples are injected. An example of a blank LC Column Log in use at UCHealth Toxicology and TDM Laboratory is presented in Fig. 7.1. Completed logs are reviewed by the section supervisor and stored with maintenance records for 2 years.

uchealth University of Colorado Hospital - Clinical Laboratory

Instrument ID________________ **Stream ___ LCMS Column Log**

Method:____________________ Flow @ 2 min. into equilibration:

Column type:__________________________ Install Date:_______________ Buffer A:_______mL/min

Size:__________ Void volume:_______________ Buffer B:_______mL/min

Lot #:________________ Temp:__________

Serial #:________________ Pressure:_______

Date													
Start pressure after equ.													
Daily Injections													
# of serum injections													
Total Column Injections (Running Total)													
Guard column changed													

Date													
Start pressure after equ.													
Total Injections													
# of serum injections													
Total Column Injections (Running Total)													
Guard column changed													

Reviewed by Date & Initials:______________________________

Approved and current. Effective starting 9/20/2019. 51480.3756 (version 1.0). Printed on 12/3/2024 8:42 AM (MST). Page 1 of 1

Fig. 7.1 Example of LC column log. Each log is specific to a column, instrument, and method. Columns are identified by their type, size, lot, and serial number. Daily observations of LC back pressure and the number of samples injected per day of operation are recorded with the running total of injections. The log contains a signature line to document review by the laboratory director or designee

The Pressure Trace

Many chromatography software will display real time pressure changes during the run. This pressure trace is unique to each method but reproducible between samples. It can be observed by the operator for information on HPLC performance during the run. If the chromatography software provides the option of saving the pressure trace, it should be stored electronically to aid troubleshooting, especially if the analysis was run unattended.

Mass Spectrometer Maintenance

In an LC-MS/MS system, the mass spectrometer serves as the detector, providing the identifying and quantitative information for analyte measurement. The most important aspects of mass spectrometer performance are mass accuracy and sensitivity. Modern mass spectrometers are robust and have stable electronics, requiring a mass accuracy check and recalibration once every six to 12 months. Follow the manufacturer's instructions to perform the required calibrations, if it is done by laboratory personnel, or have it done by the manufacturer's field service personnel during scheduled preventative maintenance (PM).

MS sensitivity, on the other hand, can change gradually during use and requires constant monitoring and remedial actions. Peak height, peak area, and signal-to-noise ratio (s/n) of internal standards or low concentration analytes are markers of changing sensitivity. The observed parameters, expected values, and frequency of monitoring must be described in the maintenance SOP, along with the corrective actions to return the instrument to optimal performance. The most common cause for loss of sensitivity is contamination of the ion source, the capillary electrode, or the curtain plate from deposits left behind by the samples; therefore, the best MS maintenance practice is careful sample preparation. If the instrument is equipped with a diverter valve, it should be used to direct the outflow from the HPLC into waste when the mass spectrometer is not acquiring data (outside of the acquisition window). Cleaning of the source and the curtain plate is routine maintenance. Flushing the electrode with LCMS grade water and methanol and washing and wiping the curtain plate with methanol and isopropanol after removal from the mass spectrometer, are required periodically, depending on sample cleanliness and the number of injections. Source, electrode, and curtain plate cleaning is usually part of the daily or weekly maintenance. Each laboratory should develop its source cleaning schedule based on operating experience. Deeper cleaning of the mass spectrometer, such as the ion optics or quadrupoles, requires training and is better left to field service.

Maintenance of the ancillary equipment such as the roughing pump or the gas generator should be part of the annual maintenance, although oil change on the rough pump can be easily performed in-house. Gas generator maintenance by laboratory personnel should be limited to monitoring pressure gauges and verifying gas pressure each day of use. Other maintenance, which commonly consists of mechanical and electronic parts replacement, is better left to be performed by the manufacturer either within the scope of the maintenance contract or as a fee-for-service action.

Software Maintenance

The chromatography, acquisition and quantitation methods were finalized during method validation and should not be changed without appropriate revalidation. If the software manufacturer updates acquisition or quantitation software, revalidation or performance verification should be performed before resuming patient testing to assure continued data quality. The extent of verification or revalidation should depend on the nature of the software changes. Actions can include verifying the performance of the acquisition or quantitation methods by reanalyzing previously completed batches or proficiency test samples. LIS interface performance can be revalidated by uploading results from test samples and QCs to the LIS. During regular use, LC-MS/MS software maintenance consists of creating regular data backups of the data or the full computer. Off-site data backup or archival on a thumb drive or an external hard drive is preferred and will provide insurance against catastrophic hardware failure and ransomware attacks.

Maintenance Contract

Daily, weekly, and monthly maintenance are performed by laboratory personnel, but semiannual and annual preventative maintenance (PM) and certain on-demand maintenance may be outside of the laboratory's expertise. The instrument manufacturer or a third party can provide those services on an as-needed, fee-for-service basis, or under a service contract. Instrument manufacturers have the advantage of faster parts availability and software updates, while third-party service may be less costly. If possible, HPLC, autosampler, mass spectrometer and gas generator, and software should be covered under a single service contract, although the actual service of the various hardware may be performed by engineers of manufacturers of those components. Maintenance contracts are expensive, but guaranteed response time, access to up-to-date software, parts availability and service personnel expertise are the advantages, contributing to shorter downtime and increased productivity.

Regardless of the availability of a maintenance contract, the laboratory should maintain an inventory of commonly needed parts, such as valves, rotors, stators, tubing, ferrules and such for speedy completion of maintenance or repair. The hardware manufacturer can provide the list of the necessary items.

Assay Maintenance

The vast majority of clinical LC-MS/MS assays are LDTs, therefore often lack ready-to-use reagents, calibrators or quality controls. Unique analytes also lack commercially available proficiency test samples, requiring the laboratory to manufacture these components in house periodically, or to contract with a reagent manufacturing company to produce them for a fee. Reagent and calibrator manufacturing procedures were established during method development and finalized during method validation. Reproducible production of these assay components requires the same solvents, sample matrices, analytical standards, and certified standard material to be used as defined during development and validation. Once a material has been validated, the same brand should be used from the same manufacturer in future batch productions. Minor differences between trace materials from different manufacturers may adversely impact LC-MS/MS methods. The laboratory must educate institutional purchasing department personnel on the importance of brand fidelity to prevent arbitrary changes of assay components dictated by ill-conceived frugality.

Sample matrices, such as analyte free serum or urine are critical components and frequent source of trouble. Serum or plasma devoid of endogenous analytes such as hormones, are either artificially mixed from individual components, manufactured from recombinant proteins, or pooled from human or animal blood and then stripped of the analyte of interest. Each new batch of such matrices must be tested for purity before spiking them with the desired analytes and tested again after completion of the working reagents to verify expected performance. The required testing and acceptable performance criteria may be described in a separate manufacturing SOP or in the method SOP, but the results of testing and the acceptance or rejection must be recorded in a designated document separately for each batch as a part of the assay maintenance practice.

Native or isotope labeled analytes, standards and matrices must be tested for accuracy of labeling, potential contamination and suitability. Working solutions of internal standards, derivatizing reagents, calibrators and QC samples are prepared by spiking solvents or other matrices with the required analytes or internal standards. Procedures for testing and criteria for acceptability must be defined in written procedures, and the results must be documented and stored along with other QC records regardless of whether the assay component was manufactured in-house or by a contracted agency. Assay calibrator concentrations should be assigned for each new batch according to published methods [1, 2]. New lots of commercially available certified calibrators, if available, should also be verified before use. Calibrator acceptability can be assessed by patient comparison, linearity assessment, or by using proficiency samples from CAP or other sources can verify the performance of the new lot of calibrators. The required testing and acceptability criteria should be documented in an SOP, and the results of each batch should be recorded in a dedicated log and then maintained for the life of the calibrator lot plus 2 years. An example of Reagent Check-out Log in use at UCHealth Toxicology and TDM Laboratory is presented in Fig. 7.2.

Testosterone Internal Standard Checkout Log

File Analyst printouts behind log.

					T-13C Transition 1							
					RT		Peak Height					
IS Lot #	Date Made	Expiration Date	T-^{13}C Lot #	MTBE Lot #	Old Lot	New Lot	Old Lot	New Lot	Contamination? Y/N	OK to use? Y/N	Initials	Date In Use

Reviewed by:____________________ Date:____________________

Fig. 7.2 Example of reagent check-out log. Each new lot of reagents is recorded with the date of manufacture and, expiration date. The starting chemicals are also recorded by lot number. Results of the acceptance testing are also documented

System Suitability Test

Optimal data quality of LC-MS/MS measurement depends on optimal performance by each of the system's components, such as the HPLC, reagents, and mass spectrometer. The performance of each individual component may be monitored separately, but a more economical approach is to use special samples that stress the performance of the system. If the expected response derived from these samples has been previously established under known faultless working conditions, monitoring a carefully chosen group of parameters can inform of deviation from optimal performance. The samples used for this purpose are called system suitability test samples (SST samples) and the process of employing these samples is called system suitability testing (SST).

System suitability testing is "a test to verify the adequate working of the equipment used for analytical measurements," [3] and as such, is essential for instrument and assay maintenance and must be an integral component of each batch or run. SST samples are prepared in a batch, ready to be injected on the LC-MS/MS. They don't get processed with the samples of the batch run; therefore, their results depend only on the LC-MS/MS instrument's state and on the currently used mobile phases.

SST samples usually contain the most critical analyte at close to LLOQ concentration and the IS if the method measures a single analyte. SST samples for multi-analyte panels should contain two or more of the most error-prone or labile analytes. Adding critical isobaric compounds to the SST samples should also be utilized if the method requires it. It is good practice to select an analyte from the beginning and one from the end of the chromatogram. If polarity switching is used in the method, an analyte from the group of positive and one from the negative ions should be incorporated in the SST samples.

Commonly monitored parameters of SST samples are RT, peak height or area, peak width, peak symmetry, signal to noise (s/n) ratio, or selectivity for assessing adequacy of chromatography (LC, column, mobile phases). Peak height or area, s/n ratio, and ion ratio could be monitored to assess the mass spectrometer's performance [3–5]. Parameters that reflect the operation of the HPLC, reagents, and mass spectrometer would be selected and acceptable limits calculated from multiple measurements. The actual daily results then would be compared to those limits before batch run acceptability decision is made. It is good maintenance practice to record and track SST sample results in time as changes can signal the need for maintenance. Figure 7.3 is an example of an SST Log used at UCHealth Toxicology Laboratory.

As such SST is essential for error free operation as well as for instrument and assay maintenance, SST samples should be analyzed before the calibrators and quality control samples. If their results meet the criteria, they provide assurance that the calibration and quality controls can be relied upon [5].

Stream______

Testosterone by LCMS System Suitability Test Log

		Testosterone (Transition 1)					Internal Standard (Transition 1)					EpiTesto		
Assay Run Date	Tech	RT 0.85-- 0.95	Peak Area >1.50E4	Peak Shape OK (Y/N)	Ion Ratio >0.852	S/N >98	RT 0.84-- 0.95	Peak Area >3.30E5	Peak Shape OK (Y/N)	Ion Ratio >0.848	S/N >974	RT	ΔRT (EpiT-T) (>0.2)	Comments

Reviewed By Date & Initials______________________

Fig. 7.3 Example of SST Log. The monitored analyte(s) and acceptability criteria are used to evaluate each SST sample on the day of run

Return-to-Service Testing

Maintenance, especially when performed on major components of the LC-MS/MS system, may adversely affect method parameters, such as accuracy, precision, selectivity, carryover or interferences, therefore, performance verification is necessary following completion of maintenance. This is called return to service testing (RST) and its goal is to verify that the full testing system (hardware, software, and reagents) was not adversely affected by the maintenance (maintenance induced failure), the previously detected deficiency has been eliminated, and the LC-MS/MS instrument and method are capable to produce results to specifications. Return to service testing should be focused on the potentially affected aspects of the LC-MS/MS instrument and method for all tests performed on the recently maintained instrument. Polypropylene glycol (PPG) or specific mixtures of chemicals are routinely analyzed under standardized conditions to assess LC performance and/or mass spectrometer mass accuracy, instrument sensitivity, and other performance metrics. Additionally, instrument performance evaluation should incorporate user specific methods as part of return-to-service testing. Include SST samples, previously resulted patient samples, or CAP proficiency samples or perform linearity and AMR assessment before the LC-MS/MS method is returned to service.

Return to service testing documentation after major maintenance must be completed with an indication of result adequacy and the date the instrument was returned to service. All relevant documentation must be retained in the instrument maintenance log. Table 7.1 is a summary of recommended maintenance practices of clinical LC-MS/MS systems.

Table 7.1 Suggested LC-MS/MS maintenance schedule

Instrument maintenance check list		
Components	Recommended maintenance and frequency	Comments
Chromatography		
Autosampler needle, needle seats	Replace annually or biannually per the manufacturer's recommendation	Frequency also depends on the testing volume and the cleanness of the samples. Back pressure, peak area, or height are good indicators
Autosampler needle wash	Regularly (daily, or at least weekly)	
Pumps: check valves	Replace on condition	Back pressure, peak area, height, or RT shift are good indicators
Pumps: pistons, piston seals	Replace biannually or annually per the manufacturer's recommendation	
Seal rinse	Replace regularly (daily to weekly)	Monitor the fluid volume of closed-loop rinse set up
Rotary valves: rotor, stator	Replace regularly per the manufacturer's recommendation	On condition replacement may be needed, depending on time in service or number of injections
Analytical column	Monitor daily, replace on condition	Peak height, area, symmetry, and RT are indicators Use column log to track usage and performance
Guard column, filter	Monitor daily, replace on condition	Column back pressure is good indicator. Use column log to track usage and performance
Tubing, fitting hardware	On condition	Use factory pre-cut stainless steel tubing Beware of fitting hardware differences
Mobile phases	Regularly	Monitor daily, replace at least weekly
Mass spectrometers		
Mass accuracy, sensitivity	Biannually or annually	Per manufacturer's recommendation
Ion source, capillary electrode	Clean on condition or at least weekly	
Curtain plate	Clean on condition or at least weekly	
Ion path cleaning	As needed or annually	Consider contracted service

(continued)

Table 7.1 (continued)

Instrument maintenance check list		
Components	Recommended maintenance and frequency	Comments
Roughing pump (oil change)	Annually	Per manufacturer's recommendations
Gas generator	Monitor pressure daily	
	Replace parts regularly	Per manufacturer's recommendations Consider contracted service
Software		
Updates	As needed	
Calculation verification	Annually	
LIS interface	As needed	Following a software change or update.
Data backup	Regularly	Weekly and monthly backups are recommended
Full system backup	Regularly or after a significant software update	
Assay maintenance		
Buffers, reagents	Regularly	
Glassware cleaning	After each use	Treat separately from other labware cleaning. Avoid detergents.
Instrument purge and rinse	Every day of use	
AMR and linearity	Every 6 months	
SST	Every day of use	
Return to service		
Return to service testing and performance verification	As needed	Perform after each maintenance. The scope of testing should match the maintenance performed

Maintenance actions must be performed at least as frequently as required by the instrument manufacturer, but may be required more frequently as instrument wear depends on time in service and on the number of injections. Sample and reagent cleanness significantly impacts the maintenance schedule

Summary

LC-MS/MS instrument and method maintenance is a planned, ongoing process. Its goals are assurance of continuous high-quality results, trouble-free instrument operation, and extended instrument lifetime while keeping maintenance costs reasonable. Instrument manufacturers may provide recommendations regarding frequency of maintenance, but custom hardware and software, combined with LDT methods, require the laboratory director and personnel to develop practical and effective maintenance procedures in-house. To achieve all of the above goals, a comprehensive, written maintenance SOP must be drafted, addressing the specific needs of all components of the LC-MS/MS instruments and methods, and the timing when or under what conditions maintenance must be performed. This article is intended to help clinical laboratory practitioners using LC-MS/MS instruments and methods in creating their maintenance SOP and help them run a successful maintenance program at their institutions.

References

1. Lasky FD. Achieving accuracy for routine clinical chemistry methods by using patient specimen correlations to assign calibrator values. A means of managing matrix effects. Arch Pathol Lab Med. 1993;117(4):412–9.
2. Schlain B. A stochastic approximation method for assigning values to calibrators. Clin Chem. 1998;44(4):839–48.
3. Hund E, Vander Heyden Y, Massart DL, Smeyers-Verbeke J. Derivation of system suitability test limits from a robustness test on an LC assay with complex antibiotic samples. J Pharm Biomed Anal. 2002;30(4):1197–206. https://doi.org/10.1016/s0731-7085(02)00470-3.
4. Mutton I, Boughtflower B, Taylor N, Brooke D. The design and use of a simple System Suitability Test Mix for generic reverse phase high performance liquid chromatography-mass spectrometry systems and the implications for automated system monitoring using global software tracking. J Chromatogr A. 2011;1218(23):3711–7. https://doi.org/10.1016/j.chroma.2011.04.033.
5. Briscoe C, Stiles M, Hage D. System suitability in bioanalytical LC/MS/MS. J Pharm Biomed Anal. 2007;44:484–91. https://doi.org/10.1016/j.jpba.2007.03.003.

Troubleshooting for LC-MS/MS

8

Anthony Maus and Paul J. Jannetto

Introduction

LC-MS/MS testing is an extremely powerful tool due to the exceptional sensitivity, specificity, versatility, and costeffectiveness of the technique. However, implementing and maintaining LC-MS/MS workflows is not without challenges. Among the greatest challenges is troubleshooting problems as they arise. Even with the best laboratory practices and preventative maintenance procedures, troubleshooting is an inevitability. The causes, effects, and observations associated with the totality of possible problems are innumerable, but the goal of this chapter is to provide a guide for some common problems and outline general approaches that apply to the various manifestations of issues that can arise.

The first step in troubleshooting LC-MS/MS testing is to identify the component of the process that is responsible for the issue. Generally, LC-MS/MS workflows can be broken down to five steps or components that can be the sources of problems:

1. Preanalytical
2. Sample preparation
3. Liquid chromatography
4. Mass spectrometry
5. Data processing

A. Maus · P. J. Jannetto (✉)
Division of Clinical Biochemistry and Immunology, Department of Laboratory Medicine and Pathology, Mayo Clinic, Rochester, MN, USA
e-mail: jannetto.paul@mayo.edu

Y. V. Zhang, U. Garg (eds.), *Practical Guide to Implementing Liquid Chromatography Mass Spectrometry in Clinical Laboratories*, https://doi.org/10.1007/978-3-032-03852-4_8

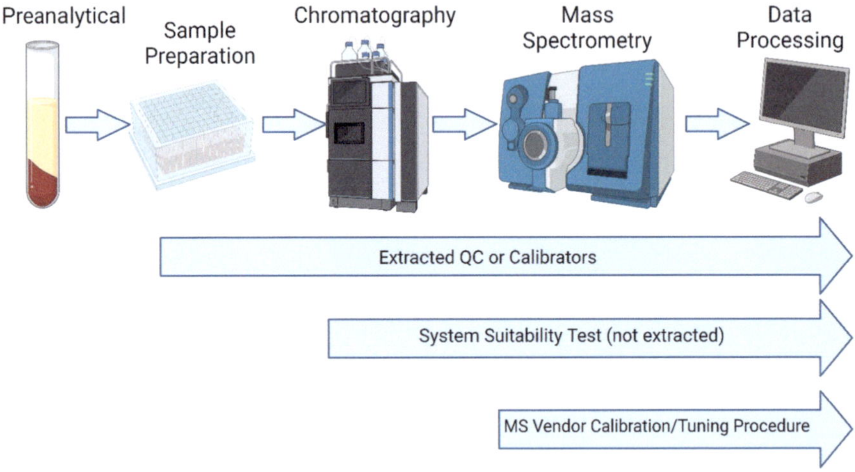

Fig. 8.1 General LC-MS/MS testing process along with basic strategies for testing components of the process. (Created in BioRender. Maus (2025) https://BioRender.com/tepab72)

Whenever a problem is encountered, the first step is identifying which component is the likely source of the issue. This may seem obvious, but it can be difficult in practice, and even the most experienced laboratory scientists can misidentify the source of a problem. Identifying any components of the system that have been modified or new variables introduced is often a beneficial way to determine the source of an issue. If no significant changes have been made, isolating the possible source component and doing targeted experiments to address the observed issues is generally the best approach. Figure 8.1 depicts the general LC-MS/MS testing process along with basic strategies for testing components. For example, extracted quality control samples assess all steps in the process except the preanalytical phase. The first step in most troubleshooting scenarios is differentiating between extraction/sample preparation and LC-MS/MS instrument issues. A strategy commonly deployed to decouple these two facets and test performance of the LC-MS/MS instrumentation daily is system suitability testing, which can be done by analyzing pre-prepared solutions containing target molecules. [2] This could be performed utilizing pooled residual extracts or simply a solution with the analyte or internal standard (IS) spiked in. It is recommended that you perform this before every batch and whenever a problem occurs during batch acquisition. It is best to inject system suitability solutions when the instrument is performing properly to establish acceptance criteria and then store it properly so that it can serve as a benchmark for instrument performance. When executed properly, this can be used to isolate problems to the instrumentation. If the LC-MS/MS instrument is determined to be the source of a problem, the system can be further parsed down by testing the mass spectrometer using the vendor calibration and tuning procedure, which typically utilizes infusion of a stable solution and removes the LC as a variable. We will caution that *passing the vendor-recommended testing does not definitively prove that the instrument is fully functional,* as these procedures cannot fully assess all application-specific parameters. If an operator has isolated a problem to the mass spectrometer, but the calibration and tuning procedures are meeting specifications, placing a service call with the manufacturer or cleaning the mass spectrometer is still appropriate.

Once the source of the problem is identified, the process of addressing it can begin. In the following sections, we apply these basic principles to some commonly observed issues, but the best general advice we can give is no matter how complex the problem, do not forget the basic premises within the scientific method of forming hypotheses, isolating variables, and performing experiments.

Issues with Signal

No Chromatographic Peaks

A wealth of information can be gleaned from a blank injection. It is imperative that operators differentiate between very low signal versus no chromatographic peaks and typical noise in the chromatograms because the troubleshooting steps are different for these scenarios. An example of the difference is shown in Fig. 8.2. Similarly, when troubleshooting low sensitivity, it is important to note the level of noise compared to batches with expected/normal sensitivity.

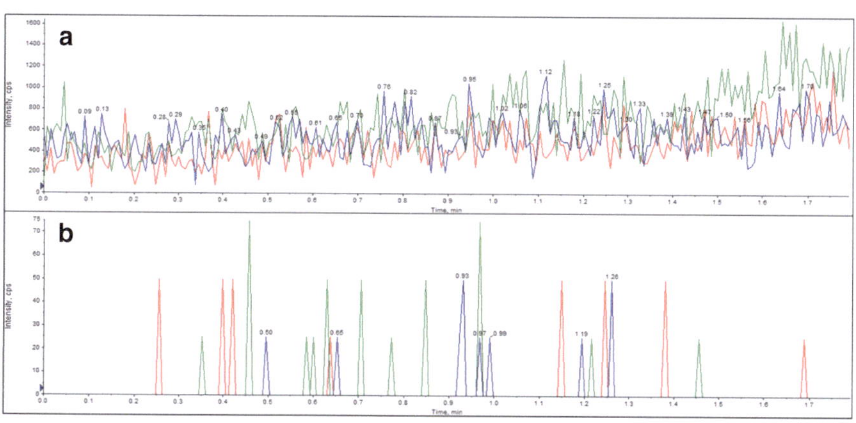

Fig. 8.2 (**a**) typical baseline and noise observed when a blank is injected, and LC flow is going into the mass spectrometer (**b**) Low baseline/noise indicative of a problem. In this example, the LC was not connected to the mass spec

Very Low Signal or No Signal at All

The three most likely scenarios that cause this observation are:

1. No LC flow is reaching the mass spectrometer
2. Problem with the ionization process within the source
3. Hardware failure within the mass spectrometer

Recommended troubleshooting procedure:

1. Check LC for leaks, blockages of the flow path, and ensure the LC is connected to the mass spectrometer.
2. Inspect the source and especially the ESI process. Visually check for inconsistent spray.
3. Perform the mass spectrometer vendor's recommended calibration and performance check procedure.

Normal Baseline and Noise, but no Chromatographic Peaks

There are many possible root causes of no chromatographic peaks at the expected retention time. When this occurs, it is imperative to isolate system components to determine where the failure is occurring. There are many potential causes, including:

1. Extraction issues
   (a) Technologist error
   (b) Lot/reagent issue
2. Autosampler issues
   (a) Inadequate sample volume for injection
   (b) Injecting out of the incorrect vial or plate position
3. LC issues
   (a) Leaking in the flow path
   (b) Column issues
      (i) Incorrect column
      (ii) Poor performing column
   (c) Mobile phase issues
      (i) Past expiration date
      (ii) Incorrectly prepared
      (iii) Lot/reagent problem
   (d) Retention time shift outside of the mass spec acquisition window
4. Mass spectrometer hardware issues

Recommended troubleshooting procedure:

1. System suitability test and/or reinject previous extraction with adequate results (if stability allows) to differentiate between extraction and LC-MS/MS problems
   (a) If the system suitability test/reinjection of the previous extract is acceptable and suggests extraction

   (i) Re-extract to determine if it was an isolated/anomalous problem
   (ii) Exchange lots/preparations of critical reagents
 (b) If system suitability test/reinjection of previous extract is not acceptable and suggests a LC-MS/MS instrument issue
   (i) Ensure that the correct mobile phase is being used and the lines are in the appropriate solvents (i.e., A and B are not reversed)
   (ii) Watch the autosampler to ensure it is aspirating the sample from the correct vial
   (iii) Analyze the pressure trace and compare it to historical batches with acceptable performance
   (iv) Check the LC system for leaks
   (v) Replace the mobile phase with a new preparation
   (vi) Replace the mobile phase with a new preparation using different lots of reagents
   (vii) Test new analytical column
   (viii) Replace autosampler washes with the correct wash strength of solvent.
   (ix) Widen mass spec acquisition window to check for significant retention time shift.
   (x) Perform the mass spectrometer vendor's recommended calibration and performance check procedure.

Drop in Signal and Sensitivity

Sensitivity issues are among the most common in LC-MS/MS testing, but they are difficult to address because there are many potential causes. A drop in sensitivity is typically characterized by a drop in signal-to-noise, which most frequently corresponds to a decrease in signal intensity but can be due to an increase in background/noise as well. When troubleshooting signal intensity issues, the first consideration is whether *the drop in signal has been a gradual decrease or a sudden drop*. We will discuss all these scenarios in the following sections.

Gradual Decrease in Signal

Potential causes of a gradual in signal include:

1. Mass spectrometer
   (a) Mass spectrometer becoming contaminated/dirty
   (b) Mass shift
2. LC
   (a) Mobile phase stability/pH changes over time
   (b) Hardware/pump problems
   (c) Degradation of analytical column performance

Recommended troubleshooting procedure:

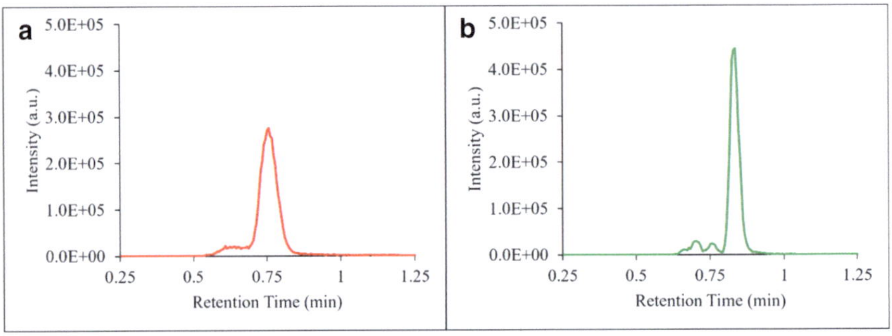

Fig. 8.3 Comparison of chromatographic peak shape and intensity before (**a**) and after (**b**) changing the analytical column. After changing the analytical column, the resolution increased, which resulted in a corresponding increase in signal intensity

1. Perform vendor calibration and tuning procedure
   (a) Check for a decrease in mass spectrometer performance by comparing to specifications or previous calibrations
      (i) Degradation in performance is likely due to the mass spectrometer ion optics becoming contaminated or dirty. This is frequently rectified by cleaning the mass spectrometer, ideally by the vendor. Some mass spectrometers allow for operator cleaning, but this is dependent on the vendor, model, and experience of the user.
   (b) Calibrate and see if the mass shifted significantly. Note that if successive mass shifting is occurring, necessitating atypically frequent calibration, the problem should be escalated to the vendor.
2. Analyze the pressure trace and compare it to historical batches with acceptable performance to assess LC hardware functionality
3. Prepare fresh mobile phases
4. Replace analytical column
   (a) Degradation in column condition due to usage can cause a decrease in signal-to-noise ratio (S/N) and often a corresponding decrease in chromatographic resolution or increase in peak width is observed. If any of these symptoms are observed, comparing it to a new analytical column is the best course of action. An example of this is shown in Fig. 8.3.
5. Perform maintenance on the pump per the manufacturer's recommendation, which typically entails changing piston seals and check valves, but this can vary with the pump manufacturer and model

Sudden Decrease in Signal

If there is a sudden significant decrease in signal intensity it is important to determine if their background/noise is normal as shown in Fig. 8.2.

The following are potential explanations for a sudden decrease in signal:

1. Extraction issues
   (a) Technologist error
   (b) Lot/reagent issue

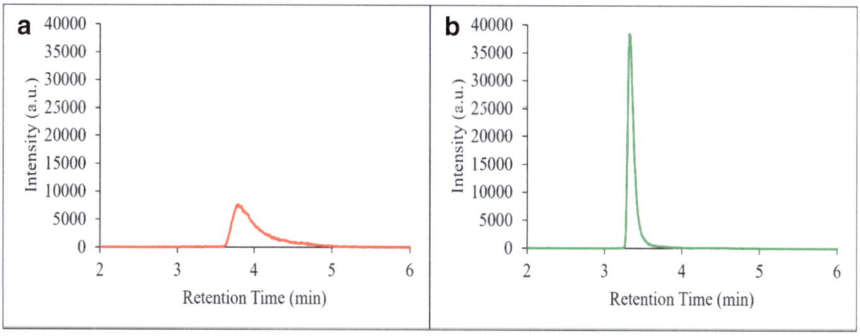

Fig. 8.4 Differences in peak shape and intensity from replicate injections of monoclonal antibody light chains with different preparations of mobile phase. In this case, the issue was determined to be an underperforming lot of formic acid, which was used as the mobile phase modifier

2. LC issues
   (a) Bad mobile phase due to prep error, contamination, or an underperforming reagent lot. An example of an improperly performing reagent lot is shown in Fig. 8.4.
   (b) LC system is leaking
   (c) Degradation in analytical column performance
   (d) The autosampler is not drawing sample properly due to a clogged injection needle or other malfunction
3. Mass spectrometer
   (a) Mass shift
   (b) Failure of hardware component

We would recommend the following troubleshooting steps in this scenario:

1. Test instrument performance using system suitability testing or a previously injected extraction that met acceptance criteria (if stable)
   (a) If system suitability test/reinjection of previous extract is acceptable and suggests extraction
      (i) Re-extract to determine if it was an isolated/anomalous problem
      (ii) Exchange lots/preparations of critical reagents
   (b) If system suitability test/reinjection of previous extract is not acceptable and suggests a LC-MS/MS instrument issue
      (i) Test the mass spectrometer with the vendor's recommended calibration and tuning procedure. Note that if successive mass shifting is occurring, necessitating atypically frequent calibration, the problem should be escalated to the vendor.
      (ii) One caution with many mass spectrometer vendor calibration/tuning procedures is they typically use source conditions that do not simulate clinical LC-MS/MS parameters. The easiest way to test the source is to use a backup or alternative source from another instrument if available to run clinical methods and samples. If this is not possible, consider visually inspecting the electrospray in the source or replacing the electrode.

(iii) Analyze pressure trace and compare it to historical batches with acceptable performance
(iv) Check LC system for leaks
(v) Replace mobile phase with a new preparation
(vi) Replace mobile phase with a new preparation using different lots of reagents
(vii) Test new analytical column
(viii) Watch autosampler to see if it is performing properly or perform autosampler testing procedure

High Background/Noise

Atypically high background/noise causing a decrease in S/N is most likely due to an extraction issue or contamination. More specifically, potential causes of this are:

1. Extraction issues
   (a) Contaminated reagent
   (b) Problem with enrichment step
2. LC issues
   (a) Mobile phase
      (i) Contamination
      (ii) Lot problem
3. Contaminated autosampler washes
4. Contaminated gas supply for mass spectrometer

   This procedure will help diagnose and overcome this issue:

1. System suitability test/reinject previous extraction with adequate results (if stability allows) to differentiate between extraction and LC-MS/MS problems
   (a) If system suitability test/reinjection of previous extract is acceptable and suggests extraction
      (i) Replace relevant reagents
      (ii) There is a problem with the enrichment step, troubleshooting this would be dependent on the sample preparation methodology
   (b) If system suitability test/reinjection of previous extract is not acceptable and suggests a LC-MS/MS instrument or mobile phase contamination
      (i) Mobile phases are the most likely cause, so replace the mobile phases. [8] An example of this type of contamination is shown in Fig. 8.5. In this figure, the S/N was exceedingly low with the initial preparation of mobile phase (A). However, after repreparing the mobile phase with different reagents and glassware, the background/baseline dropped significantly and there was a coinciding increase in S/N.
      (ii) Contamination of bottles of solvent due to improper handling is also possible, so starting with brand new, previously unopened reagents is often helpful when troubleshooting

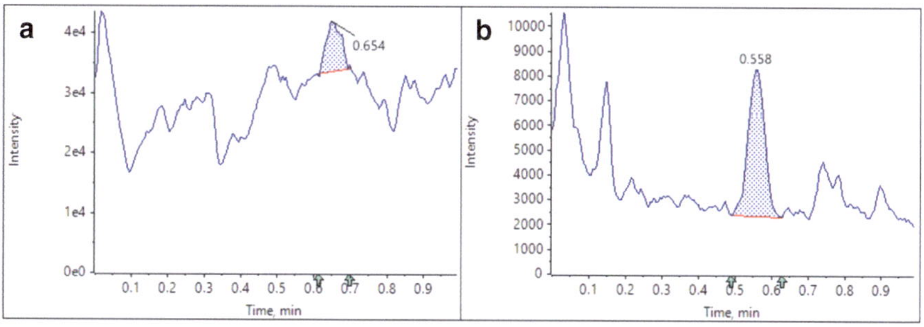

Fig. 8.5 The impact of mobile phase contamination. (**a**) Injection with an initial preparation of mobile phase (**b**) Same sample injected after changing the mobile phase and glassware. Note the drop in background/baseline and the improvement in S/N. All retention times are verified with isotopically labeled internal standards

(iii) Contamination or suboptimal performance can also be due to the manufactured lot of reagents, so try different lots or lots that were previously determined to result in normal performance
(iv) The same process can be used to test autosampler wash solutions if mobile phases are not the root cause
(v) Consider testing gas supply as a potential source of contamination using a new tank

Issues with Chromatographic Performance

Asymmetrical Peaks

Figure 8.6 shows different peak shapes encountered when performing chromatographic separation. The ideal peak has a high S/N, is perfectly symmetrical and Gaussian, which makes integration reproducible and accurate. In contrast, asymmetrical peak shape is an indication of suboptimal chromatographic performance. [4] Peak fronting is shown in the left panel and potential causes include incorrect mobile phase conditions, such as pH or the solvent strength of the injected solution being too strong, both of which hinder focusing on the head of the column. [5] Overloading the column is also a possible explanation. Peak tailing is shown in the right panel. Some of the causes, such as incorrect mobile phase conditions, column overloading, and injection solvent strength, are shared with peak fronting; additional issues capable of causing peak tailing include inadequate retention on the analytical column. [6] We have specifically observed this when trying to inject polar molecules on reversed-phase columns. Improper connections of fittings or lines are another underappreciated consideration when troubleshooting peak tailing or other chromatographic performance issues. Poor cutting of PEEK tubing or improperly seating lines when forming connections is common and the resulting void can have

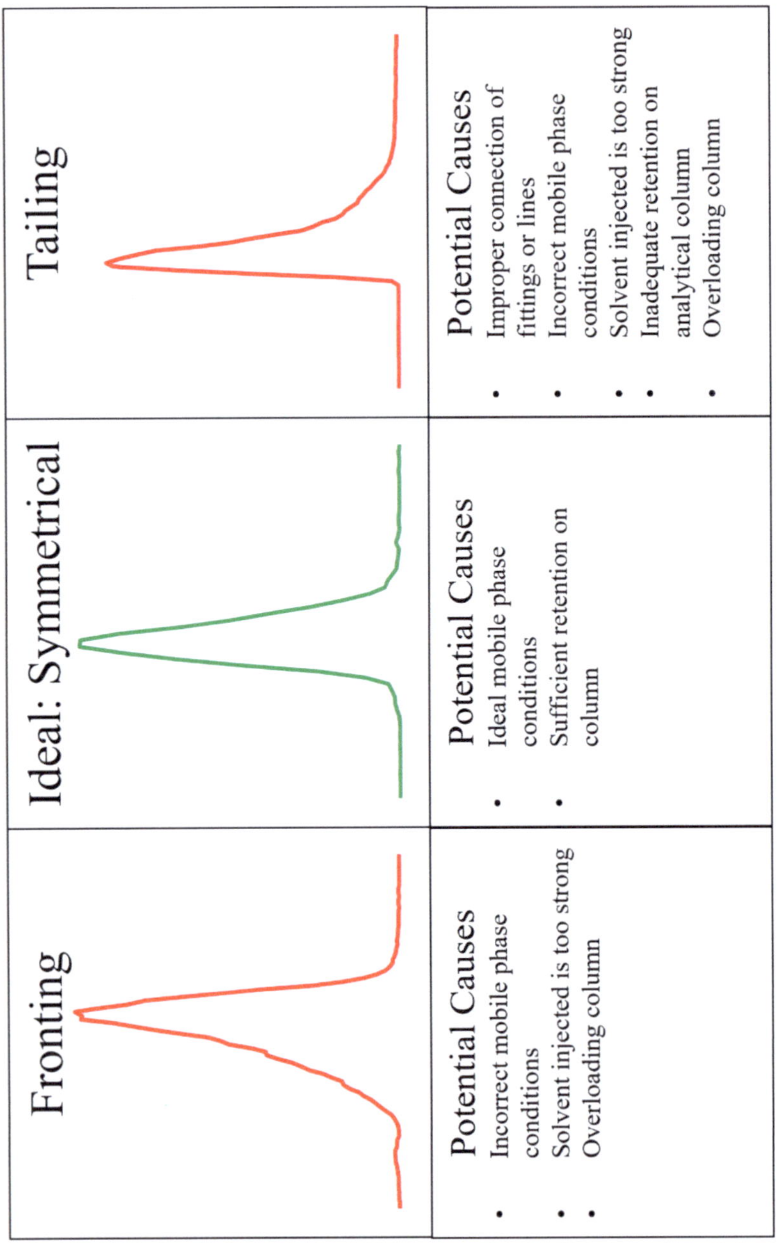

Fig. 8.6 Common peak shapes seen when performing LC-MS/MS and associated causes

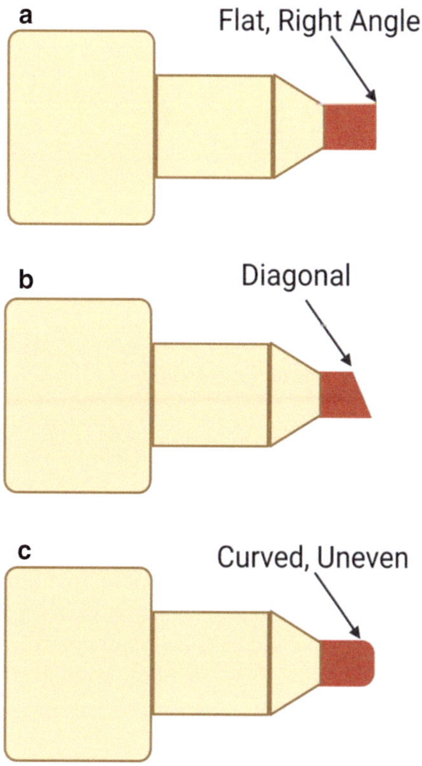

Fig. 8.7 (**a**) properly cut PEEK tubing is flat, has a right-angle (**b**) improperly cut tubing with a diagonal end (**c**) improperly cut tubing with a curved and uneven end

deleterious effects on chromatography. When using PEEK tubing, *it is especially important to verify that the tubing is cut at a flat, right angle and is properly seated.* [3] The importance of properly (Fig. 8.7a) cut PEEK tubing and negative implications of improperly (Fig. 8.7b, c) cut PEEK tubing is widely underappreciated. If peak shape problems persist after this, replacing every line/tubing through the flow path is often beneficial as it provides an opportunity to ensure proper cutting and fitting as well as eliminating any unwanted chemical interactions with the lines due to build-up of particulates over time.

Choppy Peaks

When chromatographic peaks are splitting at the top, noisy, or choppy like those shown in Fig. 8.8, the cause is most often suboptimal electrospray ionization performance. If the method is new to the mass spectrometer being used and the peak is noisy, then it is possible that the source parameters are suboptimal. This can be alleviated by optimizing the source parameters for the analytes of interest by tee infusion or injection. An important point to keep in mind is that peaks will often appear very noisy if you are making too many measurements within a peak due to

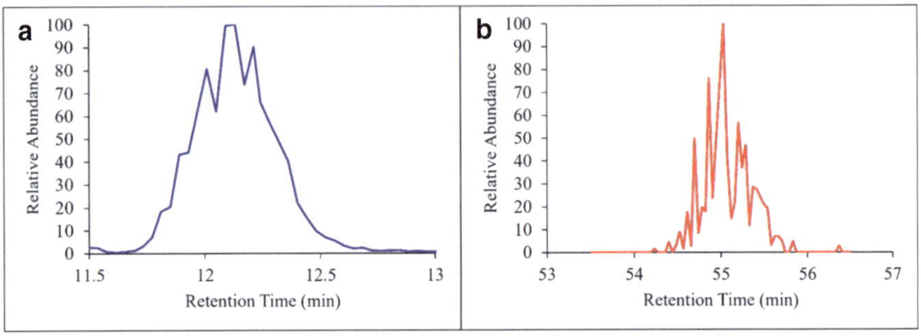

Fig. 8.8 Noisy/choppy peaks from LC-MS/MS measurements of tryptic peptides due to an improperly performing electrode

inappropriately set dwell times. When performing quantitation, 10 measurements within a chromatographic peak are widely regarded as the minimum, with 15 considered ideal [9]. However, if more than 15 measurements are being taken within a chromatographic peak, it is often beneficial to increase the dwell time so that at least 15 measurements are occurring. Increasing the dwell time improves the precision of each measurement, making the peaks appear smooth.

If the method has historically performed well and the peak issues are an atypical phenomenon, then it is likely an ionization problem. We recommend these steps to assess this issue:

1. Visually inspect to ensure consistent flow at approximately the right flow rate is reaching the mass spectrometer.
2. Reprepare mobile phase, ideally with different lots of reagents if a new one has been put into use.
3. Replace the electrode/needle/probe.
4. Try an alternative source housing if one is available.
5. Place a service call with the vendor.

Peak Splitting

Peak splitting occurs when suboptimal chromatographic performance causes the peak to widen and in extreme cases, begin to split into two peaks. An example of this is shown in Fig. 8.9. In this example, it can be determined that the peak is splitting and there is no coeluting interference because the phenomenon is occurring for both transitions of the isotopically labeled internal standard and the analyte, as well as with the calibrators that are not in matrix (calibrator data not shown).

Explanations for this include:

1. Mobile phase conditions
   (a) Improperly prepared

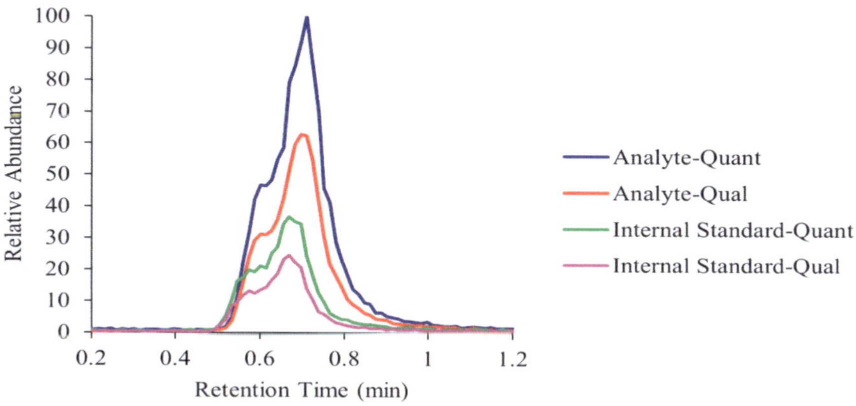

Fig. 8.9 Peak splitting due to the elution strength of the injected solvent

   (b) Incorrect pH
   (c) Wrong modifier
   (d) Problem with reagent lot

2. Inappropriate elution strength of the solution being injected
3. Inappropriate elution strength of LC method starting conditions (not focusing on column)
4. Dead volume
5. Partially clogged or improperly performing guard cartridges or analytical columns

To address this issue, we recommend the following:

1. Mobile phase
   (a) Reprepare with same lots of reagents
   (b) Reprepare with new lots of reagents
2. Lower the organic composition of the injected solution (Fig. 8.9)
3. Lower the organic composition at the beginning of the LC method
4. Visually inspect connections, stators, rotors, and PEEK lines (Fig. 8.7) for potential introduction of dead volume and replace as necessary
5. Replace guard cartridge and/or analytical column

Retention Time Shift

Most know that the LC separation is a significant contributor to the specificity of LC-MS/MS measurements, therefore, retention time of the chromatographic peaks is relied upon as a compound identifier and quality monitoring tool. [1] Thus, maintaining consistent retention times is imperative, but there are many contributing variables that must be controlled to ensure consistency. Defining a general unacceptable shift in retention time is difficult because it would depend on application-specific factors such as length of the method and chromatographic conditions. The best general estimation we can provide for clinical LC-MS/MS methods using reversed-phase conditions would be 0.1 min, but it is best to establish data-based criteria for each method.

Whenever a significant retention time shift is encountered on a locked method (no change in method parameters like flow rate), the pressure traces are very useful to guide subsequent steps. If atypical pressure phenomena are occurring, proceed to the appropriate section below. If the observed pressure trends align with normal performance, potential causes include:

1. Mobile phase
   (a) Improperly prepared
   (b) Contaminated reagent
   (c) Problem with reagent lot
   (d) Past expiration date
2. Incorrect column temperature
3. Leaking in the flow path (especially post-column if pressure trace is normal)
4. Degradation in guard cartridge or analytical column performance
5. LC pump not performing properly

Recommended troubleshooting steps for this scenario would be:

1. Mobile phase
   (a) Reprepare with same lots of reagents
   (b) Reprepare with new lots of reagents, ideally that have not been used previously to rule out the possibility of contamination
2. Verify that the column compartment/sleeve is maintaining the correct temperature
3. Carefully check the flow path for leaks
4. Replace guard cartridge and/or analytical column
5. Perform maintenance on the pump per the manufacturer's recommendation
6. Verify pump performance by setting the pump to deliver 100% mobile phase A and directing the flow into a graduated cylinder for a predetermined amount of time. Based on the flow rate and time, one can calculate the intended solvent volume and compare it to the measured volume in the graduated cylinder. This should be done with 100% A and 100% B settings to fully assess the pump performance.

Increased Prevalence of Chromatographic Interferences

Despite the exceptional specificity of LC-MS/MS techniques, interferences from coeluting molecules with similar structures and masses is possible. It is more common for certain classes of molecules than others and is also dependent on the matrix. Thus, much effort must be taken during the method development stage to minimize the impact of interferences. It is imperative to note the frequency of interferences during method validation, as an increase in the prevalence of interferences is an indication of suboptimal performance of the test. Interferences can be identified visually by poor chromatographic peak shape and/or resolution, nonlinearity upon dilution, or by discrepancies with quantifier/qualifier ratios.

The most likely sources of such issues are:

1. Extraction
   (a) Technologist error
   (b) Contaminated reagent
   (c) Lot issue with a critical material, such as a solid phase extraction cartridge
   (d) Problem with the enrichment step
2. LC
   (a) Mobile phase
      (i) Improperly prepared
      (ii) Contaminated reagent
      (iii) Problem with reagent lot
      (iv) Past expiration date
   (b) Analytical column
      (i) Degradation in performance
      (ii) Issue with a lot of columns, Fig. 8.10 exemplifies a recent interference issue experienced in our lab, which was identified by an atypical number of quantifier/qualifier ion ratio discrepancies and degradation of chromatographic performance that was ultimately determined to be an issue with the column lot
   (c) Improperly performing LC hardware

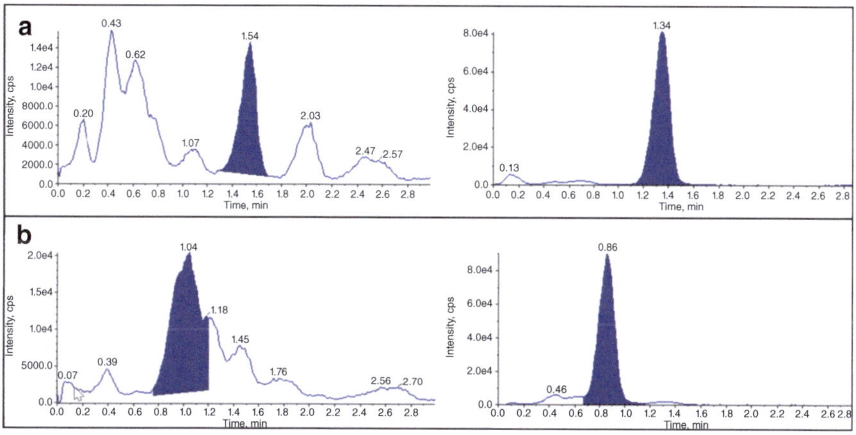

Fig. 8.10 Interference problem that was determined to be due to an issue with a column lot. In addition to the apparent chromatographic interferences, there was an atypically large discrepancy in quantifier/qualifier ion ratios as well. The analyte is shown in the left panel and the IS is shown in the right panel for each injection (**a**) Properly performing column lot (**b**) Improperly performing column lot

Steps to address such issues are:

1. System suitability testing could be helpful to assess the performance of the instrument, but often the system suitability sample does not have the matrix and interference diversity that is encountered in patient samples; therefore, injection of a previously satisfactory batch of patient matrix-based extractions is the best way to differentiate between instrument and extraction.
   (a) If system suitability test/reinjection of previous extract is acceptable and suggests extraction
      (i) Repeat to determine if an error occurred
      (ii) Replace critical reagents with new lots if possible
      (iii) There is a problem with the enrichment step, troubleshooting this would be dependent on the sample preparation methodology
   (b) If system suitability test/reinjection of previous extract is not acceptable and suggests the problem is with the LC-MS/MS measurement
      (i) Mobile phase
         1. Reprepare with same lots of reagents
         2. Reprepare with new lots of reagents, ideally that have not been used previously to rule out the possibility of contamination
      (ii) Analytical column
         1. Replace analytical column with the same lot
         2. Replace analytical column with a new lot
      (iii) Perform maintenance on the pump per the manufacturer's recommendation

Pressure Problems

Arguably the most powerful single tool when troubleshooting LC problems is the plot of back pressure vs. time of the chromatographic separation, which is commonly referred to as the pressure graph or trace. Some examples are shown in Fig. 8.11. Although the entire flow path contributes to measured back pressure, it is helpful to begin with an understanding of the variables that determine column back pressure, which can be calculated using the following equation: [6]

$$P = f\frac{u_v \eta L}{\pi r^2 d_p^2}$$

where u_v is volumetric flow rate, η is the viscosity of the solvent, L is the length of the column, r is column radius, and d_p is the particle diameter, and f is an empirical constant based on physical characteristics of the packing material. This equation clearly demonstrates the major contributing factors to column pressure, which is typically the largest contributor to overall pressure. However, the same variables dictate pressure throughout the entire LC system, so the pressure contribution from tubing diameter and length should be considered as well when troubleshooting. It is imperative to determine an acceptable range for observed pressure for every method.

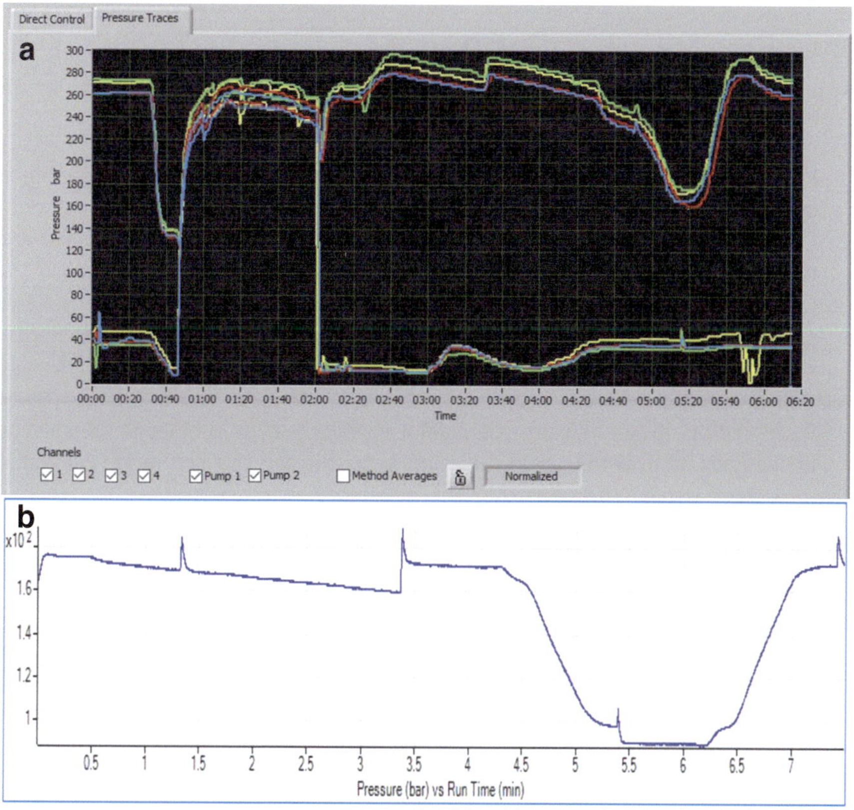

Fig. 8.11 Example pressure graphs (**a**) Example pressure graph from Aria MX. The pressure graph shows pressure from the loading and eluting pumps across all 4 channels. (**b**) Example pressure trace from Agilent MassHunter

Although the equation above can be used as a general guide, it is best to establish criteria based on monitoring of pressure traces over time, which accounts for the contributions of all the components within the LC system and allows for establishing criteria based on relating pressure to chromatographic and assay performance. The following sections will provide recommendations for troubleshooting when pressure falls outside of the normal operating conditions.

Low Pressure

There are numerous potential causes of low pressure, such as:

1. Incorrect mobile phase
2. Incorrect column
3. Leaking in the flow path

4. Air in the LC system
5. Improperly performing LC hardware

Strategies to address this include:

1. Ensure that the correct mobile phase is being used because viscosity is a major contributor to system pressure.
2. Ensure the correct column is being used because column characteristics are major contributors to system pressure.
3. Check LC system for leaks. The extent to which the pressure has dropped can guide where to look for leaks because pre-column leaks generally drop the pressure much more than post-column leaks, because the column is the single biggest source of pressure.
4. Purge the pumps and ensure you cannot visually see air bubbles in the solvent intake lines. If air is frequently an issue, degassing solvents before use can minimize these issues.
5. In some cases, purging is not sufficient and it is necessary to manually draw solvent through the system using a syringe.
6. It can be helpful to monitor pressure while setting the pump to deliver 100% mobile phase A and then 100% mobile phase B because this can allow one to isolate the problem to the A or B pump components.
7. Perform maintenance on the pump per the manufacturer's recommendation.

High Pressure

As mentioned in the previous subsection, an easy first step is ensuring that the correct mobile phase and column are being used. It is important to maintain a log of high-pressure issues to obtain a frame of reference for typical incidence rates of this issue because an increase in the frequency of high-pressure issues likely indicates an issue with the test, such as extraction issues or contaminated reagents. Generally, high-pressure issues correspond with a buildup of protein on the head of the column, so if a method is exhibiting an unacceptable frequency of pressure issues, it is best to improve the sample preparation to minimize the amount of protein and other matrix components injected onto the LC-MS/MS instrument. When troubleshooting high pressure, it is helpful to maintain solvent flow and actively monitor pressure as you remove LC connections. If the pressure is prohibitively high, it can be helpful to simply lower the flow rate so that tests can be conducted to isolate the component that is causing the high pressure.

The column is the single biggest contributor to back pressure and the most likely source of high-pressure problems, so it is logical to initially focus troubleshooting there. This troubleshooting process is outlined in Fig. 8.12. First, disconnect the connection from the column and see if the pressure drops significantly. If yes, the problem is the column OR a component post column. If not, the problem

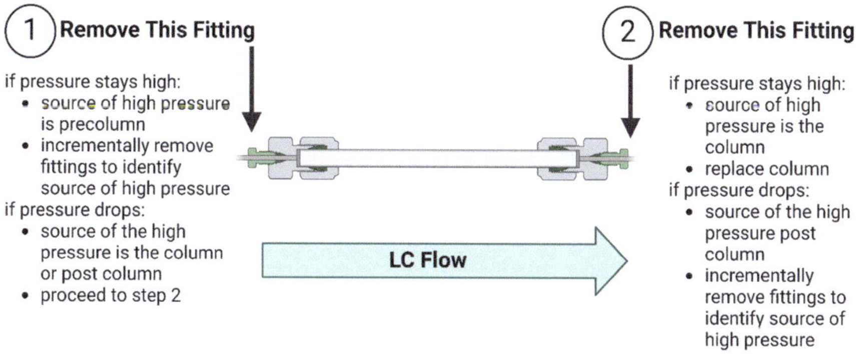

Fig. 8.12 Procedure for initial steps of troubleshooting high-pressure problems

is a component before the column. If the pressure did drop, reconnect the column and disconnect the post column connection. If the pressure is still high, you have isolated the pressure contribution to the column. If the pressure now drops, the issue is with a post-column component. If you have isolated the problem to the column, this can be easily rectified by replacing the column. If the frequency of replacement is unsustainable, introducing a precolumn guard cartridge or filter can prolong column life in some cases; however, this is not universally beneficial and if not carefully selected and utilized, there can be negative implications of guard cartridge usage, such as increased carryover or broadening of chromatographic peaks. Therefore, we recommend only using guard cartridges when necessary and when the benefits are readily apparent (i.e., the pressure drops when the cartridge is replaced, indicating that it is preventing buildup on the column head).

The testing above should have determined if the column was the problem and if not, isolated the problem to pre- or post-column. It is then necessary to incrementally remove LC connections and monitor pressure to determine which component is responsible for the increased pressure. Nearly every component in the LC system can be a source of increased pressure, but common components that cause these issues include electrodes in the mass spectrometer source, valve rotors and stators, and tubing. It is typically easy to eliminate the problem by replacing the necessary part, but finding the source can be time consuming.

Fluctuating Pressure

An example of inconsistent or fluctuating pressure compared with method averages is shown in Fig. 8.13. The most common causes of this observation are:

1. Air in the LC system
2. Faulty check valve or piston seal in the pump

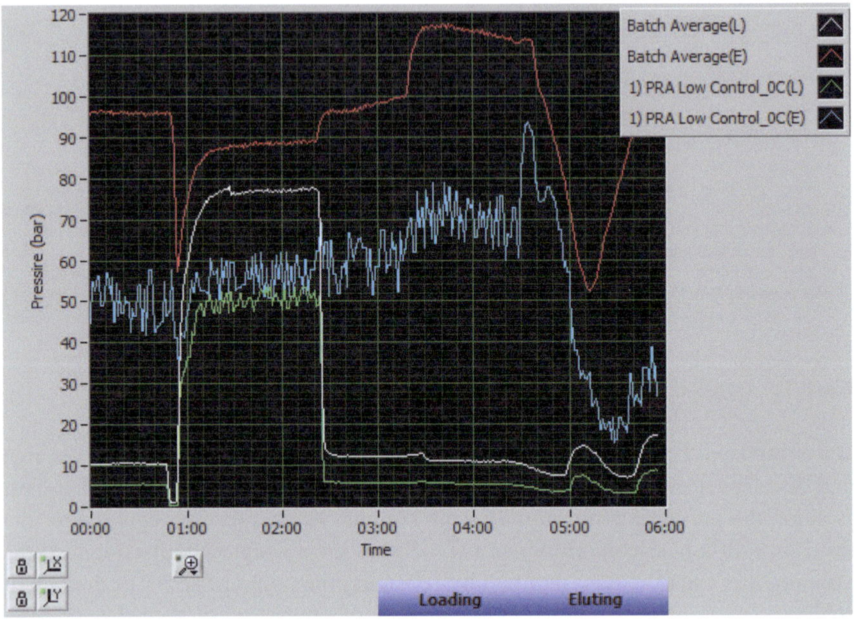

Fig. 8.13 Inconsistent pressure trace due to air in the lines (blue and green) compared to method averages (red and white). The issue was resolved by extensive purging

These situations can be rectified by:

1. Purge the pumps and ensure you cannot visually see air bubbles in the solvent intake lines. If air is frequently an issue, degassing solvents before use can minimize these issues.
2. In some cases, purging is not sufficient and it is necessary to manually draw solvent through the system using a syringe
3. Perform maintenance on the pump per the manufacturer's recommendation, which typically entails changing piston seals and check valves, but this can vary with the pump manufacturer and model

Carryover Issues

Quantitatively assessing carryover and ensuring that the carryover is appropriate for the clinical application is a critical part of validation, but validation cannot be the end of carryover evaluation. These validation studies and knowledge of the clinical implications of carryover must be used to establish acceptance criteria for the subsequent routine testing, and carryover must be constantly monitored because a plethora of variables can cause a change in carryover performance over time. [7] When carryover exceeds the established acceptance criteria, the issue must be addressed much like would be the case with a QC failure.

Sources of carryover include:

1. Autosampler
   (a) Incorrect composition of wash solvents
   (b) Wash solvent pumps are not performing properly
2. LC system
   (a) Increased retention of analytes on columns or guard cartridges due to degradation of performance with use or lot-to-lot variability in chemical properties
   (b) Analyte retention in injection port(s)
   (c) Dead volume in the LC system

Troubleshooting steps for these issues include:

1. Change columns and guard cartridges. Carryover issues can be related to the amount of packing material, so if carryover persists after initial replacement with the same lot it is ideal to use a lot that was previously proven to yield acceptable carryover. However, in some cases, a previously tested lot is not available, and it is necessary to test an alternative lot to try to determine if lot-to-lot chemical properties of the packing material are causing the carryover.
2. If the LC systems use mixing columns, consider changing those as well, as they can be harbingers of unwanted chemical interactions
3. Replace autosampler wash solvents and verify solvents are being directed to the correct pumps
4. Test autosampler wash function per the manufacturer's instructions
5. Replace injection port(s)
6. Incrementally check and reseat or replace every LC connection in the flow path to ensure minimal dead volume

Reproducibility Issues

Irreproducibility or imprecision can manifest in many ways, but most frequently it is detected by insufficient QC performance and violation of Westgard rules. Regardless of the exact issue observed, it is beneficial to think about the precision of measurements like a pyramid, as outlined in Fig. 8.14. Whenever an imprecision issue is encountered during method development or routine use, we recommend taking a step back and performing a few simple experiments to determine what step in the procedure is introducing the variability. The foundation of the pyramid and the coinciding measurements is reproducibility from the same extraction. The reason this foundation is so important is if the CV target for a clinical test is 10% and the CV from a single extraction is 7%, then it will be very difficult to achieve the ultimate goal of 10% because there is very little margin as error is propagated with the addition of inherent variables such as different laboratory technicians, mobile phase preparations, lot-to-lot variability of materials, fluctuations in mass spectrometer performance, etc. It is imperative that the foundation be solid to enable achieving long-term precision goals.

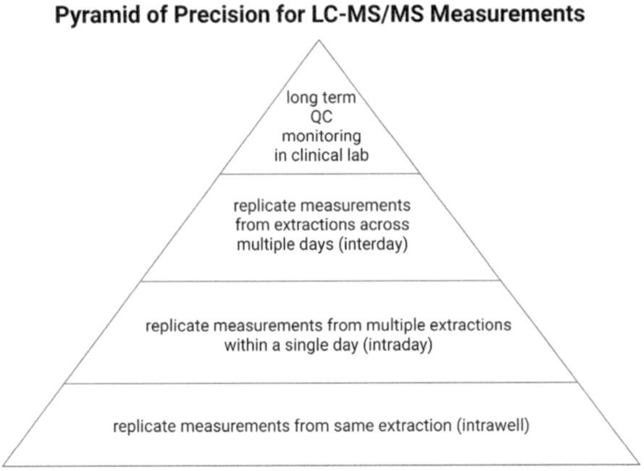

Fig. 8.14 Pyramid of precision of LC-MS/MS measurements

The performance of replicate measurements can be tested by conducting five to twenty replicate measurements of a single pool of extracted samples from the same plate well or vial. When doing this, it is best practice to use authentic patient extracts to ensure you are assessing the totality of the matrix effects and to perform testing at a minimum of two different and clinically relevant concentration levels within the analytical measuring interval to determine if there is concentration dependency to the imprecision. Although to some extent the acceptance criteria for these experiments would depend upon the clinical utility of the testing, typically a CV of less than 5% from the replicate measurements is a reasonable threshold. If the CV from the pooled samples is greater than 5%, it can be concluded that a significant portion of the imprecision is coming from LC-MS/MS separation or measurement. Thus, troubleshooting efforts should focus on reducing the variability within this process. Examples of sources of irreproducibility within the measurement include inadequate retention of the analyte(s) on the column, ion suppression/enhancement, or suboptimal source or mass spectrometer parameters. These can generally be addressed by improving chromatographic conditions or re-optimization of mass spectrometer parameters. In contrast, if the CV was less than 5%, then the conclusion is that the LC-MS/MS measurement is performing properly, and it is time to consider other sources of variability, such as the extraction.

After conducting the replicate measurement experiment and ensuring a solid foundation, one can then move incrementally up the pyramid to intraday and interday imprecision experiments. Intraday and interday imprecision experiments are a cornerstone of method validation, with each introducing a new set of variables that can be isolated if a precision problem is encountered. After meeting method validation acceptance criteria, methods will be moved to the pinnacle of the pyramid, which is routine clinical use. Over time methods will be exposed to a plethora of new variables. If imprecision increases at any point after implementation of a method and no obvious source of the variability can be identified, it can be helpful to step down the pyramid and perform the necessary experiments to determine the root cause of the issue.

Another strategy for addressing imprecision problems is analysis of the individual components that yield a calculated concentration result. Traditionally LC-MS/MS measurements rely on IS correction and determination of results based on an external calibration curve spanning the analytical measuring range. When imprecision is encountered, it can be helpful for troubleshooting to eliminate the calibration curve from the equation and recalculate the CVs over a short period of time based on IS corrected signal. This is obviously inappropriate long term, but if the IS is consistent (same preparation) within the time period studied, this can allow for isolation of the calibration curve as the source of variability. If the CVs are similar for IS corrected signal and the calculated results derived with the calibration curve, it can be concluded that the calibration curve is not the source of variability. However, if the CVs significantly improve when eliminating the calibration curve component, then the issue is likely derived from issues with calibration. There are myriad potential issues with the calibration scheme. It can be helpful to determine if the variability is coming from a subset of the calibrators or the entire curve by manipulating the data to include/exclude calibration points. If the issue is not isolated to a subset of calibration levels, then assess the calibrators holistically. Common issues with calibrators include stability issues, storage conditions, and matrix effects. Finding an appropriate matrix for calibrators can be very time consuming. Also, details like the type of vials that calibrators are stored in can have tremendous impacts on the long-term viability of calibration materials.

If the calibrators are performing properly, it can be beneficial to carefully analyze the signal from the internal standard, which is another critical component of the measurement. Analyzing trends in the internal standard within a batch or within a preparation of the internal standard can yield a great deal of useful information about test and instrument performance, which can be useful to identify sources of imprecision. [10] IS signal intensity is subject to many variables such as extraction efficiency, instrument performance, and ion suppression/enhancement. Therefore, prior to implementing a LC-MS/MS method, it is necessary to establish limits for acceptable IS intensity to ensure the quality of results. In cases where precision is inadequate, it can be helpful to calculate the CV of IS intensity within a batch, with a 20% CV across the batch being a general benchmark or a comparison with properly performing batches being helpful as well. Excessive variability of IS intensity across the batch or individual samples with large differences in IS intensity from the norm indicates suboptimal performance of the testing, as shown in Fig. 8.15. Figure 8.15a shows ideal IS performance within a batch, with very little variability of the IS through the course of analysis. Figure 8.15b also has minimal variability, except for one point that drops below the −3 SD confidence interval shown, suggesting atypical ion suppression or an extraction error. Therefore, it is best practice to repeat the sample neat and at dilution in an effort to bring the IS signal within the predetermined acceptance criteria. Figure 8.15c shows a downward trend of IS through the course of analysis of the batch; this typically means that the mass spectrometer ion optics are becoming contaminated, which is commonly referred to as "charging."

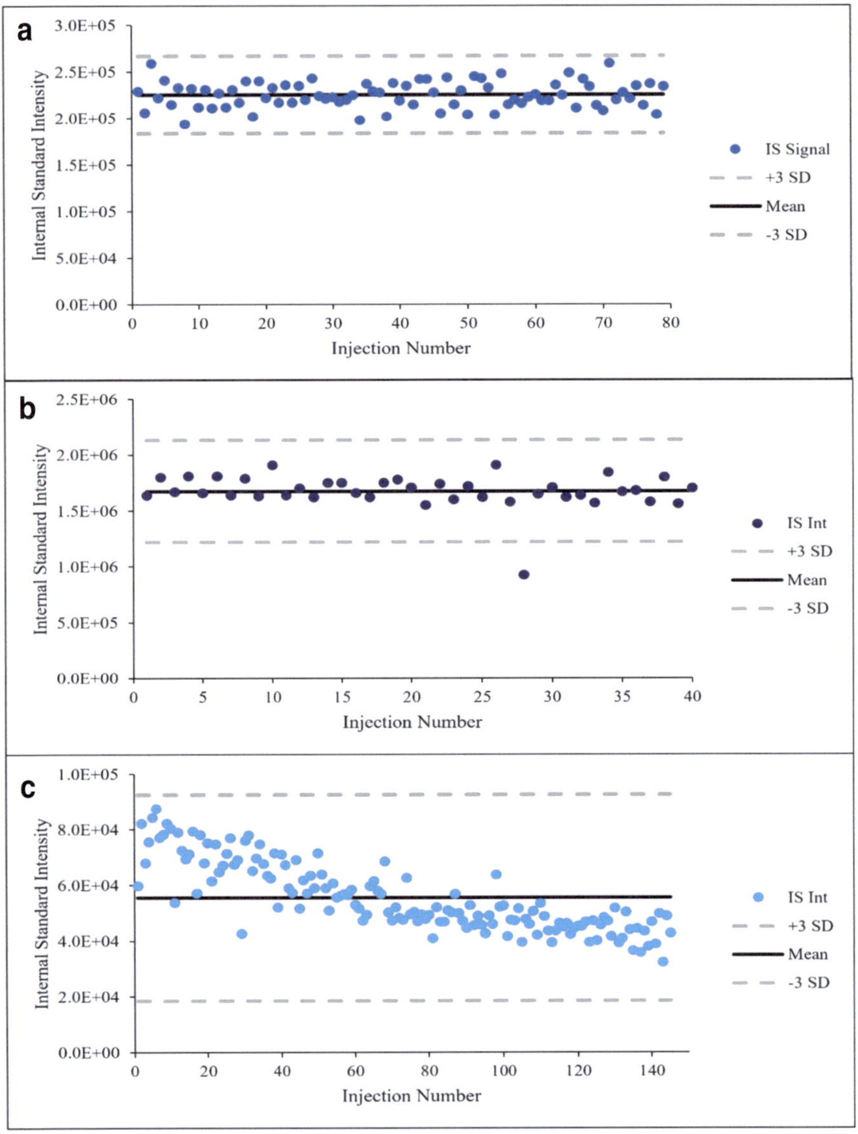

Fig. 8.15 Internal standard intensity plots within LC-MS/MS batches. (**a**) Ideal IS signal intensity with very little variability in intensity within the batch (**b**) IS intensity plot with a single sample outside the +/– 3 SD range. This sample is exhibiting insufficient IS signal and would need to be repeated. (**c**) IS intensity plot with a downward trend, likely due to contamination of the ion optics through the course of the batch

This must be addressed by cleaning the mass spectrometer. If this phenomenon is observed frequently, improving the sample purification process is likely necessary. In summary, the internal standard plots can be used to identify sources of irreproducibility, which can be leveraged to address the root cause of the issue.

Conclusions

It is impossible within the space of one chapter to thoroughly address all the possible issues that can be encountered when utilizing LC-MS/MS for clinical testing; however, the themes and practices discussed here can be applied to every problem. As alluded to in the introduction, the recurring theme throughout this chapter is performing experiments that isolate variables until the source of the problem can be identified and then addressed. This idea is not unique to LC-MS/MS, it is just an application of the scientific method. The goal of this chapter was to demonstrate how the scientific method can be applied to LC-MS/MS troubleshooting. No matter how complex the problem may seem, the best course of action is to break the system down into smaller components until the problem can be characterized and resolved. Sometimes this means you have to start at the foundation of the method and build back up to the apex of performing robust, high-quality LC-MS/MS measurements.

References

1. Boswell PG, Abate-Pella D, Hewitt JT. Calculation of retention time tolerance windows with absolute confidence from shared liquid chromatographic retention data. J Chromatogr A. 2015;1412:52–8. https://doi.org/10.1016/j.chroma.2015.07.113.
2. Briscoe CJ, Stiles MR, Hage DS. System suitability in bioanalytical LC/MS/MS. J Pharm Biomed Anal. 2007;44(2):484–91. https://doi.org/10.1016/j.jpba.2007.03.003.
3. Diagnosing Chromatography Problems & Troubleshooting. https://www.ssi.shimadzu.com/service-support/faq/liquid-chromatography/knowledge-base/diagnosing-chromatography-problems-troubleshooting/index.html. Accessed 15 May 2024.
4. Dolan J. Troubleshooting basics, part IV: peak shape problems. LCGC. 2012;30:564–9.
5. Dolan J. Peak fronting … some of the time. LCGC. 2013;31:992–7.
6. Harris DC. Quantitative chemical analysis. 9th ed. W. H. Freeman and Company; 2016.
7. Jogpethe A, Jadav T, Rajput N, Kumar Sahu A, Tekade RK, Sengupta P. Critical strategies to pinpoint carryover problems in liquid chromatography-mass spectrometry: a systematic direction for their origin identification and mitigation. Microchem J. 2022;179:107464. https://doi.org/10.1016/j.microc.2022.107464.
8. Lenk A. Solvents: an overlooked ally for liquid chromatography–mass spectrometry. The Column. 2018;14:19–21.
9. Saito Y, Kuss H-J, Kromidas S, editors. Quantification in LC and GC. A practical guide to good chromatographic data. Anal Bioanal Chem. 2010;397(2):407–8. https://doi.org/10.1007/s00216-010-3613-z.
10. Tan A, Hussain S, Musuku A, Massé R. Internal standard response variations during incurred sample analysis by LC–MS/MS: case by case trouble-shooting. J Chromatogr B Analyt Technol Biomed Life Sci. 2009;877(27):3201–9. https://doi.org/10.1016/j.jchromb.2009.08.019.

Data Analytics for LC-MS/MS Platform

9

Stephen R. Master and Randall K. Julian Jr.

Introduction

Understanding Chromatographic Peaks

Chromatographic peaks represent compounds of interest when detected above background noise. While this sounds simple, precisely defining "detection" and "noise" presents challenges. Peaks have specific characteristics determined by both the separation process and the mass spectrometer itself.

Key Peak Characteristics

The fundamental features of a chromatographic peak include:

- *Apex intensity and apex retention time*: The highest point of the peak and retention time.
- *Peak width*: Typically measured at 50% of the maximum height (FWHM—full width at half maximum).

S. R. Master
Department of Pathology and Laboratory Medicine, Children's Hospital of Philadelphia, Philadelphia, PA, USA

Perelman School of Medicine, University of Pennsylvania, Philadelphia, PA, USA

R. K. Julian Jr. (✉)
Indigo BioAutomation, Inc., Carmel, IN, USA

Purdue University, West Lafayette, IN, USA
e-mail: rkjulian@indigobio.com

Y. V. Zhang, U. Garg (eds.), *Practical Guide to Implementing Liquid Chromatography Mass Spectrometry in Clinical Laboratories*,
https://doi.org/10.1007/978-3-032-03852-4_9

- *Peak symmetry*: Measured by comparing the front and back slopes (fronting vs. tailing).
- *Peak area*: Related to the concentration of the detected compound.
- *Start and end times*: Where the signal rises significantly above baseline noise and returns to it.

Baselines

All the peak characteristics described above are in relative reference to the background signal on which the analyte signal is superimposed. This background, routinely described as the baseline, is often a complex mix of electronic and chemical noise. Detectors and separation methods can generate curved, sloping, or elevated baselines that all distort peak measurements. Several algorithms exist to estimate and correct for baseline effects, with the asymmetric least squares approach being particularly effective for LC-MS data [1, 2].

Peak Detection Methods

Detecting true analytical peaks, particularly against a noisy background, can be a challenging problem. In many routine laboratory settings, peaks are identified solely based on chromatographic retention time and/or coelution with a suitable internal standard. For low-intensity peaks, human visual assessment has sometimes been used to determine the presence of an appropriate peak for quantification. However, this may lead to subjective and inconsistent analyses. To address this issue, as well as situations where many peaks need to be quickly evaluated, a variety of mathematical techniques have been developed to detect analytical peaks within baseline noise. In the following section, we provide a brief overview of the principles of these techniques that may be useful in evaluating their results. Please note that some of the descriptions below assume a general knowledge of signal processing; for more background, please consult a general textbook such as *A digital signal processing primer* by Steiglitz [3] or *Signals, Systems, and Signal Processing* by Jankowski [4]. Although readers may skip those details if desired, it is worth noting that the details of the mathematics are often reflected in certain parameters (such as smoothing parameters) that can be adjusted within common mass spectrometry software packages.

Derivative-Based Approach: Finding Critical Points in Smoothed Data

The derivative-based approach to identifying peaks is one of the most common methods for peak detection and is used by many commercial quantification packages. It relies on basic principles from calculus, such as the derivative (slope) of the apex of a peak is zero. Rising edges have a positive slope, and falling edges have a negative slope. The second derivative (the rate of change of the slope) can also be used since the slope rate starts to slow down as a normal chromatographic peak approaches the mid-point of the amplitude. The beginning and end of a peak can be identified where both derivatives meet specific conditions [5] (Fig. 9.1).

While simple in principle, a significant challenge emerges when applying this conceptually simple approach to real data: calculating the derivative of noisy data dramatically amplifies the noise. As Carl Lanczos [6] eloquently noted, this limitation potentially renders the numerical differences useless for analysis. Smoothing is normally thought of as a way to make data "look better," but in this case, smoothing is what makes numerical difference methods usable.

Smoothing is often performed before derivative-based peak detection. By applying appropriate smoothing filters before calculating derivatives, the underlying chemical signal can be recovered from noisy data, allowing the derivatives to reveal the true peak structure rather than noise artifacts. In analytical chemistry, the most well-known solution for smoothing is to use a smoothing technique first published by Savitzky and Golay (S-G) [7]. S-G smoothing has technical advantages over

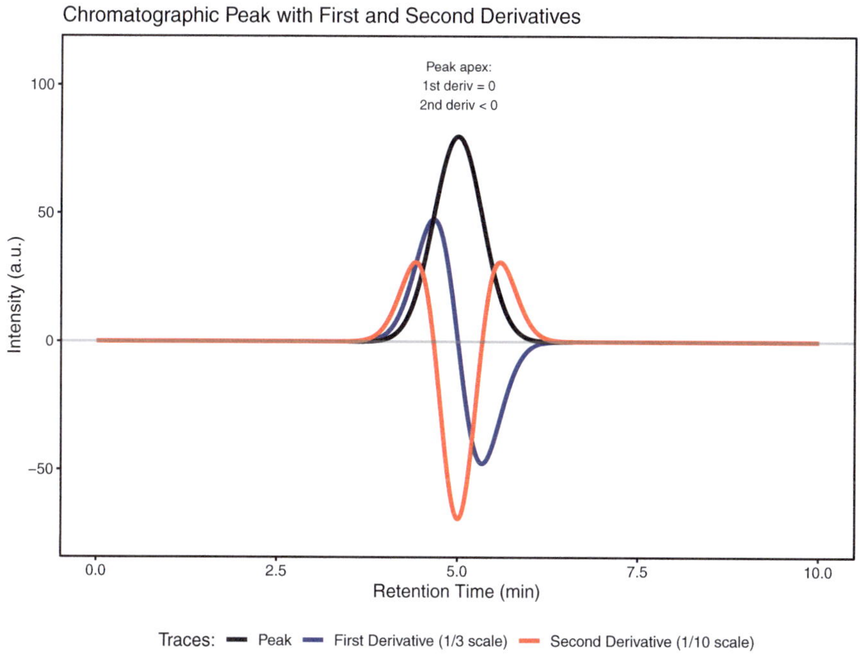

Fig. 9.1 Chromatographic peak with first and second derivatives. The plot displays a chromatographic peak intensity profile with its mathematical derivatives used for peak apex determination. The solid black line represents the chromatographic trace, with the first derivative (blue, scaled by 1/3) and second derivative (red, scaled by 1/10) overlaid. The peak apex is identified where the first derivative equals zero and the second derivative is negative, occurring at approximately 5 min retention time

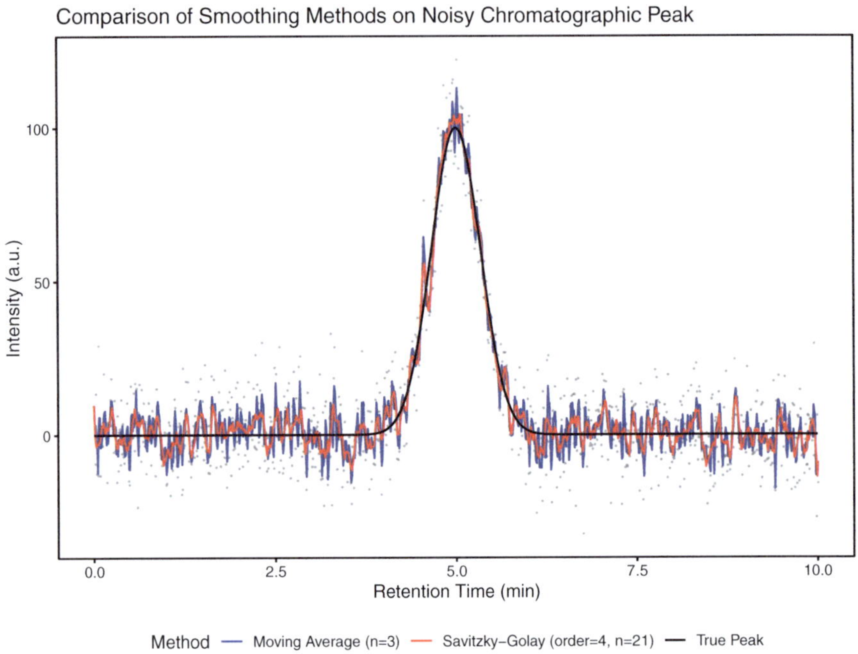

Fig. 9.2 Comparison of smoothing methods on noisy chromatographic peak. The plot demonstrates the effectiveness of two smoothing algorithms applied to chromatographic data with significant baseline noise. The gray dots represent raw noisy data, with three traces shown: (1) moving average smoothing with $n = 3$ window (blue); (2) Savitzky–Golay smoothing with fourth order polynomial and $n = 21$ window (red); (3) the true underlying peak profile (black). Both methods effectively reduce noise while preserving peak shape, with Savitzky–Golay providing slightly better peak fidelity

simple moving-average or boxcar smoothing, which are outside the scope of this chapter, but they are available in most data systems and very easy to implement (Fig. 9.2).

S-G Filters:

1. Fit a polynomial locally to a set of data points.
2. Use the polynomial's analytical derivatives rather than numerical differences.
3. Can combine smoothing and differentiation in a single operation.

The two parameters which must be selected for the S-G filter are is the polynomial degree and the length or window-width. The window is critical and should be selected based on the peak's characteristics—typically related to the peak width at half-maximum (FWHM). This approach ensures the filter preserves the peak shape while eliminating high-frequency noise.

By establishing appropriate statistical thresholds for the derivatives (considering the noise characteristics), analysts can identify where a peak begins and ends with precision.

Optimal Filtering: Beyond Savitzky-Golay

While S-G filters provide an effective practical solution, they may not solve specific noise problems. There is a more advanced method for designing smoothing filters based on Fourier analysis that can be used to deal with specific noise issues outside the ability of the moving average and S-G [8]. Optimum filters based on the Fourier Transform work by:

1. Transforming time-domain data to the frequency domain.
2. Directly observing which frequencies carry chemical information and which represent noise.
3. Designing a shape in the frequency domain that precisely separates the signal from noise based on frequency content.
4. Apply the filter shape to the raw data in either the frequency domain or convert it to the time domain and treat it in the same fashion as the S-G filters.

A key insight is that Fourier analysis does not assume that peaks are Gaussian—it only assumes that the deterministic chemical signal (i.e., the signal derived from an analyte of interest) is composed of predominantly low-frequency components, while noise dominates at higher frequencies. This is true regardless of the specific peak shape, making the approach more universal.

Using Fourier analysis allows the design of optimal filters like the Kaiser filter, which:

1. Precisely targets the frequency boundary between signal and noise.
2. Minimizes artifacts (specifically "ringing") common in simpler filters.
3. Preserves peak shape integrity while maximizing noise reduction.

The result is smoother data that more accurately represents the underlying chemical process, enabling more precise differentiation and peak boundary determination. With these optimally smoothed derivatives, the beginning and end of chromatographic peaks can be identified with statistical rigor, rather than arbitrary thresholds.

Practical Implications

The choice between peak picking approaches often depends on the specific analytical goals:

- If the primary objective is rapid peak detection of a peak apex, the wavelet approach offers computational efficiency and excellent detection sensitivity.
- If precise boundary determination is critical (as in quantitative analysis), the derivative approach with optimal filtering provides superior results.

Understanding the mathematical principles behind these techniques empowers analysts to make informed choices about processing parameters and to interpret results with appropriate confidence, ultimately leading to more accurate quantification in chromatographic analysis.

Continuous Wavelet Transform: A Shape-Matching Strategy

Wavelet transformations via the continuous wavelet transform (CWT) [9] have been used for years in packages like xcms [10] and other mass spectrometry-specific applications. The wavelet approach to peak detection leverages the observation that chromatographic peaks inherently resemble bell-shaped Gaussian curves due to the physical and chemical processes that generate them. Rather than using general mathematical operations to find peaks, CWT employs a shape-matching strategy using a specially designed wavelet, which is a small and localized curve designed (in this case) to correspond to the general form of the data that we expect.

One such curve, the "Mexican hat" wavelet (also called the Ricker, or Marr wavelet) is the negative of the second derivative of a Gaussian function. This specific mathematical form creates a shape resembling a cross-section of a sombrero—a central positive peak flanked by smaller negative valleys. This shape is particularly significant because:

1. It acts as a matched filter for chromatographic peaks, producing maximum response when encountering shapes that match its profile. The profiles of commonly used wavelets have characteristics of the underlying signal. In the case of LC-MS, chromatographic peaks have a Gaussian component. Other mass spectrometry data, like FTMS or TOF data, will have a different underlying signal, and are better represented by other wavelet families, including complex wavelets that generate coefficients which are complex numbers.
2. The wavelet can be scaled to match peaks of different widths, allowing detection of both narrow and broad peaks in a single analysis. The scaling factor applied to any one wavelet before performing the transform defines the width of the wavelet and is simply called its *scale*.
3. For CWT, the convolution operation (corresponding to matching the wavelet across the range of the chromatographic trace) inherently performs smoothing as a side effect, reducing noise interference without requiring a separate smoothing step. Depending on the wavelet used, amplification or attenuation of different frequency components in the raw signal can create artifacts that should be evaluated. For example, the Mexican Hat wavelet has negative coefficients on either side of the main lobe. When the coefficients are used directly, these negative

lobes will create ripples in the transformed data. If the coefficient is converted to power (which involves squaring the magnitude), then the negative lobes will become positive, Gaussian-shaped artifacts, which can easily be confused with real peaks. Taking care in how raw data is smoothed is an essential element to analyzing LC-MS data. This will be covered in more detail below.

When applied to LC-MS data, the CWT generates a two-dimensional matrix: retention time versus scale, with each value in the matrix representing the CWT coefficient at a given time and scale. High coefficient values at specific time-scale coordinates indicate the presence of peaks with widths corresponding to those scales.

The wavelet approach works very well for locating peak maxima and approximating their widths, but it has limitations when it comes to other characteristics of a peak. While the Mexican hat wavelet effectively captures the Gaussian central portion of peaks, it performs less optimally at determining precise peak boundaries where the signal transitions into noise.

Most applications that use wavelets to detect peaks use a secondary method to determine peak start and end as well as the other essential parameters of the peak. Many applications use threshold methods, which start at identified peak maxima and set the peak start and stop at the time point where the intensity reaches some value relative to the baseline.

Quantification

Once peaks are properly detected, the next step is quantification—translating peaks into concentrations. This first requires integration to compute the peak area, followed by normalization, and then back calculation to concentration via a calibration equation.

Numeric Integration

The area under a chromatographic peak relates to concentration. Thus, one of the most important computational tasks for mass spectrometry is to accurately calculate this peak area. There are a variety of methods that have been used to perform this calculation, and they differ in their degree of complexity and in their susceptibility to noise.

The simplest, and perhaps most initially attractive, way to calculate peak area is to use the traditional trapezoidal rule, as is presented in any numerical methods textbook [11]. Briefly, this method takes the height of the curve above baseline at every time point, and it assumes that the area of the peak can be calculated by adding up the area of the trapezoid strips constructed by connecting any two adjacent points to their baseline. While the trapezoidal rule provides a basic approach, a better approximation of area is provided by the "Simpson's Rule" calculation, which better matches the curved shapes of chromatographic peaks. Most vendor software and most publications for quantification rely on numerical integration using Simpson's rule [11]. Guidance documents such as CLSI C62 [12] and others discourage the use of trapezoidal integration for applications where accuracy and precision are required (Fig. 9.3).

While trapezoidal and Simpson's Rule approaches make minimal assumptions about what a peak "should" look like, even better results can be obtained by modeling the chromatographic (or mass spectrometric) peak shape based on the underlying physical processes. Many models of chromatographic and mass spectrometric peaks have been published over the years. The two most important models in these domains are the exponentially modified Gaussian (EMG) equation for LC-MS/MS, [13] the Lorentzian equation for FTMS [14] and the Gaussian equation for time-of-flight [15]. In the case of chromatographic peaks derived from LC-MS or LC-MS/MS, the EMG provides a function that captures most of the expected Gaussian character of the peak while also robustly fitting certain common artifacts, such as chromatographic tailing. By constraining the peak to this mathematical form, it is

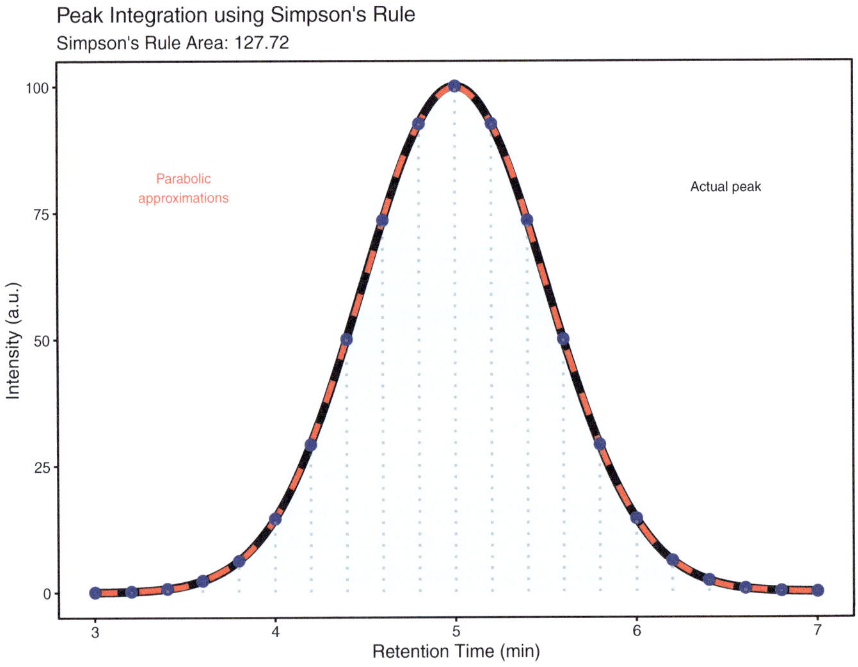

Fig. 9.3 Peak integration using Simpson's Rule. The plot illustrates the numerical integration of a chromatographic peak using Simpson's Rule approximation method. The black line represents the actual peak profile, with blue dots indicating the evenly spaced points used for integration. Red parabolic curves show the quadratic approximations between each set of three consecutive points. The shaded blue area represents the integrated region, yielding a total area of 127.72 arbitrary units

possible to derive very precise values for peak area and location that are more robust in the presence of noise.

Normalized Instrument Response

To control for run-to-run variation, internal standards (typically isotope-labeled versions of the target compound) are added. Dividing the analyte peak area by the internal standard peak area yields a normalized instrument response that reduces systematic variability. Performing calculations using these normalized responses has major advantages, since it can correct (at least partially) for many common mass spectrometry artifacts such as ion suppression and spray instability.

Calibration and Weighting Strategies

The goal of quantitative mass spectrometry is to generate an accurate value of analyte concentration. As was discussed above, the peak area (or response factor derived from dividing analyte peak area by internal standard peak area) reflects this concentration; however, translating that peak area or response factor to the concentration itself requires calibration. Calibration in chromatographic analysis bridges instrument response to analyte concentration, but the relationship between these variables requires careful modeling due to the complex nature of analytical measurements.

Broadly speaking, calibration schemes are referred to as "internal" or "external." Internal calibration denotes the use of the internal standard (IS) itself—spiked into a sample at a known concentration—to derive a concentration for the analyte of interest. In such cases, the data analysis is relatively straightforward: Analyte concentration = IS concentration * analyte peak area/IS peak area.

While this approach is used for some applications, it is generally less reliable than external calibration [16], which utilizes a separate curve derived from known concentrations of analyte. After measuring the analyte peak area (or, better, the response factor derived by dividing the analyte peak area by the IS peak area, with a constant IS spiked into each sample) at a variety of known concentrations, a low-order (typically first- or second-order linear) equation that forms a linear or quadratic curve of response factor (or peak area) vs. concentration can be fit to the data. After generating this curve, the measured values of unknown samples can be converted into concentration values. In the following sections, we discuss specific data analysis issues such as how to choose the weighting factor for the curve, the number of calibration points, and the adequacy of the curve fit to the calibrator data.

Understanding Heteroscedasticity and the Need for Weighting

Mass spectrometry data typically exhibits heteroscedastic behavior, which (in this case) means that measurement variance increases with concentration. In many cases, this means that the ratio of the standard deviation to the concentration (SD/mean, also known as "coefficient of variation" or "relative standard deviation") remains somewhat constant through much of the curve (note that—conversely—at low concentrations the standard deviation might be small in absolute terms when expressed as a percentage of the signal). Without accounting for this variance structure, ordinary least squares regression would disproportionately prioritize high-concentration data points during fitting. Because the variance is high at these high concentrations, this can significantly compromise the accuracy of the global curve fit.

Weighting schemes address this imbalance. Rather than treating all data points equally, weighted regression assigns importance inversely proportional to their expected variance. That is to say, as the variance increases (with increasing concentration), the measured point will have less of an influence on the curve fit. Common weighting functions include:

- $1/x$: Assumes standard deviation increases proportionally with concentration.
- $1/x^2$: Assumes variance increases proportionally with concentration (the most common case).
- $1/y$ *or* $1/y^2$: Similar concepts but based on response rather than concentration.

The most accurate weighting function can be determined empirically by plotting the standard deviation of replicates against concentration. LC-MS and LC-MS/MS commonly show variance (sd^2) that varies with concentration, so $1/x^2$ weighting usually provides the best results, particularly improving accuracy at the lower end of the calibration range. This effect can be seen clearly in Fig. 9.4.

Optimal Number of Calibration Points

While regulatory guidelines often specify minimum requirements, the optimal number depends on several factors:

- *Calibration range span*: Wider ranges generally require more points.
- *Expected response function*: Linear relationships can be characterized with fewer points than non-linear ones and if a calibration can drift to become non-linear, calibrators in the concentration range where non-linearity can occur can detect drift.
- *Regulatory requirements*: Bioanalytical and forensic applications often have requirements for the minimum number and placement of calibrators.

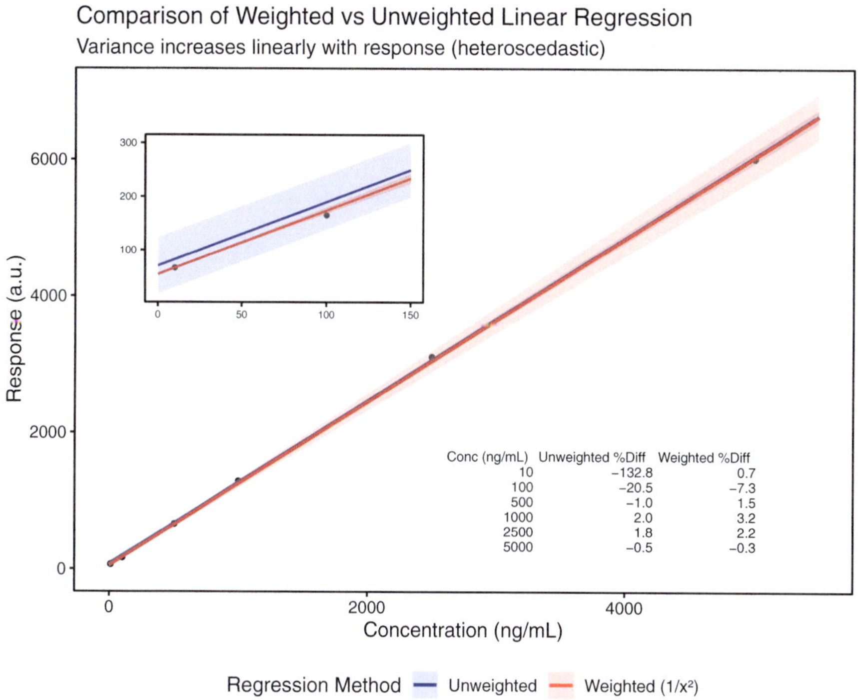

Fig. 9.4 Comparison of weighted vs unweighted linear regression. The plot demonstrates calibration curve fitting for heteroscedastic data where variance increases proportionally with response. Two regression methods are shown: unweighted least squares (blue line with confidence band) and weighted least squares using $1/x^2$ weighting (red line with confidence band). The embedded table displays percent differences between measured and predicted values at six concentration levels (10–5000 ng/mL), showing improved accuracy at low concentrations with weighted regression

The distribution of calibration points matters as much as their number. Points should be spaced to adequately characterize the response function, with particular attention to regions where the curve changes most rapidly. For quadratic calibrations, placing more points in regions of higher curvature improves model fitting.

Goodness of Fit Metrics

Traditional coefficient of determination (R^2) values [17] can be misleading in analytical calibrations, particularly with weighted regression. A high R^2 doesn't necessarily indicate an accurate calibration across the entire range [18].

More meaningful metrics include:

1. *Residual analysis* Plotting residuals (observed minus predicted values) against concentration reveals systematic deviations from the model. Random distribu-

tion of residuals around zero suggests an appropriate model, while patterns indicate model misspecification.

2. *Percent difference analysis* Computing the percent difference between known and back-calculated concentrations provides an intuitive measure of calibration performance:

$$\text{Percent difference} = \left[\left(\text{back} - \text{calculated} - \text{known}\right) / \text{known}\right] \times 100\%$$

   For reliable quantification, these differences should typically fall within ±15% (±20% at the lower limit of quantification) [12].

3. *Sum of relative errors* The sum of relative errors (SRE) or sum of squared relative errors (SSRE) focuses on relative rather than absolute deviations, making it more appropriate for heteroscedastic data:

   $SRE = \Sigma[(\text{Back-calculated} - \text{Known})/\text{Known}]$

   $SSRE = \Sigma[(\text{Back-calculated} - \text{Known})/\text{Known}]^2$

Calibration Model Selection Process

The optimal calibration approach should follow these steps:

1. Plot the calibration data to visually assess linearity
2. Fit multiple candidate models with appropriate weighting
3. Examine residual plots for systematic patterns
4. Calculate back-calculated concentrations and percent differences
5. Select the simplest model that meets accuracy requirements across the entire range

The chosen model should satisfy accuracy requirements at all concentration levels, with attention paid to the lower and upper limits of quantification. Most guidelines require that back-calculated concentrations fall within ±15% of nominal values (±20% at LLOQ).

Calibration isn't just a mathematical exercise—it directly impacts the accuracy and precision of all unknown and quality control sample measurements. A well-designed calibration strategy balances statistical robustness with practical considerations of the analytical method.

Another aspect of calibration is related to the instrument itself. Before exploring the assay calibration, we must establish an absolute foundation: every mass spectrometer must be appropriately calibrated to give correct mass-to-charge ratio (m/z) values. Mass calibration is not optional and should be checked routinely—it is the basis for all other quality considerations. For tandem mass spectrometers, each analyzer requires individual calibration since they operate independently and can drift at different rates.

Quality Control

Understanding quality control in mass spectrometry requires recognizing a fundamental principle: your measurement results exist to support statistical analysis, whether hypothesis testing, regression modeling, or clinical decision-making. The specific statistical application determines not just what level of analytical performance you need but exactly which quality control measures will give you confidence that your conclusions are valid.

We will examine how quality control design evolves across three distinct contexts: research applications focused on hypothesis testing, quantitative studies requiring regression and prediction capabilities, and clinical practice where classification decisions directly impact patient care. Understanding this progression will help you see why clinical laboratories implement such extensive quality control systems and how to design appropriate controls for your specific analytical goals.

Research Applications

- *Hypothesis testing statistical goal*: Determine whether experimental treatments produce statistically significant changes in analyte levels compared to controls.
- *Primary risk*: Misidentification of compounds due to mass accuracy drift or false statistical conclusions arising from poor measurement precision and chromatographic instability.
- *Quality control focus*: Monitoring mass accuracy, retention time stability, and signal intensity reproducibility through replicate quality control injections.

In most hypothesis testing applications, an experiment compares analyte concentrations between classes of samples (disease-positive or disease-negative, for example) primarily through MS-based techniques such as proteomics and metabolomics. The statistical analysis centers on hypothesis testing—specifically, determining whether observed differences in analyte intensities represent genuine biological effects rather than random analytical variation.

A primary concern in hypothesis testing is accurate analyte identification, which fundamentally depends on matching observed m/z to known or theoretical m/z values within acceptable tolerances. However, consistent chromatographic separation and stable ionization efficiency are also needed in addition to mass accuracy. Poor precision in these areas introduces noise that can obscure meaningful biological differences or create false positives.

Unlike quantitative studies, hypothesis tests compare relative analyte levels between conditions rather than measuring exact concentrations. This fundamental difference allows you to use simpler quality control approaches than what absolute quantification applications demand, but precision and reproducibility remain critical for valid statistical inference.

Quantitative Studies

- *Statistical goal*: Build predictive models or establish dose–response relationships where analyte measurements are either predictor variables or quantitative endpoints.
- *Primary risk*: Measurement error introduces bias in regression coefficients (attenuation bias) and reduces predictive power; systematic errors compromise model validity across different analytical batches.
- *Quality control focus*: Stable isotope-labeled internal standards for normalization, external calibration curves using weighted regression, and multi-level quality control pools to monitor precision and accuracy over the analytical range.

When your research questions evolve toward quantitative modeling—investigating dose–response relationships or building predictive algorithms based on analyte concentration patterns—your quality control requirements become substantially more sophisticated. The relationship between measured intensities and actual biological concentrations now directly influences your statistical conclusions.

The crucial statistical insight is that measurement error in your independent variables (the analyte concentrations) leads to attenuation bias in regression analysis. Your estimated relationships become systematically weaker than genuine biological relationships, and your predictive models perform poorly on new data. Internal standards provide the most powerful tool for controlling this problem.

Stable isotope-labeled internal standards represent your analytical insurance policy. These compounds differ from your target analytes only in mass due to incorporated heavy isotopes, so they behave nearly identically during sample preparation, chromatographic separation, and ionization. By monitoring the ratio between your analyte signal and its internal standard, you effectively normalize for extraction efficiency variations, matrix effects, and instrument drift that would otherwise compromise your regression models.

You should also implement external calibration curves that plot the response ratio (analyte signal divided by internal standard signal) against known concentration ratios. Using weighted regression for these calibration curves accounts for the fact that measurement precision typically varies across the concentration range, ensuring that your quantitative results meet the assumptions of your downstream statistical analyses.

Multi-level quality control samples are essential in quantification studies. Unlike single-level controls, which primarily monitor precision, multi-level controls spanning your analytical range help detect systematic bias and verify linearity—both critical for maintaining regression model validity across different analytical sessions.

Clinical and Bioanalytical Practice

- *Statistical goal*: Support decisions by measuring analyte concentrations for populations as a routine operation.
- *Primary risk*: Measurement bias near decision thresholds leads to misclassification; imprecision creates uncertainty zones around critical cutoff values.
- *Quality control focus*: Levy-Jennings plots for trend detection, Westgard rules for systematic error detection and total allowable error specifications that link analytical performance to clinical risk.

Clinical and bioanalytical mass spectrometry represents the most demanding application because your measurements can directly influence patient care or drug efficacy and safety decisions. An analyte measurement that places a sample just above or below a decision threshold might change the determination of potency, toxicity, or drive a therapeutic change. This decision-making process makes measurement uncertainty near decision thresholds critically important.

One of the main tools for monitoring analytical systems in clinical and bioanalytical applications is the Levey-Jennings plot. These plots track quality control sample results, detecting gradual trends or sudden shifts that could systematically bias results toward or away from decision points.

In practice, when an analytical system is running under control, Levey-Jennings plots will show QC results clustering around the target value in a way that follows basic statistical patterns—most results fall close to the center, fewer fall further out, and very few are in the extreme ranges. You can predict this behavior mathematically and use it to your advantage. Once you establish where your control limits should be based on historical data, any unusual patterns tell you something's going wrong before it affects patient samples.

Westgard rules provide a systematic way to interpret what you're seeing on those plots and decide whether to keep running or stop and investigate. For an introduction to Westgard rules, see the work of James Westgard [19–21].

The Westgard 1–3s rule states that if any QC value is greater than 3 SD from its pre-determined mean value over time, the batch should be rejected, and troubleshooting should be initiated. Different problems create different patterns, and the Westgard approach utilizes a variety of rules to catch these problems. For convenience, control values are typically plotted over time in a form (the Levey-Jennings plot; see Fig. 9.5) that allows easy application of Westgard rules. Some errors are sudden and dramatic, and these are readily identified. Others, such as slow drifts in bias over time or changes in precision that do not shift the mean, require different detection strategies. The 1–3s rule (reject when one quality control result exceeds three standard deviations) catches large random errors with high specificity; the probability of exceeding three standard deviations by chance alone is less than 0.3%.

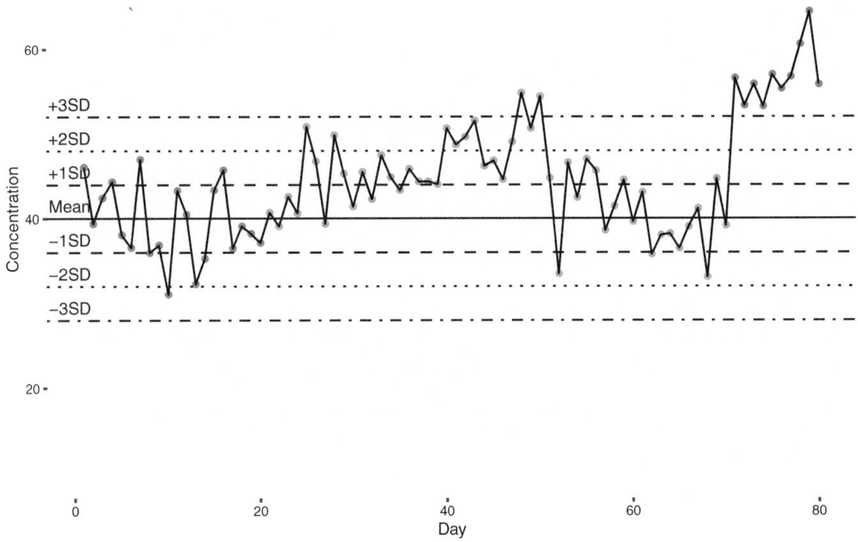

Fig. 9.5 Levey-Jennings plot. The Levey-Jennings plot represents measured values for control materials measured for each batch or each day. The solid line represents the expected mean, with 1SD (dash), 2SD (dot), and 3SD (dot-dash) lines indicated. Three conditions are shown: (1) normally distributed control data with the assay performing as expected (red, blue); (2) assay drift over time (green); (3) assay shift of 4SD (purple)

The 2–2s rule (reject when two consecutive control results exceed the same two-standard-deviation limit on the same mean) targets systematic accuracy shifts that gradually bias measurements in one direction. This error can be hazardous because it systematically misclassifies patients near decision thresholds. The R-4s rule (reject when one control is > +2s and the other is < -2s within the same runt, making the range between quality control levels exceed four-standard-deviations) detects an increased random error that widens uncertainty around clinical decision points.

The concept of total allowable error (TEa) [22] links analytical performance specifications directly to clinical requirements: TEa is the maximum combined error from bias (b) and imprecision (σ) that can be tolerated without compromising clinical decision. A quality control system design should ensure the probability of exceeding TEa remains acceptably low.

Because mass spectrometry is ideally suited to measuring a large number of analytes simultaneously (multiplexed assays), it is important to note some caveats related to the use of traditional statistical quality control. For normally distributed errors, we would expect to see a value that is 3SD from the mean by chance 0.3% of the time (that is, if there is no true change in the underlying performance of the assay). This means that 0.3% of the time we would *falsely* reject a batch when using a 1–3s rule; however, this is rare enough that it is acceptable in practice. However, if we are testing 10 analytes, the probability that one of them fails the rule by chance alone rises to ~3%. If we create a multiplex assay of 50 analytes, at least one will fail the 1–3s rule ~14% of the time. Thus, the multiple testing problem creates some fundamental limitations on the use of traditional Westgard approaches for highly multiplex assays. There are potential solutions to this problem, including determining the absolute amount of change that would be clinically significant; if a 4SD rule ("1–4s") provides sufficient assurance of assay performance, a 50-analyte assay would only fail QC ~0.5% of the time, thus restoring a practical level of performance.

Connecting Quality Control Design to Statistical Purpose

This progression from research to clinical applications illustrates how statistical requirements drive analytical requirements. Research applications focused on hypothesis testing can often tolerate higher measurement uncertainty because they typically examine large effect sizes and make relative comparisons. Quantitative modeling applications demand sophisticated normalization approaches because measurement error directly degrades predictive performance.

Clinical decision-making requires the most rigorous quality control because measurement errors immediately affect patient care. Understanding this connection helps you design efficient and fit-for-purpose quality control systems. Rather than implementing generic quality control procedures, you can select specific measures that address the statistical risks most relevant to your application. This approach avoids under-control (compromising statistical validity) and over-control (wasting resources without improving decision-making).

Accessing Mass Spectrometry Data

While most of the data analytics discussed in this chapter are performed on the output from mass spectrometer data systems, there are situations where an analyst may be required to use the raw data produced by an instrument. For those situations, it is helpful to know more about how mass spectrometry data is stored and can be accessed.

As a rule, the raw binary files created by instrument acquisition software systems cannot be read directly without the use of a vendor-supplied library used from within a programming language. Instrument vendors have many reasons for using a binary format, which is sometimes even encrypted, as the native format for a mass spectrometer. Besides using a software library to extract data directly from the native binary format, several file formats have been created as either formal or de facto open file formats. Some instrument vendors also provide a feature in the acquisition software to generate an export file. In this section, the most common export file formats will be discussed. Direct access to the vendor binary files will not be covered. For information on using instrument vendor software libraries, refer to the instrument vendor documentation.

Mass spectrometry data can take a 1-D (intensity of a single ion) or 2-D (intensity of multiple ions forming a spectrum) form. Instruments often report data using flat files; this is especially true for 1-D data, but flat files can be used for 2-D data as well. The oldest flat file for spectra is the format called JCAMP-DX [23–25] used by groups like the National Institute of Standards and Technology (NIST) and the US Environmental Protection Agency (EPA). It is relatively straightforward to read flat text files containing either 1-D or 2-D data from the types of instruments mentioned for purposes of machine learning. One common application for 2-D spectra is the look-up of an unknown spectrum from a spectral library.

When some form of chromatographic separation is introduced into a mass spectrometry system, 3-D data (spectra over time) are available. The mass spectrometer is sometimes configured to repeat an acquisition for a period of time. As described earlier, the intensity of a single m/z value could be monitored over time as in Single Reaction Monitoring (SRM), which produces 2-D data (intensity vs. time for a specific m/z or precursor-product m/z pair) to form a chromatogram or when there is no chromatographic separation, a *chronogram*. It is also typical to monitor several m/z values during the sample introduction period, which produces a three-dimensional data set representing a collection of 2-D data sets. In this 3-D data, the x-axis is usually time, and the y-axis is used to represent the individual m/z values monitored, and the z-axis represents the intensity observed. Common applications of chronograms include inductively coupled plasma mass spectrometry (ICP-MS) analysis of metals, flow injection, more recently, ambient ionization systems such as desorption electrospray ionization (DESI), and the various derivatives of paper-spray. Chromatograms are routinely used in clinical applications for a variety of analytes.

Some instrument software can export 3-D data in a flat-file format, which, as mentioned, is easy to read. While JCAMP-DX does not formally support the extra time dimension, there have been extensions proposed to allow the standard to be used for chromatography data. To represent the time dimension, a format called "analytical data interchange format for mass spectrometry" (ANDI-MS) was created by the Analytical Instruments Association (AIA) based on the Network Common Data Format (netCDF) developed and maintained by the Unidata program at the University Corporation for Atmospheric Research (UCAR). AIA/ANDI-MS was adopted as a standard by the ASTM International organization [26]. The format has been known variously as ANDI-MS, AIA, or netCDF. The ASTM standard uses netCDF [27] which is a machine-independent binary file format that can hold almost any array-like data. The format can be used to hold single spectra, chronograms, and full chromatographic data. Programming libraries are needed to access netCDF, but they are not dependent on an instrument vendor or specific computer operating system. There are many language libraries for netCDF data, and the format is extremely well documented. The specific variables stored in the netCDF file, according to the ASTM specification, however, are limited. The most significant limitation is the lack of a way to store higher dimensions of mass spectrometry. This is not an actual limitation of the UCAR netCDF format, but rather the way the format was used by AIA to store mass spectrometry data.

It is now common to collect mass spectrometry data using one or more liquid chromatographic stages combined with two stages of mass spectrometry. This has typically been called LC-MS/MS. Since the ASTM netCDF format makes no provision for tracking the extra information of the product/precursor pair, it cannot be used to store data for SRM measurements. New formats have been created, primarily based on the eXtensible Markup Language (XML) [28] standard, to represent tandem mass spectrometry data. XML is essentially a well-defined specification for a flat text file, which improves machine readability.

The first XML format to be developed for mass spectrometry data was mzXML, [29] which is well supported and is an extremely practical format for all types of mass spectrometry data analysis. The mzXML format was developed at the Institute for Systems Biology (ISB) to support the first proteomics applications. As such, it is under the control of the ISB, which has the benefit of a very long-running support team and widespread use through the distribution of ISB open-source tools. It does, however, change as needed to support the ISB tools. It also uses some non-XML features to improve performance. To establish a more robust exchange data format, the Human Proteome Organization (HUPO) created an open, multi-vendor standards body along with processes to approve changes to the format. The standard produced is now called mzML [30] and has the support of vendors, developers (including the ISB), and journal editors. The mzML format deliberately trades performance for completeness. Unlike mzXML, which uses a fixed collection of elements and attributes to describe complex mass spectrometry measurements, mzML uses a small set that must be combined with a controlled vocabulary [31, 32]. The schema for mzML has not changed in many years, ensuring that software designed to read the data will not be broken by changes. The controlled vocabulary, called psi-ms, however, is being constantly updated as new instruments and new experiments are invented. Both the format and the controlled vocabulary are under the control of an editorial board, and both are supported by a very active community.

The XML formats described above can be used for almost any mass spectrometry experiment. They are designed to handle very high-dimensional data, such as the type collected for data-dependent and independent acquisition, as well as multiple stages of mass spectrometry (sometimes referred to as MS^n) and spectra collected with a variety of system settings, such as multiple collision energies and other parameters.

The data produced by mass spectrometers can range from single numbers to very high-dimensional data. Through the work of many groups and with the collaboration from instrument vendors, there are now several ways to access everything from raw spectral data to computed results.

References

1. Eilers PHC. A perfect smoother. Anal Chem. 2003;75(14):3631–6. https://doi.org/10.1021/ac034173t.
2. Julian RK. R programming for mass spectrometry: effective and reproducible data analysis. 1st ed. Newark: Wiley; 2025.
3. Steiglitz K. A digital signal processing primer: with applications to digital audio and computer music. Mineola: Dover Publications, Inc; 2020.
4. Jankowski M. Signals, systems, and signal processing: a computational approach, First in Wolfram etextbook series. Champaign: Wolfram Media, INC; 2024.
5. Felinger A. Peak detection by derivatives. In: Data analysis and signal processing in chromatography, Data handling in science and technology, no. v. 21. Amsterdam/New York: Elsevier; 1998. p. 185–9.
6. Lanczos C. Chapter 5: Data analysis. Section 5: the difficulties of a difference table. In: Applied analysis. New York: Dover Publications; 1988. p. 313–5.
7. Savitzky A, Golay MJE. Smoothing and differentiation of data by simplified least squares procedures. Anal Chem. 1964;36(8):1627–39. https://doi.org/10.1021/ac60214a047.
8. Felinger A. Fourier-domain filtering. In: Data analysis and signal processing in chromatography, Data handling in science and technology, no. v. 21. Amsterdam/New York: Elsevier; 1998. p. 167–76.
9. Addison PS. The illustrated wavelet transform handbook: introductory theory and applications in science, engineering, medicine and finance. 2nd ed. Boca Raton: CRC Press; 2020.
10. Smith CA, Want EJ, O'Maille G, Abagyan R, Siuzdak G. XCMS: processing mass spectrometry data for metabolite profiling using nonlinear peak alignment, matching, and identification. Anal Chem. 2006;78(3):779–87. https://doi.org/10.1021/ac051437y.
11. Press WH, editor. Numerical recipes: the art of scientific computing. 3rd ed. Cambridge/New York: Cambridge University Press; 2007.
12. C62, Liquid chromatography-mass spectrometry methods, 2nd edn. CLSI, June 21, 2022.
13. Grushka E. Characterization of exponentially modified Gaussian peaks in chromatography. Anal Chem. 1972;44(11):1733–8. https://doi.org/10.1021/ac60319a011.
14. Scigelova M, Hornshaw M, Giannakopulos A, Makarov A. Fourier transform mass spectrometry. Mol Cell Proteomics. 2011;10(7):M111.009431. https://doi.org/10.1074/mcp.M111.009431.
15. Schmid RP, Weickhardt C. Designing reflectron time-of-flight mass spectrometers with and without grids: a direct comparison. Int J Mass Spectrom. 2001;206(3):181–90. https://doi.org/10.1016/S1387-3806(00)00311-0.
16. Grant R. Everything you wanted to know about internal standards, but were too afraid to ask [Online]. Available: https://www.labcorp.com/providers/resources/publications/everything-you-wanted-know-about-internal-standards-were-too. Accessed 15 Nov 2023.
17. D'Agostino RB, Stephens MA, editors. Goodness-of-fit techniques, Statistics, textbooks and monographs, no. vol. 68. New York: M. Dekker; 1986.
18. Tellinghuisen J. Goodness-of-fit tests in calibration: are they any good for selecting least-squares weighting formulas? Anal Chem. 2022;94(46):15997–6005. https://doi.org/10.1021/acs.analchem.2c02904.
19. Westgard JO, Carey RN, Wold S. Criteria for judging precision and accuracy in method development and evaluation. Clin Chem. 1974;20(7):825–33.
20. Westgard JO, Barry PL, Hunt MR, Groth T. A multi-rule Shewhart chart for quality control in clinical chemistry. Clin Chem. 1981;27(3):493–501. https://doi.org/10.1093/clinchem/27.3.493.
21. Westgard Rules | Multirules by James Westgard – Westgard QC. [Online]. Available: https://westgard.com/westgard-rules.html. Accessed 28 May 2025.

22. Sharma LK, Datta RR, Sharma N. Sigma metric evaluation of drugs in a clinical laboratory: importance of choosing appropriate Total allowable error and a troubleshooting roadmap. J Lab Phys. 2021;13(1):44–9. https://doi.org/10.1055/s-0041-1726572.
23. Lampen P, Hillig H, Davies AN, Linscheid M. JCAMP-DX for mass spectrometry. Appl Spectrosc. 1994;48(12):1545–52. https://doi.org/10.1366/0003702944027840.
24. McDonald RS, Wilks PA. JCAMP-DX: a standard form for exchange of infrared spectra in computer readable form. Appl Spectrosc. 1988;42(1):151–62. https://doi.org/10.1366/0003702884428734.
25. Hau J, Lampen P, Lancashire RJ, et al. JCAMP-DX v.6.00 for chromatography and mass spectrometry hyphenated methods. Pure Appl Chem. 2005:77.
26. ASTM E2078-00(2016). Standard guide for analytical data interchange protocol for mass spectrometric data, ASTM International, West Conshohocken.
27. Unidata | NetCDF. [Online]. Available: https://www.unidata.ucar.edu/software/netcdf/. Accessed 30 Aug 2022.
28. Extensible Markup Language (XML) 1.0 (Fifth Edition). [Online]. Available: https://www.w3.org/TR/2008/REC-xml-20081126/. Accessed 12 Mar 2020
29. Keller A, Eng J, Zhang N, Li X, Aebersold R. A uniform proteomics MS/MS analysis platform utilizing open XML file formats. Mol Syst Biol. 2005;1:1–8. https://doi.org/10.1038/msb4100024.
30. Martens L, et al. mzML—a community standard for mass spectrometry data. Mol Cell Proteomics. 2011;10(1):R110.000133. https://doi.org/10.1074/mcp.R110.000133.
31. Mayer G, et al. The HUPO proteomics standards initiative- mass spectrometry controlled vocabulary. Database. 2013;2013:bat009. https://doi.org/10.1093/database/bat009.
32. Controlled Vocabularies | HUPO Proteomics Standards Initiative. [Online]. Available: http://www.psidev.info/controlled-vocabularies. Accessed 12 Mar 2020.

Quality Assurance for LC-MS/MS Measurement Systems

10

Lorin M. Bachmann, Deborah French,
J. Grace van der Gugten, and Jacqueline A. Hubbard

Introduction

Liquid chromatography-tandem mass spectrometry (LC-MS/MS) measurement procedures are considered among the most sensitive and specific assays for quantification of clinically relevant analytes [27]. However, the development and implementation of an effective quality assurance (QA) system is necessary for ensuring the accuracy of LC-MS/MS results.

There are many reasons why erroneous patient sample results may be obtained during LC-MS/MS testing. Most spectrophotometric and immunoassay-based measurement systems have sophisticated error detection mechanisms and automatic alerts that are sent to the operator in the form of warnings or flags when the reaction profile or kinetics are abnormal, or when system operational errors are present. Unfortunately, most current LC-MS/MS systems lack comparable integrated internal sensors and automated alert flags to inform the operator when there are problems with the measurement system [2]. For example, LC-MS/MS systems typically

L. M. Bachmann (✉)
Department of Pathology, Virginia Commonwealth University, Richmond, VA, USA
e-mail: lorin.bachmann@vcuhealth.org

D. French
Department of Laboratory Medicine, University of California San Francisco, San Francisco, CA, USA

J. G. van der Gugten
BC Provincial Toxicology Centre, Vancouver, BC, Canada

J. A. Hubbard
Department of Pathology, Beth Israel Deaconess Medical Center, Harvard Medical School, Boston, MA, USA

Y. V. Zhang, U. Garg (eds.), *Practical Guide to Implementing Liquid Chromatography Mass Spectrometry in Clinical Laboratories*,
https://doi.org/10.1007/978-3-032-03852-4_10

do not inform the operator when the performance of the extraction reagent, mobile phase, or column is abnormal. Most LC-MS/MS systems do not automatically provide an alert when an insufficient volume of sample extract is injected by the autosampler or the overall analyte signal is low due to column issues. Small leaks or blockages in the LC system that cause inaccurate analyte quantification may go undetected. Often, there is no alert generated when the background signal in a chromatogram is high, or the wrong peak is integrated by the analyzer software, or if ion suppression is present in an individual patient sample. These types of assays or system errors, also called "error conditions," can lead to reporting of erroneous results for patient samples. Therefore, the laboratory's LC-MS/MS QA program should be designed to identify quality issues and to provide an alert to the operator when an error condition may be present.

Quality Assurance Metrics for Evaluation of Individual Sample Results

Evaluation of the quality of each individual peak included in the analytical run is critical for reporting accurate LC-MS/MS measurements [29]. The quality of the peaks should be evaluated for every sample, including calibrator, quality control (QC), and patient samples. Careful assessment of QA metrics for each peak ensures that the measured analyte peak is fully separated from interferences, the peak area is correctly integrated by the instrument software, and the measurement system is functioning properly. Failure of a QA metric (or multiple metrics) to meet acceptability criteria indicates a need to investigate further to determine if a reagent or instrument problem, or underlying interference is present that could result in reporting of erroneous results.

Key metrics that should be included in the laboratory's QA program for evaluating individual peak quality include peak shape, peak retention time, and peak resolution from nearby peaks [6]. Assessment of the peak area ratio for a quantifier and qualifier ion (called "ion ratio"), and monitoring of the recovery of the internal standard, offers additional insights related to the measurement selectivity, the potential presence of matrix effects, and the overall functionality of the measurement system. Failure of one or more of these QA metrics may indicate the presence of an analytical error or measurement system issue. The following sections provide a discussion of each QA metric and the common causes of metric failure. Approaches for establishing acceptability criteria for QA metrics are discussed in section "Selection of QA Metrics and Establishment of Acceptability Criteria".

Peak Shape

The peak is generated from the recorded responses when the product ions of the mass transition used for analyte measurement elute from the chromatography column and reach the mass spectrometry detector [24]. The response is typically expressed in ion counts per second (cps) or percent of ion counts per second [24, 32]. The peak area represents the area under the curve (AUC) of an integrated peak and is calculated using various mathematical algorithm approaches, depending on the manufacturer. The peak height is the maximum response value for the peak, measured from the peak baseline to the apex of the peak, which usually occurs at the retention time. Measurement of the peak area is generally considered more reproducible for quantifying analyte signal for quantitative methods than peak height, especially for wide peaks or peaks that are not perfectly symmetrical. However, multiple QA metrics include peak height; therefore, both measurements should be obtained for all samples included within an analytical run.

Metrics used to assess peak shape are a critical component of the laboratory's QA program and should be evaluated for every analytical run. Recognition of poor peak shape enables identification of a broad array of analytical problems for LC-MS/MS measurement procedures. The ideal peak is narrow, symmetrical about the apex of the peak, and Gaussian in shape, resulting in a peak that can be accurately integrated and quantified by automated peak integration algorithms [30] (Fig. 10.1).

Identifying poor peak shape is critical because abnormalities can adversely impact the accuracy and precision of quantification [12]. Peak shape abnormalities decrease the ability of the instrument software models to distinguish the peak inflection points, resulting in inappropriate peak integration. Aberrations in peak shape can also indicate other problems that contribute to erroneous results such as poor chromatography system tubing connections, the use of the incorrect solvent or mobile phase compositions, or the presence of underlying interfering peaks. Peaks that are too wide, or "broad" can cause poor separation from closely eluting compounds, poor precision and accuracy, and sensitivity loss due to reduced ability to distinguish the peak from background noise.

There are three primary metrics used to evaluate the peak shape: (1) calculation of the peak area-to-height ratio, (2) calculation of the peak width at 50% of the peak height, and (3) calculation of a factor that represents peak symmetry [6]. The calculation and reporting of these metrics are often provided by the instrument system manufacturer's software. *Peak shape parameters may be calculated differently for different instrument systems, therefore, the general concepts for the calculation of each parameter are presented below.* The laboratory should review the manufacturer's software user's manual for specific details.

The peak area-to-height ratio (area/height) is calculated by dividing the peak area by the peak height. An example of the peak area/height calculation is shown in

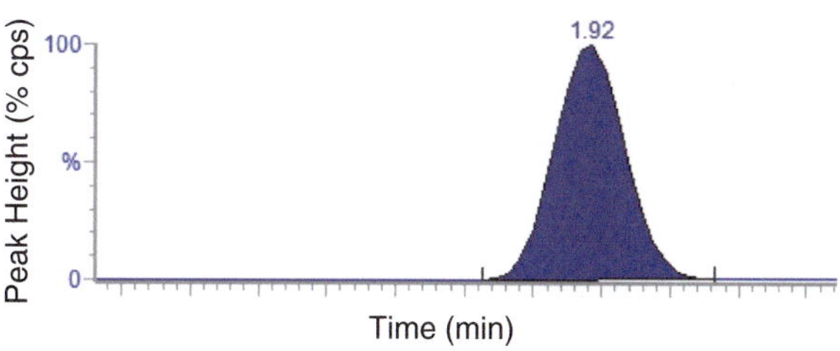

Fig. 10.1 The ideal peak shape is narrow, symmetrical and displays a Gaussian shape

a

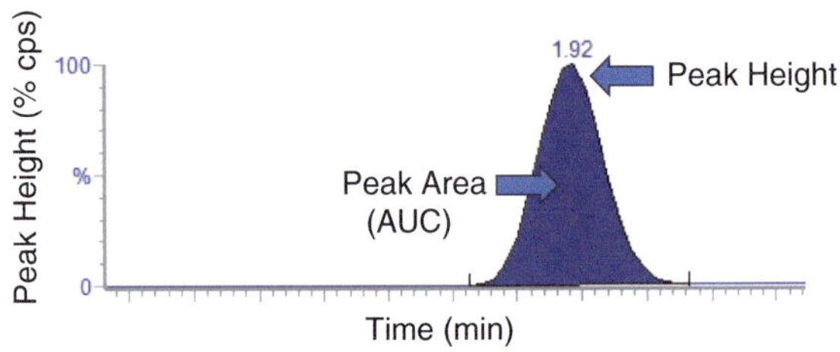

Peak Area (cps)	Peak Height (cps)	Area/Height
760	25031	**0.03**

b

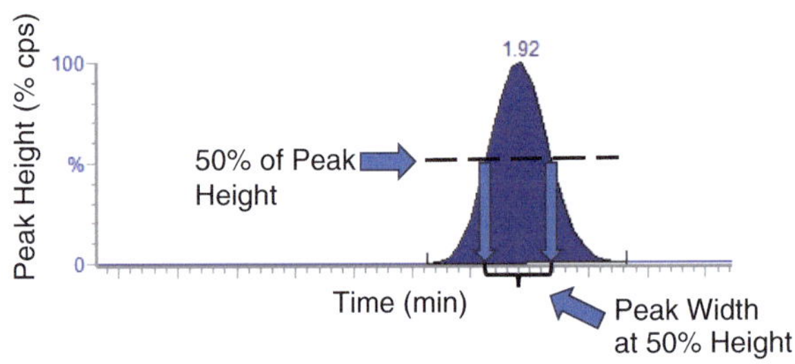

Peak Height (cps)	Width at 50% Peak Height (min)
25031	**0.373 min**

c

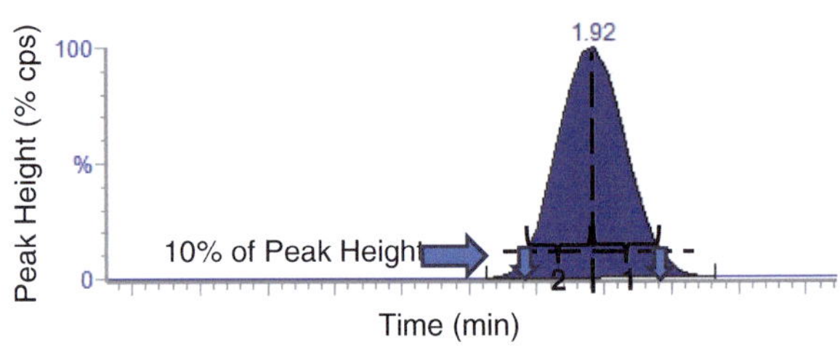

[1]Width from middle to end of peak (min)	[2]Width from middle to beginning of peak (min)	Peak Symmetry Factor
0.253	0.270	**0.937**

Fig. 10.2 (**a**) Calculating the peak area/height (*Note*: the peak area is less than the peak height in this example because the instrument software uses the average area of summed segments of the peak, rather than the total AUC of the peak). (**b**) Calculating the peak width at 50% height, (**c**) Calculating the peak symmetry factor

Fig. 10.2a. The peak width at 50% height is typically calculated by measuring the peak width in units of time at the response equivalent to 50% of the maximum response peak value, relative to the peak baseline [30] (Fig. 10.2b). The peak width is measured at 50% of peak height because the middle section of the peak is the most reproducible when measured between different samples and different analytical runs. Peak symmetry can be assessed by calculating the peak symmetry factor, also called the "peak asymmetry factor" or the "peak tailing factor." The peak symmetry factor is expressed as a ratio of two measurements of peak width in units of time at a specified height (usually 10% peak height). The ratio is obtained by measuring the width from the middle of the peak (measured at the maximum peak height) to the end of the peak, and from the middle of the peak to the beginning of the peak (Fig. 10.2c). Another common way to calculate the symmetry factor is to divide the total peak width (at a specified height) by 2 times the distance from the middle of the peak to the front of the peak [24]. Perfectly symmetrical peaks will have a symmetry factor of 1.0, while peak tailing will result in a ratio > 1.0 and peak fronting will result in a ratio < 1.0. See section "Laboratory-Specific Strategies for QA Program Design" for establishing an acceptable range for the symmetry factor.

Ideal, narrow, Gaussian-shaped peaks typically will result in smaller peak area/height, smaller peak widths at 50% height, and peak symmetry factors near 1.0. In any given assay, calculated peak shape QA metric values should remain within an acceptable range if the peak is identified correctly, if the chromatography conditions do not va,ry and if there are no underlying interfering peaks. Abnormalities in peak shape commonly reflect problems with the sample itself (e.g., presence of an interference), or problems with the processing procedures, reagents, column, or instrument system [19] (Fig. 10.3). Additional common causes of peak shape abnormalities can be found in Table 10.1. All of these common peak shape issues can adversely impact the quality of the results; therefore, the laboratory's QA metrics should sufficiently identify them.

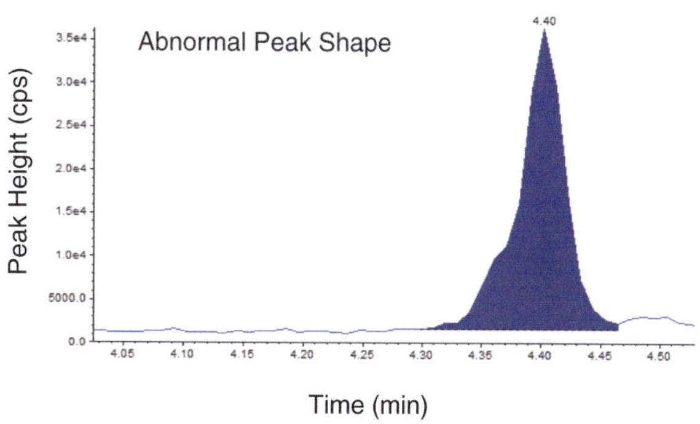

Peak Area (cps)	Peak Height (cps)	Area/Height (Normal is 2.33)	Symmetry Factor
96800	34700	**2.79**	**0.599**

Fig. 10.3 Abnormal peak shape—The peak area/height is inconsistent with normal peaks for the analyte, and the symmetry factor is significantly lower than 1.0, indicating fronting or possibly an underlying interfering peak

Table 10.1 Common causes of quality assurance metric problems related to chromatographic peaks

Type of QA metric problem	Common causes
Peak shape	
Increased peak width (also called "band-broadening")	Incorrect injection solvent composition too high (for reversed phase chromatography) The injection volume on the column too large Excess dead volume due to long tubing length Incorrect composition or pH of mobile phases
Distorted peaks	Dirty guard columns, dirty frits, dead volume caused by improper chromatography tubing connections, or worn LC fittings
Peak tailing	Unoptimized gradients or a degraded column stationary phase [11].
Peak fronting	Amount of analyte injected exceeds the capacity of the column (such as when using narrow-bore or fused-core columns)
Peak fronting or tailing, or abnormal peak spikes or shoulders	Underlying interfering peaks
Retention time	
Absolute retention time shift	Changes in mobile phase flow (such as leak, clogs, and partial blockage in columns, frits, or valves) Variation in mobile phase composition, temperature, and mixing Mobile phase delivery problems (such as improper mobile phase preparation, pump failure, and inadequate LC system maintenance) Inadequate column equilibration, column degradation, and accumulation of matrix components on the column
Relative retention time shift	Mis-integration of wrong peak Presence of an underlying interference
Peak resolution	
Resolution loss	Old or dirty column Improper injection solvent Improper mobile phase (due to LC instrument issues, loss of mobile phase pressure or flow rate due to a leak or blockage, increased dead volume due to improper LC connections)
Ion ratio	
Ion ratio failure	The presence of interfering peaks (due to prescription or over-the-counter drugs or drug metabolites, disease-related metabolites, collection tube additives, mobile phase contaminants, or impurities from plastics in tubes, plates, filters, or tips [4])

Retention Time

The absolute retention time is a useful QA metric to monitor LC system quality. The absolute retention time, reported in units of time, is the time between injection of the sample and the maximum height of the chromatographic peak [24] (Fig. 10.4). Absolute retention time acceptability should be established by the laboratory (See section "Laboratory-Specific Strategies for QA Program Design"). It is important to monitor absolute retention time because analyte peaks are identified according to a

a

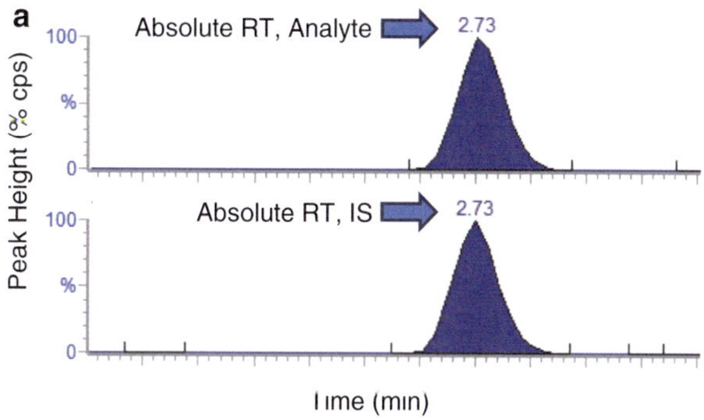

RT, Analyte Peak (min)	RT, IS Peak (min)	Relative RT
2.73	2.73	**1.000**

b

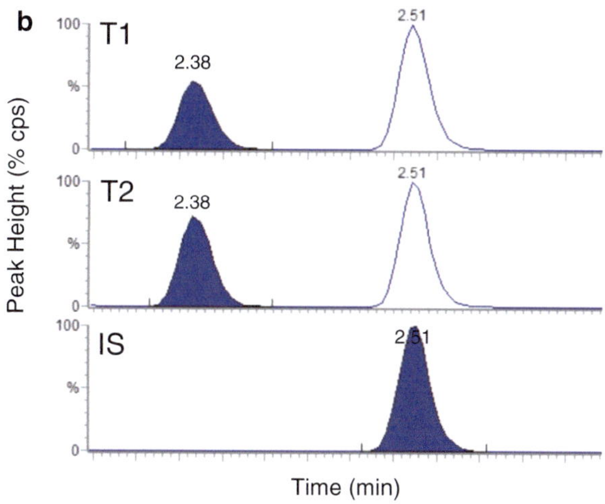

RT, Analyte Peak (min)	RT, IS Peak (min)	Relative RT
T1	2.38	**0.948**
T2	2.38	**0.948**
IS	2.51	

Fig. 10.4 (**a**) Determining absolute retention time (RT) and calculating relative RT. (**b**) Two transitions for an analyte (transition 1 (T1) and transition 2 (T2) and the internal standard (IS) are shown. The analyte peaks should co-elute with the IS in this measurement procedure, and therefore, the relative RT should be 1.000. However, the LC-MS/MS software has integrated the incorrect peaks for T1 and T2, resulting in a relative RT of 0.948

retention time window that is defined by the user within the instrument software. A shift in the retention time could result in the inability of the manufacturer's software to locate the analyte peak or could result in the integration of the incorrect peak. Conditions that adversely affect the LC system flow rate or pressure may cause changes in the absolute retention time. Common causes for absolute retention time shifts are shown in Table 10.1.

The relative retention time is defined as the ratio of the retention time of the analyte peak to that of a reference peak, which is typically an exogenously added internal standard (Fig. 10.4a). If an isotopically labeled internal standard is used as the reference peak, the relative retention time is usually not affected by minor variations in the LC system or minor matrix build-up on the column. The relative retention time is a key QA metric used to support the identification of an analyte peak. The relative retention time for the analyte should not exceed ±2.5% from the average relative retention time for the calibrators (within-run) [6]. If the integrated peak is found at the correct relative retention time, the likelihood that the peak represents the correct analyte is increased. A failure in the relative retention time frequently indicates mis-integration of the wrong peak or the presence of an underlying interference (Fig. 10.4b).

Resolution

The chromatographic resolution of two peaks describes their degree of separation on a chromatography column. Chromatographic resolution depends on analyte-specific column retention characteristics, column selectivity, and the extent of analyte dispersion within the column (also called column efficiency). The degree of resolution is affected by other chromatographic system characteristics such as column length, column particle size, mobile phase flow rate, mobile phase temperature, and amount of dead volume, or amount of extra-column mobile phase volume. Resolution can be calculated as the difference (measured in units of time) between the RTs of two peaks divided by the average width at baseline of the two peaks using the following equation [6]:

$$\text{Resolution}(\text{R}) = \frac{2\left(\text{RT}_{\text{peak } B} - \text{RT}_{\text{peak } A}\right)}{\text{Width}_{b\,\text{peak } A} + \text{Width}_{b\,\text{peak } B.}}$$

The width of the peak is typically measured as the time obtained by drawing a tangent line from the inflection point on either side of the peak to the baseline. Another equation to calculate resolution uses the peak width at 50% height (United States Pharmacopeia 2021):

$$\text{Resolution}(\text{R}) = \frac{1.18\left(\text{RT}_{\text{peak } B} - \text{RT}_{\text{peak } A}\right)}{\text{Width}_{h\,\text{peak } A} + \text{Width}_{h\,\text{peak } B}}$$

It should be noted that different manufacturers' software programs may calculate resolution using a different fixed factor, or may measure peak widths at different peak heights. Baseline resolution is generally considered accomplished when the calculated resolution is greater than or equal to 1.25 [6] or 1.5 [13]. Larger resolution factors indicate better separation between the analyte peak and a closely eluting peak. Typically, the use of the peak resolution as a QA metric requires a closely eluting peak to be identified in each test sample to enable the manufacturer's software to automatically perform the calculation. Alternatively, the laboratory may calculate resolution manually if the components used in the calculation of resolution are available from the manufacturer's software. Confirmation of baseline peak resolution by visual inspection is less preferred, however may be the only option available for the laboratory.

Baseline resolution (Fig. 10.5a) of the analyte peak from closely eluting peaks is necessary for optimum quantification accuracy. See section "Laboratory-Specific Strategies for QA Program DesignS11" for recommendations on how to establish

Fig. 10.5 (**a**) Baseline chromatographic resolution, $R > 1.25$. (**b**) Inadequate chromatographic resolution, $R \leq 1.25$

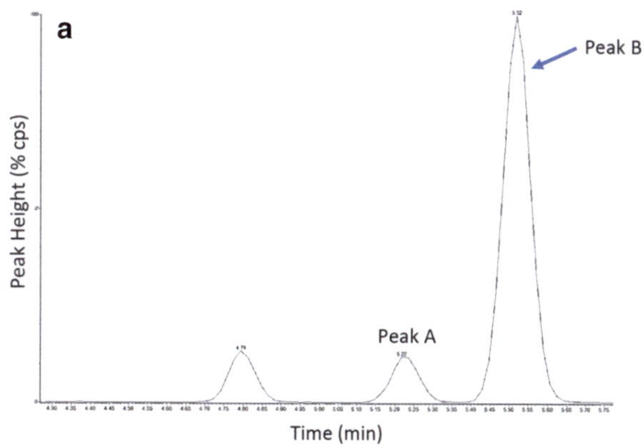

RT, Peak A (min)	RT, Peak B (min)	Width, Peak A (min)	Width, Peak B (min)
5.22	5.52	0.17	0.22
Resolution = 2* (5.52 – 5.22)/(0.17 + 0.22) = **1.54**			

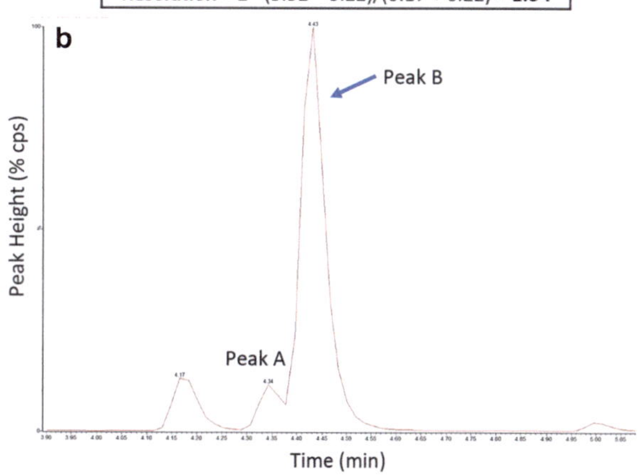

RT, Peak A (min)	PT, Peak B (min)	Width, Peak A (min)	Width, Peak B (min)
4.34	4.43	0.10	0.19
Resolution = 2* (4.43 – 4.34)/(0.10 + 0.19) = **0.62**			

acceptability criteria for the resolution factor. Inadequate resolution (Fig. 10.5b) may occur when there is a closely eluting peak resulting from an interfering substance in the sample, or when the chromatographic efficiency declines such that closely eluting peaks are no longer resolved. Common causes of resolution loss are shown in Table 10.1.

Ion Ratio

The ion ratio is utilized as a QA metric to ensure correct identification and integration of an analyte peak [6, 16]. The ion ratio is calculated by dividing the peak area of a product ion used to quantify the analyte ("quantifier ion") and the peak area of a product ion used to qualify the identification of the analyte ("qualifier ion"), or vice versa [21]. The quantifier ion is the unique product ion used to calculate the peak area ratio to determine the final analyte concentration from the calibration curve equation, while the qualifier ion is a second unique product ion used to confirm the identity of the analyte. A typical approach is to calculate either the fixed or percent difference of the ion ratio of the test sample versus a target ion ratio calculated using the average ion ratio of the calibrators (Fig. 10.6). A minimum of one ion ratio should be monitored for each analyte reported, although the laboratory may choose to monitor more than one ion ratio for each analyte. A commonly used ion ratio criterion is that the ion ratio calculated for the test sample should be within ±20% of the ion ratio calculated from the calibrators. However, the laboratory should establish its own acceptability criteria (See section "Laboratory-Specific Strategies for QA Program Design").

If no analytical performance issues or interferences are present, the ion ratio difference should fall within a pre-established acceptable range. If the ion ratio

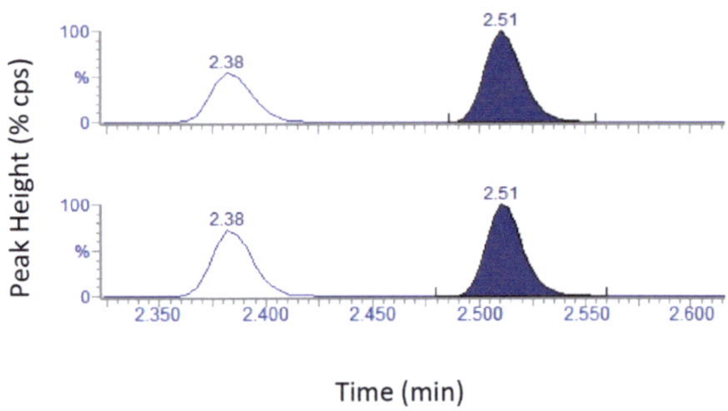

Peak Area, Quantifier (cps)	**Peak Area, Qualifier (cps)**	**Ion Ratio,** Quantifier/ Qualifier	**Target Ion Ratio,** Avg Ion Ratio of Calibrators
11594	7109	**1.631**	**0.780**
Ion Ratio (%Diff) = ((Ion Ratio-Target Ion Ratio)/Target Ion Ratio)*100; Acceptability Criteria: ±20% = **109%** (FAIL)			

Fig. 10.6 Ion ratio—The percent difference of the ion ratio, calculated as the ratio between a quantifier and qualifier analyte ion vs. a target ion ratio, is shown. The target ion ratio was calculated as the mean ion ratio for the calibrators. According to the acceptability criteria, the ion ratio for the analyte should be ±20% of the target ion ratio obtained using the mean ion ratio of the calibrators. In this case, the ion ratio failed criteria, indicating the likely presence of an underlying interfering peak

difference exceeds the acceptability criteria, the peak may be mis-integrated or an interfering substance may be present. Examples of sources of interfering peaks are shown in Table 10.1. It should be noted that isobaric and isomeric compound interference will not be detected by use of ion ratios; therefore, these interfering compounds must be chromatographically separated.

Internal Standard Recovery

A standard practice for clinical LC-MS/MS measurement procedures is the addition of a fixed amount of internal standard to each test sample prior to sample extraction. The purpose of the internal standard is to normalize for minor analyte recovery differences between individual samples related to differences in ion suppression, extraction efficiency or other matrix-related effects. Use of a stable, isotope-labeled analyte as the internal standard is recommended to ensure that the chemical behavior of the internal standard approximates that of the analyte [6]. Analogs should be used as internal standards only if stable isotope-labeled compounds are not available.

The recovery of the internal standard peak area for each sample should be monitored as part of the laboratory's QA program [20]. To quantify the internal standard peak area recovery, the percent difference of the internal standard peak area for each test sample vs. the average internal standard peak area for the calibrators should be calculated and compared to pre-established acceptability criteria. A commonly used acceptability criterion is the ion ratio for the test sample within ±20% of the mean internal standard calculated for the calibrators. However, the laboratory should establish its own acceptability criteria (see section "Laboratory-Specific Strategies for QA Program Design"). Common causes of internal standard recovery failure are shown in Table 10.2. An example of a mis-injection of a sample from the autosampler is shown in Fig. 10.7.

Table 10.2 Common causes of quality assurance metric problems related to analytical runs

Type of QA metric problem	Common causes
Internal standard	
Internal Standard Recovery Failure	Sample extraction error, such as internal standard not added, extraction reagent not added, or improperly prepared Mis-injection of the extracted sample by the autosampler Charging of the mass spectrometer quadrupoles indicates the need for maintenance Excess ion suppression for an individual sample
Signal-to-noise ratio	
Signal-to-noise ratio failure due to low signal	Leaks or clogs in the LC system Aspiration problems in the autosampler Use of the wrong column Use of the incorrect LC gradient or MS data analysis settings Lack of sufficient LC or MS system maintenance
Signal-to-noise ratio failure due to high noise	Inadequate sample preparation leading to a high background signal Interferences from disposables, collection containers, or mobile phases

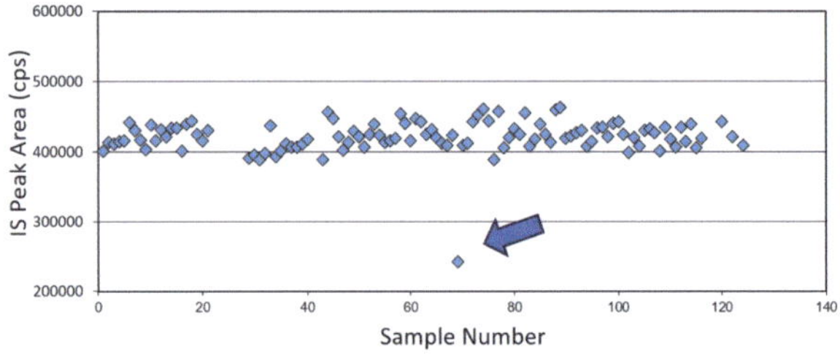

IS Peak Area (cps)	Avg Peak Area of the Calibrators (cps)	% Diff, IS Peak Area vs. Avg Calibrator Peak Area	PASS/FAIL? ± 20% Diff is Acceptable
423000	422524	1.1	PASS
242000	422524	43.0	FAIL

Fig. 10.7 Internal standard (IS) recovery—The IS peak area for each sample is shown. The arrow depicts a mis-injection from the autosampler, resulting in failed IS peak area recovery

Signal-to-Noise Ratio

The signal-to-noise ratio (S/N) is typically calculated as the ratio of the analyte peak height to an estimate of the nonspecific background signal, or noise, at the baseline of the chromatogram [6]. Noise in a chromatogram can arise from sources such as sample matrix interferences, collection tube additives, mobile phase additives or contaminants, contaminants from plastics and disposables, and electronic noise. A large S/N means that the noise does not represent a significant percentage of the analyte peak measurement, therefore, its contribution to measurement error is small. Conversely, a low S/N indicates that nonspecific interferences comprise a significant source of measurement error.

Different manufacturers' software programs calculate the S/N using different approaches, and some manufacturers may offer multiple approaches for calculation that the user may choose from. The signal for a peak is typically calculated as the maximum peak height, measured from the apex of the peak to an extrapolation of the baseline [24]. The noise may be calculated by multiplying the average standard error of residuals computed by linear regression of the baseline drift within a specified time frame. Another common approach to calculate noise is to measure the maximum difference range in noise values over a specified time period. For the calculation of the S/N, the United States Pharmacopeia recommends that the height of the peak be multiplied by two and the result be divided by the maximum difference range of the noise measured over a time span of 5–20 times the peak width at half-height. Each laboratory should investigate the calculation used to calculate the signal, the noise, and the S/N. Unfortunately, published studies investigating the impact of different approaches for S/N calculations on clinical laboratory LC-MS/MS assay performance are lacking, therefore, the laboratory may wish to directly compare each available calculation approach.

The S/N for each analyte should be optimized during method development and pre-validation and then routinely monitored during routine laboratory operation.

The CLSI C62, *Liquid Chromatography-Mass Spectrometry, 2nd edition* document recommends a S/N of at least 20:1 for a sample with a concentration at the lower limit of quantification for best practice, or minimally 10:1, to ensure good sensitivity, reproducibility, and assay robustness over time [6]. It is not uncommon for the assay S/N to decrease over time due to aging of the LC-MS/MS system components. For example, the assay S/N may start out at 20:1 when the system is new, but then decrease to a lower value after a few years of routine operation, even if the manufacturer's recommended maintenance procedures are followed. Therefore, the S/N should be as close to ideal as possible during initial method development.

The S/N can be monitored and compared to acceptability criteria for each quantifier and qualifier ion during an analytical run. A low S/N may result from an error condition that decreases the analyte signal or increases the noise. The most common analyte or matrix-related causes of a low signal for an individual sample during a run are that the concentration of the analyte is too low for quantification or ion suppression is present. Common measurement system-related reasons for low signal or increased noise are shown in Table 10.2.

Prior to each day's run during routine testing, the S/N of a reference sample, referred to as the system suitability test (SST) sample should be monitored. A more comprehensive discussion of the utility of the SST can be found in section "QA Metrics Applied to the Run (Batch)". If the S/N of the SST sample fails in a particular run, then a problem with the LC or MS system is likely, and testing should be discontinued until the issue is resolved. Frequent failure of the S/N may indicate that the assay needs to be redeveloped or reoptimized or that a more frequent maintenance schedule is needed.

Selection of QA Metrics and Establishment of Acceptability Criteria

The primary design goal for an effective and efficient LC-MS/MS QA program is not only to identify error conditions that could adversely affect patient care, but also to avoid labor time spent on unnecessary investigations and interventions. The program should employ QA metrics that identify potentially significant errors to enable the laboratory staff to investigate and implement corrective action prior to reporting patient results. However, false alerts, or alerts that do not represent error conditions, can arise from monitoring inappropriate QA metrics or implementing inappropriate acceptability criteria for the QA metric being monitored. The "false alert rate" can be calculated by dividing the number of false QA alerts by the total number of QA alerts. Studies have shown that alert fatigue in healthcare workers directly contributes to missed error conditions [1, 31], therefore efforts should be undertaken to minimize the false alert rate. The overall strategy is to develop a QA program that identifies actual measurement system failures, but that also avoids as many false alerts as possible. Therefore, false alert rate should be routinely evaluated during QA metric selection and the establishment of acceptability criteria.

The CLSI C62 document [6] provides guidelines for the implementation of QA metrics for monitoring LC-MS/MS methods implemented in the routine clinical laboratory. The document describes QA metrics applied to each individual sample, including peak shape, relative retention time, resolution, ion ratio, and internal standard recovery. Throughout the CLSI C62 document, recommendations are also provided for quality assurance activities designed to evaluate the quality of each LC-MS/MS analytical run, such as analysis of SST samples, assessment of the acceptability of calibration and quality control results, and evaluation of the response for blank samples to confirm the absence of carryover. These overall analytical run assessment QA activities will be further discussed in section "QA Metrics Applied to the Run (Batch)".

Although the CLSI C62 document provides a basic framework that defines QA metrics for monitoring and provides examples of general acceptability criteria, there is significant value in careful consideration of each QA metric in the context of the laboratory's specific measurement procedure. Generation of specific acceptability criteria for each QA metric based on the laboratory's own datasets may allow improved ability to identify real errors and, at the same time, to decrease the false alert rate. Descriptions of commonly utilized QA metrics for evaluation of individual sample results and practical approaches for selecting QA metrics and establishing acceptability criteria will be described in this section.

General Strategies for QA Program Design

QA metrics and acceptability criteria are part of the Quality Management System (QMS) for LC-MS/MS methods and should be established during the pre-validation phase of method development. Acceptability criteria should be finalized prior to the launch of routine patient testing. There are two general strategies for selecting quantitative QA metrics and establishing acceptability criteria. The first is to utilize professional practice guidelines recommendations, such as be found in CLSI C62. These recommendations serve as an excellent starting point for QA program design. However, the CLSI C62-recommended metrics and acceptability criteria may not be ideal for each specific assay. The laboratory may be able to improve the effectiveness and efficiency of the QA program by performing analysis of its own data, and then by using the findings to adjust the QA program parameters based on its assay-specific analytical performance expectations. Therefore, the second strategy for QA program design is to conduct experiments to select QA metrics and associated acceptability criteria using laboratory-generated data for each specific assay. This approach involves a laboratory "data-driven" QA design strategy [10]. Once the initial QA metrics and acceptability criteria are proposed, the laboratory can then test the effectiveness and efficiency of the program and further refine the program, if required. It should be noted that some laboratories may choose to implement a manual, *qualitative* review process for QA metrics during routine laboratory testing. For example, peak shape and resolution can be assessed using visual inspection. However, a major benefit of the use of quantitative QA metric evaluation is that the evaluation process can be automated, resulting in improved QA program accuracy and efficiency. The remainder of this Chapter will focus on the assessment of quantitative QA metrics.

The CLSI document C24, *Statistical Quality Control for Quantitative Measurement Procedures: Principles and Definitions*, details a process for establishing a statistical QC strategy for quantitative measurement procedures [5]. The same general concepts can be applied for establishing a QA program for clinical LC-MS/MS. The basic framework of a data-driven QA design program is to begin with a set of well-characterized reference samples with pre-assigned analyte concentration values. These samples can be used to test each potential QA metric to verify if the metric is useful for detection of error conditions and the results can be used to establish acceptability criteria. Both strategies (the use of professional practices guidelines and the laboratory data-driven approach) to develop the QA program are described below.

Guideline-Based Strategies for QA Program Design

The CLSI C62 document provides recommendations for monitoring of various LC-MS/MS QA metrics and provides general acceptability criteria. The basic document recommendations are summarized in the list below:

- Peak shape: peak shape should be monitored, and acceptability criteria should be established by the laboratory (see section "Laboratory-Specific Strategies for QA Program Design").
- Absolute retention time: absolute retention time acceptability criteria should be established by the laboratory (see section "Laboratory-Specific Strategies for QA Program Design").
- Relative retention time: relative retention time for the analyte should not exceed ±2.5% from the average relative retention time for the calibrators (within-run).
- Resolution factor: a resolution factor of 1.25 or greater indicates baseline peak resolution and should be used as the acceptability criteria.
- Internal standard recovery: the peak area of the internal standard should remain consistent throughout the run and should remain within a pre-defined range established by the laboratory (see section "Laboratory-Specific Strategies for QA Program Design").

Although the CLSI C62 document recommendations can serve as a basic framework for the laboratory's QA program design, the laboratory may be able to implement a more QA stringent program using a data-driven approach to select QA metrics and establish acceptability criteria. Evaluation of the laboratory's own data is also required for those metrics that lack specific CLSI C62 recommendations for acceptability criteria.

Laboratory-Specific Strategies for QA Program Design

The data-driven QA design program begins with analysis of a set of well-characterized reference samples with pre-assigned analyte concentration values. The data obtained from the reference samples will be used to evaluate each potential QA metric to verify that the 1) selected metrics and 2) proposed acceptability criteria are optimized for detection of error conditions, while avoiding undesirable false alert rates.

Selection and Analysis of Reference Samples

The reference samples selected for evaluation of QA metrics should be comprised of a sample matrix that is comparable to the matrix of the patient samples to be analyzed. If the laboratory will be performing testing using plasma samples, for example, the reference samples should consist of plasma samples collected into tubes with the same anticoagulant as patient samples. Ideally, the reference samples should be unmodified, native patient samples that have been value-assigned using a higher order reference measurement procedure. For example, if the laboratory is interested in designing a QA program for serum 25-hydroxyvitamin D (25-OH Vitamin D) testing performed by LC-MS/MS, then the laboratory can enroll in the CDC Vitamin D Standardization-Certificate Program ([22], https://www.cdc.gov/clinical-standardization-programs/php/vitamin-d/index.html). This program provides a panel of single-donor serum samples that have been value-assigned by the CDC reference method for 25-OH Vitamin D [17]. Value-assigned reference samples are available from the CDC standardization programs for analytes, including 25-OH Vitamin D, total testosterone, estradiol, total cholesterol, high-density lipoprotein-cholesterol, low density lipoprotein-cholesterol, free thyroxine, and thyroid-stimulating hormone [3]. Standardization programs serve as a preferred source of reference samples due to the availability of a relatively large number of matrix-appropriate, single-donor samples with analyte concentrations that span the analytical measurement range typical for clinical laboratory assays.

If the laboratory does not have access to a standardization program, or a standardization program is not available for the analyte, the laboratory may utilize unmodified patient samples that have been value-assigned using a validated comparator mass spectrometry-based assay. It is important to include samples with analyte concentrations that span the analytical measurement range (AMR) of the laboratory's LC-MS/MS measurement procedure to determine if values for the QA metric vary with analyte concentration. Use of materials containing analyte spiked into unmodified, native matrix samples may be included to ensure adequate coverage of the measurement procedure AMR. The performance of many QA metrics is strongly affected by the sample matrix; therefore use of surrogate matrices such as charcoal-stripped serum should be avoided whenever possible. Because QA metrics will be used to evaluate sample-specific matrix effects, the bulk majority of samples used to develop the QA program should consist of independent, single-donor samples or a large number of sample pools, each prepared using different individual patient samples. Certified reference materials, routine assay QC materials, or calibrator materials may also be utilized. However, a limitation of the use of these types of commercially prepared or surrogate-matrix materials is that they usually only include a limited number of independent samples, and the materials may exhibit different matrix effects or interferences when compared to patient samples [25].

Once the reference materials are selected, a preliminary run incorporating the proposed reference samples should be conducted to confirm that no interfering peaks are present, the background signal is low, the analyte peak shape is Gaussian, and the analyte peak is baseline-resolved from any closely eluting peaks. If any of the samples do not display these optimal chromatographic features, the sample(s) should be excluded from use as reference samples.

Once the reference samples are selected, the evaluation of QA metrics and acceptability criteria can begin. The reference samples should be analyzed over a sufficiently large number of runs to include all normal sources of within-run and between-run variation. For example, 20 runs might be expected to include many of the typical sources of variation [9]. Normal sources of variation, such as different calibration cycles, reagent lots, operators, and routine maintenance activities, should be incorporated into the experimental design to ensure the QA metric acceptable range is large enough to accommodate normal variation. If sources of normal variation are not included, the risk of establishing an acceptable range with a high false alert rate is significant. If available, multiple lots of calibrators, extraction reagents, mobile phases and columns should be included. Each run should also include the routine calibrators and QC materials utilized for the assay.

Data Analysis and Establishment of Acceptability Criteria

The retention times, raw peak areas and peak heights for the quantifier and qualifier ions for the analyte and the internal standard should be obtained for each run that is included in the reference sample evaluation. Values for QA metrics, including peak shape (peak area/height, peak width at 50% height, peak symmetry factor), retention time, relative retention time, resolution, ion ratio, and internal standard peak area are frequently calculated and available from the manufacturer's software programs. These data should be collected for each run, if available. If not available, the QA metrics can be calculated using the equations provided in section "Quality Assurance Metrics for Evaluation of Individual Sample Results". An example of a subset of QA data is shown in Table 10.3.

Once the data for the reference sample runs are obtained, the laboratory should examine the chromatograph and the final concentration result for each calibrator, QC, and reference sample to confirm the chromatography is acceptable and the expected analyte concentration is obtained. The chromatographic peak for the analyte and internal standard should be narrow and Gaussian in shape with no apparent interfering peaks. The data should be excluded from the reference sample dataset if the analyte concentration result is unexpected, if the peak shape is abnormal, or if interfering peaks are present.

Table 10.3 An example of a *subset* of 20 run's worth of QA data used to conduct the statistical analysis to determine QA metric acceptability criteria

Area / Height	IS Area / Height	RT	IS RT	Width at 50%	IS Width at 50%	Relative RT	Peak Asymmetry
1.68	1.82	1.95	1.94	0.03	0.03	1.005	1.750
1.75	1.78	1.94	1.93	0.03	0.03	1.005	1.750
1.62	1.82	1.94	1.93	0.02	0.03	1.005	1.250
1.68	1.81	1.94	1.94	0.03	0.03	1.000	2.250
1.8	1.75	1.94	1.94	0.03	0.03	1.000	1.750
1.75	1.66	1.94	1.94	0.03	0.02	1.000	2.000
1.73	1.7	1.95	1.94	0.03	0.03	1.005	0.714
1.85	1.81	1.95	1.94	0.03	0.03	1.005	1.333
1.7	1.78	1.95	1.94	0.03	0.03	1.005	1.250
1.76	1.76	1.95	1.94	0.03	0.03	1.005	1.400
1.72	1.71	1.95	1.94	0.03	0.03	1.005	1.500
1.68	1.84	1.94	1.94	0.03	0.03	1.000	1.250
1.58	1.77	1.94	1.94	0.02	0.03	1.000	2.000
1.9	1.67	1.94	1.93	0.03	0.03	1.005	1.600
1.83	1.73	1.95	1.94	0.03	0.03	1.005	1.400
1.77	1.79	1.95	1.94	0.03	0.03	1.005	1.200
1.76	1.86	1.94	1.94	0.03	0.03	1.000	2.000
1.82	1.81	1.95	1.94	0.03	0.03	1.005	1.600
1.66	1.76	1.95	1.94	0.03	0.03	1.005	1.250
1.79	1.68	1.94	1.93	0.03	0.03	1.005	1.750
1.74	1.65	1.94	1.93	0.03	0.02	1.005	0.800
1.63	1.78	1.95	1.94	0.02	0.03	1.005	1.000
1.72	1.68	1.95	1.94	0.03	0.03	1.005	0.800

The laboratory can then begin performing a statistical analysis on the reference sample dataset obtained for each QA metric to determine the range of values expected for the metric, and to decide if the metric will be useful for routine QA monitoring. Preliminary acceptability criteria can be established based on the reference dataset because the dataset represents the variation of results for each QA metric when the measurement procedure is behaving normally. The preliminary acceptability criteria may be derived by calculating the QA metric mean, standard deviation, and an expected percentile of the data distribution (e.g., central 95th percentile or central 99th percentile), or a multiple of the SD (e.g., plus or minus 3 SD). The statistical analysis can be performed using routine statistical analysis software packages, such statistical analysis functions available in Microsoft Excel or R (Microsoft; R Core Team). There are several alternative approaches for establishing acceptability criteria for QA metric data. A multi-rule approach, like that used to monitor routine QC values longitudinally [5], can be implemented to optimize the detection of errors and reduce the false alert rate. Alternatively, automated programs using custom modeling algorithms to apply peak quality evaluation criteria are commercially available [26].

The potential false alert rate should be considered when establishing acceptability criteria. For example, if the Laboratory Director chooses an acceptable range of the mean for the QA metric plus or minus 2 SD, then approximately 95% percent of patient sample QA values would be acceptable when no error condition is present [5]. In this case, approximately 5% of the values that represent normal performance will produce unacceptable results, thereby resulting in a substantial false alert rate. The Laboratory Director may choose to use a different percentile for the acceptable range, such as plus or minus 3 SD, which would reflect the central 99.7th percentile range, resulting in a false alert rate of approximately 0.3%. A rationale for the use of a larger percentile range is that multiple QA metrics may fail during a real error condition; therefore, reliance on any single metric may be less critical. Also, the original reference dataset included a process for exclusion of samples with interferences or inaccurately measured values; therefore, all samples included in the reference dataset should be interference-free.

Once the preliminary QA metrics and acceptable ranges are selected, the laboratory can test the program on an independent set of reference patient samples. Each test result should be evaluated to determine if the program correctly identified any actual error conditions that were present. All QA failures obtained from the independent reference set should be examined to determine if the metric identified a real error condition or if the metric instead produced a false alert. If an undesirable number of false alerts are identified for a particular QA metric, the Laboratory Director may consider either eliminating the QA metric or modifying the acceptability criteria to reduce the false alert rate.

It is important to note that not every QA metric may be suitable for each of the laboratory's specific LC-MS/MS measurement procedures. Selection of peak shape metrics for QA monitoring can be particularly challenging. The utility of some peak shape metrics may be limited depending on the specific measurement procedure that the laboratory uses. For example, the measurement of peak width at 50% height is very dependent on the background signal present in the chromatogram. Any increase in background signal for an individual sample will change the peak height at which the width calculation is performed. Therefore, small changes in background noise can lead to large changes in peak width measurements. If the laboratory's method-specific chromatograms exhibit small changes in background signal for patient samples, many peak width QA alerts may be obtained that do not reflect clinically significant errors. Also, low concentration samples will typically have an increased percentage of integrated background signal relative to the peak height, resulting in many peak width failures for low concentration samples. For these reasons, the laboratory may choose to discontinue use of peak width at 50% height as a QA metric for a particular assay because the false alert rate is too high. Similarly, the use of the peak symmetry factor can be very challenging if peaks are not exactly symmetrical. Slight peak tailing may occur as part of the measurement procedure's normal performance, or as the column ages, but patient results may not change by a clinically significant amount; therefore, re-development of the method is not required. In these examples, the laboratory may choose to use peak area/height as the only QA metric representing peak shape to avoid a high false alert rate and thereby save technologist labor time that would be otherwise spent responding to alerts that are not associated with an error condition.

Another commonly encountered situation is failure of ion ratio criteria at low analyte concentrations. This typically occurs because the qualifier ion peak is less intense, and therefore the peak area of the qualifier ion has larger imprecision as compared to the quantifier ion. In this case, the limit of quantification of the assay may need to be increased to ensure precise measurement of the qualifier ion.

Once the QA metrics and acceptability criteria have been implemented, each QA metric to be monitored and the accompanying acceptable range criteria should be described in the laboratory's standard operating procedure (SOP). The laboratory's SOP should also detail the appropriate response to QA metric failures, including investigation, troubleshooting, corrective action, and preventative action procedures. The metrics and/or acceptability criteria should be modified if the program is insufficient to detect true error conditions or if the false alert rate is high.

A summary of the steps for implementation of the data-driven approach for QA metric selection and establishment of acceptability criteria is as follows:

1. Select a set of reference samples.
2. Analyze the reference samples along with the method calibrators and QC materials. Include as many analytical runs and sources of normal variation as possible. For example, analyze the samples over several different days and include multiple analysts. Obtain QA metric data for each of the runs.
3. Ensure the expected analyte concentration results are obtained for the reference samples and ensure the chromatograms exhibit narrow, Gaussian-shaped peaks with no apparent interferences. Exclude QA data for samples that do not yield expected analyte concentration results or have suboptimal chromatographic peaks.
4. Review the data for each QA metric and calculate the range of values obtained from the reference sample set (e.g., central 99th percentile) to establish the acceptable range.
5. Apply the metrics to a test reference sample set.
6. Evaluate the ability of the metric and criteria to identify error conditions and determine the false alert rate.
7. Finalize the QA program by selecting metrics and criteria that alert during error conditions but minimize the false alert rate.
8. Detail corrective and preventative action responses for QA failures in the laboratory's SOPs.
9. Make sure to review the effectiveness and efficiency of the QA metrics and acceptable ranges on a routine basis.

QA Metrics Applied to the Run (Batch)

In addition to QA metrics that determine the validity of each individual sample, additional parameters must be monitored to ensure the quality of the entire run (or batch). These include evaluation of SST results, assay calibration results, carryover detection, and quality control (QC) results. Combined, these QA monitors assess overall LC-MS/MS system analytical performance. The acceptability criteria for each monitor must be established prior to assay implementation, and the results of each monitor must be reviewed with every run. Longitudinal analysis of monitors can be used to identify instrument issues that require remedial action to maintain optimal LC-MS/MS assay performance over time.

System Suitability Test (SST) Sample

An SST is conducted to provide confidence that the instrument is functioning as expected using a well-characterized sample. The SST sample may consist of an analyte and/or internal standard in solvent or a well-characterized extracted sample that is analyzed prior to starting an analytical run. Since the SST sample does not undergo extraction, sample preparation can be ruled out as the cause of an error if the SST sample result does not meet the acceptability criteria. The ideal SST sample contains all analytes performed in the method, is prepared using the assay extraction/reconstitution solvent, and has analyte concentrations near either the middle of the assay AMR or near medical decision points. Ideally, all analytes and internal standards are included in the SST because an instrument issue may affect each analyte differently, depending on the specific measurement conditions unique to each analyte. To minimize false alerts, SST stability and appropriate storage conditions should be established prior to use.

According to CLSI C62 guidelines, three to seven SST sample injections should be analyzed after instrument equilibration and priming injections have been performed, but prior to patient testing [6]. The first SST injection may be discarded. Repeat injections may be performed at the end of an analytical run to ensure instrument performance is maintained throughout the entire run. For large volume laboratories that analyze multiple consecutive runs per day, SSTs may be analyzed at the beginning and end of each day of testing.

The SST sample should pass pre-established acceptability criteria to ensure the LC and MS are operating as expected prior to the analysis of patient samples. QA metrics such as peak shape, peak intensity (peak area count), peak resolution, retention time, internal standard recovery, ion ratio, and S/N should be within acceptability criteria. Monitoring of baseline noise and/or baseline drift is a feature of some manufacturers' software programs that may be used during the SST, when available. Failure of the SSTs indicates a performance problem with the LC or MS that must be investigated and resolved prior to beginning the next run.

SSTs are also a useful tool to troubleshoot instrument issues and assess longitudinal instrument performance. If most or all patient samples fail to meet QA metric criteria during a run, then SST samples may be reviewed or re-injected to distinguish between an instrument issue and a sample preparation error as the source of the errors. SSTs may also be used to monitor instrument performance over time. It is common practice to keep a document to record the SST QA metrics such as retention time, peak intensity, and/or other characteristic metrics, each day the instrument is in use. If SST QA metric failures are frequent, then the LC or MS instrument should be serviced, and/or problems troubleshooted as necessary to avoid further degradation of performance.

Calibration Curve Acceptability

Any errors or inconsistencies in calibrator preparation or value assignment can result in inaccurate quantification of patient samples. Therefore, it is critical to set rigorous calibration curve acceptability criteria and to have a low threshold for investigation into identified issues. Like any other sample within an analytical run, each calibrator should pass all pre-established QA metric criteria, including peak shape, retention time, internal standard recovery, and ion ratio. However, additional QA metrics are required to assess the accuracy of the relationship between response and target concentration for the calibrators. These include a total allowable deviation from the target concentration (percent bias) for each calibrator and a minimum coefficient of determination (r^2) for the calibration curve equation. The CLSI 62 guidelines recommend that the allowable bias should be $\leq$15% for each calibrator above the assay lower limit of quantification (LLOQ) and $\leq$ 20% for calibrators at the LLOQ [6], although these criteria may be modified based on desired analytical performance and clinical utility of an individual assay. The r^2 value measures how much variation the independent variable (instrument signal) is contributing to the dependent value (the target concentration of the analyte in each calibrator) over the course of the calibration curve, or how well the regression equation approximates the measured calibrator concentrations. It is desirable to achieve an r^2 value of at least 0.995, although criteria may be modified as necessary for an individual assay. While not strictly required, minimum and maximum S/N criteria for each calibrator concentration may be established during method development and applied during routine analysis. Use of S/N criteria may help identify calibrator preparation issues, such as erroneously doubling the concentration of the calibrator during sample preparation. In this example, linearity may still be achieved (if detector saturation was not reached), and the error could potentially be missed by bias and r^2 metrics alone.

Each new lot of calibrators must be verified prior to use. New calibrator lot verification is usually accomplished by running replicates of the calibrators as unknowns against an already verified calibration curve. If the measured concentrations for the new calibrators meet pre-established acceptability criteria (for example, exhibit no more than 10% bias compared to the previous lot of calibrators), then the new lot of calibrators are acceptable for use. If the calibrators fail to meet acceptability criteria, then individual calibrator values may need to be reassigned or, if preparation errors were identified, the calibrators may need to be re-prepared. To avoid an additive bias over time, the difference observed between each new lot of calibrators should be monitored longitudinally, and adjustments made, if required. For example, assume that a new lot of calibrators is made in-house annually and the acceptance criteria is ± 10% bias compared to the previous lot. If an average of −6% bias was observed with each new lot of calibrators, then each lot would pass acceptance criteria, but within two years, an unacceptable −12% bias would accumulate. If, however, the next lot exhibited a +12% bias, the lot would fail the acceptance criteria but would return the assay back to its original quantification performance. Alternative approaches for verification of calibrator value assignments include quantifying calibrators by another laboratory, use of value-assigned reference samples to confirm calibrator value assignments, and/or use of accuracy-based proficiency samples. If a drift in measured calibrator concentration is noted, then storage conditions and stability criteria for stock calibrator solutions should be revisited.

Some laboratories will allow exclusion of calibrators that do not meet acceptability criteria. This practice should be avoided whenever possible. If the laboratory allows exclusion of calibrators, the exclusion procedure should be documented and strictly monitored for compliance. The procedure must include acceptable reasons for calibrator exclusion, and documentation of the rationale for each exclusion should be maintained. Arbitrarily excluding calibrator points from the calibration curve to achieve acceptability without identifying the root cause of the unacceptable calibrator value is an unacceptable practice. A way to avoid this practice is to require the Laboratory Director or Supervisor to verify the exclusion rationale and 'sign off' on each excluded value before releasing patient results. If the highest or lowest calibrator is excluded, then the reportable range of the assay may need to be adjusted to the concentration range of acceptable calibrators. Also, the maximum number of calibrators that may be excluded must be carefully evaluated according to the impact on the accuracy of the calibration curve. For example, the Laboratory Director may decide that excluding a single point from a six-point calibration curve or two single points from an eight-point calibration curve may be permitted, whereas zero points may be excluded from a four-point calibration curve. Finally, if calibrators are injected more than once, clear limitations on how many values, including replicates of the same calibrator, may be excluded must be established.

Calibrator peak areas should remain relatively constant between runs. While SST monitoring allows for an assessment of instrument performance over time, monitoring of the calibrator signal may help identify stability issues or other problems isolated to the calibrators themselves. Within a single run, any calibrator deterioration will likely go unnoticed, especially if all calibrators degrade at a similar rate, causing a proportional signal decrease over time. Longitudinal monitoring combined with pre-defined acceptability criteria can help identify any issues and avoid errors.

Matrix Blank and Carryover Assessment

Two types of blank samples are typically employed for use as QA metrics. A 'blank' sample refers to an extracted sample of the appropriate matrix that does not contain the reported analyte(s), but does contain the internal standard. A 'double blank' refers to an extracted sample of the appropriate matrix without analyte or internal standard. Each type of blank sample serves a different purpose, and both are necessary to adequately assess the performance of the analytical run.

The blank sample (matrix plus internal standard) is used to determine the contribution of the internal standard, if any, to the analyte peak area. Monitoring of this QA metric is especially important if a deuterated internal standard is used, since isotopic overlap or deuterium-hydrogen exchange may occur, causing a small percentage of the internal standard signal to contribute to the analyte peak area. If deuterium-hydrogen exchange has occurred, the signal from the internal standard will falsely increase the analyte quantifier and/or qualifier peak areas, and the internal standard peak area will concomitantly decrease. With every analytical run, a blank sample should be injected and reviewed for the absence of a peak for all analytes included in the method. If a peak is present in the quantifier or qualifier transition, the peak area must be less than 20% of the lower limit of quantification. Necessary corrective actions may include changes to the internal standard type, changes to the sample preparation method (especially if harsh conditions are used that may induce the hydrolysis of the deuterium moieties of the internal standard) or changes to the internal standard storage acceptability criteria.

The peak area of the double blank sample should be compared against pre-established acceptability criteria to assess analyte carryover. To monitor for carryover, the double blank sample should be injected after the highest calibrator and, if possible, after any sample suspected of having a high enough concentration of analyte to carry over into the subsequent sample. An alternative approach is to inject a low QC or blank sample. The double blank sample analyzed after the highest calibrator should be free of any discernible analyte peak. If a peak is detected, then the peak area contribution should be <20% of the LLOQ and ≤5% of the internal standard [6]. Sources of analyte carryover include contaminated reagents, contaminated LC components such as tubing, columns or valves, or contaminated MS components such as curtain plates, lenses, ion guides and detectors.

The analyte concentration that represents the carryover limit should be verified during method validation. The carryover limit may be established as the upper limit of the analytical measurement range (i.e., the highest calibrator) or the limit may be extended by testing for the presence of carryover at higher concentrations, such as 10x the upper limit of quantification. Use of the upper limit of the AMR is the preferred method for many laboratories because of its convenience. In this approach, carryover is adequately assessed during every run by the double blank injection after the highest calibrator, if the concentration of the highest calibrator is near the upper limit of the AMR. However, if a sample with analyte concentration exceeding the upper limit of the AMR is analyzed, samples immediately following the high concentration samples must be reanalyzed in a separate run to ensure the results are not affected by carryover. This approach is sufficient if concentrations above the AMR are unlikely, such as assays detecting endogenous compounds or therapeutic drug monitoring measurement procedures with extensive AMRs.

For assays with results that frequently exceed the AMR, such as toxicology panels, a concentration higher than the upper limit of the AMR may be used as the carryover limit. This approach has the benefit of minimizing the need to reanalyze patient samples, but also requires additional validation. Some analytes in multi-analyte panels may be more sensitive to carryover than others; therefore the carryover limit should be verified for all analytes. Carryover validation is accomplished by alternating injections of a low, mid-, and high-concentration sample and then calculating the percent carryover [8].

Evaluation of Quality Control (QC) Results

Quality control (QC) material is an essential component of the QA monitoring program. QC materials for LC-MS/MS assays should consist of the same matrix as patient samples, or the QC material matrix should be as similar to the patient sample matrix as possible. Ion suppression is common in LC-MS/MS and is due to leftover matrix in the sample extract that competes with the analyte for ionization in the mass spectrometer source. Therefore, QC materials should be matrix-matched with the patient samples to ensure the materials exhibit the same degree of ion suppression as the native patient samples used for testing. Use of pooled patient samples is generally acceptable for in-house preparation of QC materials. Patient sample pools may be spiked with exogenous analyte to achieve desired concentrations for each level of QC material. If using pooled patient samples as routine QC materials, the pools should be aliquoted and stored under conditions in which they are stable. Limitations of using pooled patient samples include limited storage stability, limited availability of appropriate samples, and the presence of endogenous analyte in the samples. Commercial QC products are available for some measurement procedures; however, their use can also be associated with numerous limitations. Commercially available QC products often have additives or preservatives and may undergo extensive manipulation during manufacturing. These manufacturing processes may cause different matrix effects for the QC material as compared to patient samples, resulting in different levels of ion suppression or the presence of interfering peaks in the chromatograms of the QC material. Charcoal-stripped matrices, such as stripped serum, are often purchased to ensure the absence of steroid hormone analytes for the preparation of QC materials for steroid measurement procedures. However, analytes in charcoal stripped materials may exhibit different ionization compared to patient sample matrices because of significant matrix removal during the manufacturing process. Therefore, use of charcoal-stripped matrices could lead to ineffective QC monitoring for signal loss.

If both calibrators and QC are made in-house, the material used to create the stock solutions for calibrators should be purchased from a different vendor than that used to make the QC materials. Alternatively, the standard material used to prepare calibrator stock solutions should be a different lot number than that used to make the QC materials. At a minimum, the QC and calibrators should be prepared independently and at staggered time intervals.

General recommendations for design of an effective QC strategy can be found in the CLSI C24 guideline [5]. CLIA requires that a minimum of two concentrations of QC materials be analyzed each 24 hours of patient testing. QC should be analyzed more frequently if the measurement procedure results are immediately clinically actionable or if the laboratory sample run size is large. Additional QC levels should be analyzed if there are multiple medical decision points or if the assay AMR spans multiple orders of magnitude. Many LC-MS/MS measurement procedures include the measurement of multiple analytes within a sample (e.g., immunosuppressant panel assays or urine drug confirmation panel assays). A minimum of two QC materials should be utilized for each analyte within a panel (a single QC material may contain more than one analyte), and QC acceptability criteria should be established for each analyte. For quantitative measurement procedures, guidelines recommend that QC materials should consist of at least a low (within 3× of the LLOQ) and a mid-to-high concentration, and additional concentrations near medical decision points. For qualitative assays, QC materials should consist of a negative and a positive concentration just below and above the cutoff, respectively.

QC materials should be analyzed at the beginning, middle, and end of each run to ensure that the measurement procedure is performing as expected throughout the entire run. If the analytical runs are less than 50 samples, analysis of QC at the beginning and end of the run is likely sufficient unless the run time is extensive. If a plate format (i.e., 96-well plate) is used, one option to assess quality over the entire plate sequence is to rotate the position of the QC within the run. Rotating the position of the QC within the plate and the position within the run ensures that the *entire* run sequence is assessed periodically. Analyzing QC in the same position in both the wells of a plate and on the instrument is more convenient and less error-prone for the laboratory technologists, but less effective at identifying errors that may exist at different time points within the run.

The QC materials should be subjected to the same procedures as patient samples including all preanalytical steps such as hydrolysis, extraction, and derivatization. If the LC-MS/MS measurement procedure includes a hydrolysis step to remove glucuronide moieties from the analyte (a common practice in toxicology assays), a QC material to evaluate the acceptability of the hydrolysis step should be included. If the QC material only contains the parent drug (e.g., morphine) and not its glucuronidated metabolites (e.g., morphine-3-glucuronide and morphine-6-glucuronide), then a hydrolysis procedure error would never be detected. The hydrolysis QC material should contain only glucuronidated metabolites, should consist of the metabolites that can be found in patient samples from patients taking the parent drugs, and should represent the drug class and hydrolysis efficiency.

For quantitative assays, the QC target mean should be established or verified with every new lot of QC materials. A minimum of 20 days of QC analysis should be conducted for each new lot to ensure sources of normal variation in the assay over time, due to factors such as minor calibrator drift, pipetting differences between users, temperature fluctuations within the laboratory, and aging of reagents and consumables are reflected in the calculated mean value.

Daily QC is typically monitored using Levey–Jennings plots that include target means, target standard deviations, and multi-rule strategies used for the detection of unacceptable measurement procedure bias and imprecision [7]. The QC approach and acceptability criteria should be established according to the clinical utility of the measurement procedure and should ensure the measurement procedure maintains pre-defined analytical performance goals established during method validation (CLSI C24).

If QC results are unacceptable, an investigation should be conducted to identify the root cause of the error. Once the root cause is identified, troubleshooting should be conducted, and corrective action implemented to correct the source of the error. Affected patient samples should be repeated and the impact on patient results should be determined. Corrected reports should be issued, if appropriate. If QC fails for one analyte within a multi-analyte panel, it is not necessary to repeat measurements for analytes that did not have unacceptable QC results. The analyte concentrations with acceptable QC results may be reported. If QC fails for either of the analytes that are directly related, such as drug parent/metabolite analyte combinations, the laboratory may report out one analyte and report the other as an "invalid result," depending on the clinical utility of the results and the discretion of the Laboratory Director. Each laboratory should determine its own procedures for analyte reporting in the case where one of a set of related analytes has a failing QC value.

Considerations for Multiplexing and Multiple Instruments

To increase sample throughput, many laboratories use multiplexed systems in which flow from two or more LC columns or systems are directed to a single mass spectrometer. Due to the potential for slight variations in LC parameters such as actual flow rate, mobile phase gradient, temperature, time of elution, and dead space, each system or column should be considered separate and should be monitored using QA metrics. Each "stream" of the LC system should include its own compliment of SST samples, calibrators, and QC materials. Similarly, if multiple instruments are running the same measurement procedure, then each instrument should be considered unique and should be independently monitored using QA metrics.

Among-instrument comparisons and among "stream" comparisons for multiplexed systems are required to ensure that each instrument system produces similar results. While current guidelines recommend among-instrument comparisons every six months, more frequent evaluation of comparability may ensure comparable results across columns and systems.

Automating and Implementing the QA Review Process

Some laboratories utilize a manual visual inspection process to evaluate peak quality. However, manual peak review is a time-consuming, subjective, and error-prone approach. The presence of interfering peaks or peak shape abnormalities may be difficult to visualize, or identification may be missed due to technologist fatigue. Automated assessment of quantitative QA metrics is recommended to achieve operational efficiency and to reduce peak evaluation errors [14]. Most LC-MS/MS system manufacturers' software packages can provide numeric quantities for select QA metrics. To implement LC-MS/MS system manufacturer's software for QA assessment for a particular assay, the laboratory typically needs to (1) select which QA metrics will be utilized for the QA program and (2) input the acceptability criteria for the QA metric results into the manufacturer's software. Then, the software can evaluate the QA metric data for each result and flag the result if acceptability criteria are not met. However, the manufacturer's software handling processes for QA metric data can have significant limitations. Some common limitations are as follows:

- There is no automated selection process offered by the manufacturer to define which QA metrics identify true error conditions, but reduce the false alert rate for a particular assay.
- The manufacturer's software may not perform the exact calculation desired by the laboratory (e.g., QA metric data is not expressed as a percentage of the response of the calibrators within a run).
- Specific QA metric calculation equations can vary among manufacturers.
- Automated quantification of some QA metrics, such as peak resolution and internal standard recovery, may not be available from the manufacturer's software.
- QA metric data may not be presented longitudinally (across runs) for evaluation of metric performance over time.

To overcome these limitations, the laboratory should implement the QA metric selection process and determine acceptability criteria according to professional practice guidelines or through the use of a data-driven approach as described in this Chapter. The laboratory may wish to seek assistance from in-house data analytics groups or information technology groups to develop automated data export approaches, to write automated functions for QA metric calculation, and to develop scripts to apply pre-defined acceptability criteria and flag unacceptable results according to the laboratory's procedures.

If the laboratory does not wish to implement the LC-MS/MS system manufacturer's software for its QA program, several alternative options for automated QA metric evaluation are available. Software programs have been developed that utilize multivariate statistical models and machine learning to develop a predictive model for each analyte peak and then compare the data to a model to identify and flag poor-quality peaks [23]. Free applications are available within the online mass spectrometry data analysis software package, Skyline, for automated peak quantification and evaluation of QA metrics [15]. Commercial services are also available that will accept raw LC-MS/MS data via flat file transfer and apply automated peak integration, quantification, and application of QA metrics based on customized machine-learning algorithms developed and validated for the laboratory's measurement procedure [26]. Some advantages of using these types of alternative approaches include:

- Vendor-neutral QA metric calculations can be used to accomplish standardization across multiple manufacturer's LC-MS/MS systems.
- Laboratory technologists only need to learn how to use one QA software package.
- Easier implementation of longitudinal monitoring of QA data.

Once the QA program is designed and validated, the laboratory can proceed to the implementation of the program into routine testing. QA metrics should be applied to each chromatographic peak, including peaks for SST samples, calibrator samples, QC samples, and patient samples during routine analysis. Each QA metric failure should be investigated to determine if an error condition is likely present. Failure of only a single QA metric can identify an error condition. For example, failure of the ion ratio can indicate an incorrect or contaminated peak even if the peak shape metrics do not fail. Failure of the absolute retention time can indicate a LC system leak in the absence of other QA metric failures. However, failure of multiple QA metrics is commonly encountered when an error condition is present. For example, integration of the wrong peak will frequently result in a combination of QA metric failures, including failure of relative retention time, peak area/height (or another peak shape metric), and ion ratio criteria. If an error condition is identified, the laboratory should determine whether the error only affected a single sample result or if the error condition potentially affected all sample results within the analytical run. The laboratory should (1) refrain from reporting all potentially erroneous results, (2) perform and document corrective action, (3) repeat patient sample analysis to determine if corrected reports should be issued, and (4) implement preventative action to prevent the error from recurring. Some examples of using the QA program to identify error conditions are shown in Fig. 10.8.

Fig. 10.8 (**a**) Relative RT passed, indicating the correct peak is integrated. However, absolute RT, peak area/height, ion ratio, peak resolution, and peak symmetry factor failed, indicating the presence of a non-baseline resolved, interfering peak. (**b**) All QA metrics passed except ion ratio, indicating the presence of an underlying interfering peak that would be missed if using visual inspection only. (**c**) Relative RT passed, but absolute RT and peak area/height failed, indicating the correct peak is integrated in the bottom chromatogram, but the analyte is not interacting with the column properly (e.g. old column) or there is a leak in the LC system

a

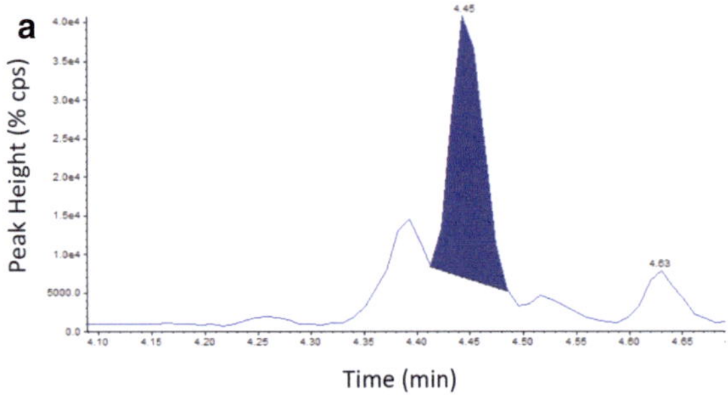

RT	Relative RT	Peak Area/Height	Ion Ratio	Peak Resolution	Peak Symmetry Factor
FAIL	PASS	FAIL	FAIL	FAIL	FAIL

b

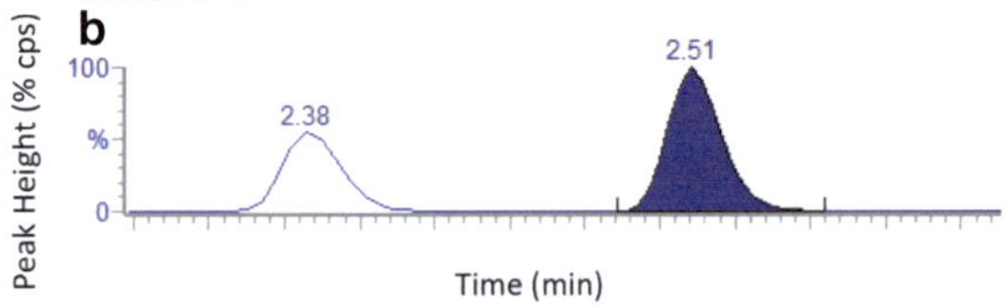

RT	Relative RT	Peak Area/Height	Ion Ratio	Peak Resolution	Peak Symmetry Factor
PASS	PASS	PASS	FAIL	PASS	PASS

c

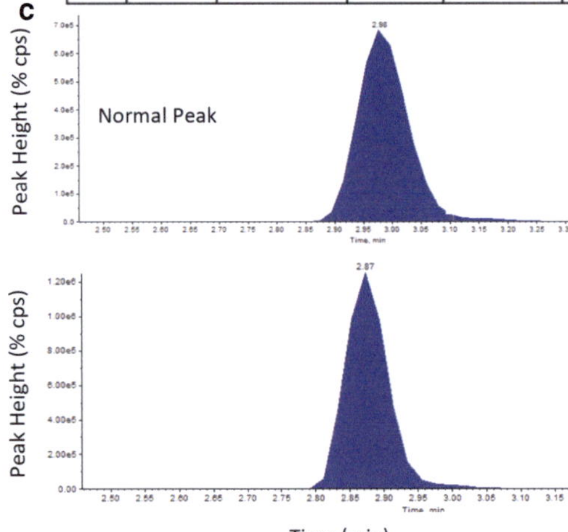

RT	Relative RT	Peak Area/Height	Ion Ratio	Peak Resolution	Peak Symmetry Factor
FAIL	PASS	FAIL	PASS	PASS	PASS

Conclusion

Development, validation, and implementation of a comprehensive, quantitative QA program is critical for ensuring high-quality results for LC-MS/MS measurement procedures. Careful selection of QA metrics and acceptability criteria can be accomplished using professional practice guidelines; however, use of a data-driven approach may result in a more effective QA program that is customized for each assay. The QA program development and validation phases should include assessment of the false-alert rate to avoid unnecessary labor time spent investigating QA flags that are not indicative of true error conditions. Options for automation of QA metric assessment should be investigated to improve the efficiency of the laboratory's QA program.

References

1. Ancker JS, Edwards A, Nosal S, et al. Effects of workload, work complexity, and repeated alerts on alert fatigue in a clinical decision support system. BMC Med Inform Decis Mak. 2017;17:36. https://doi.org/10.1186/s12911-017-0430-8.
2. Annesley T, Diamandis E, Bachmann L, et al. A Spectrum of views on clinical mass spectrometry. Clin Chem. 2016;62:30–6. https://doi.org/10.1373/clinchem.2015.250258.
3. CDC. About clinical standardization programs. In: Clinical Standardization Programs; 2024. https://www.cdc.gov/clinical-standardization-programs/about/index.html. Accessed 11 Sept 2024.
4. Clarke W. Mass spectrometry in the clinical laboratory: determining the need and avoiding pitfalls. In: Mass spectrometry for the clinical laboratory. Elsevier Inc.; 2017. p. 1–15.
5. CLSI C. C24: quality control for quantitative measurement: CLSI. In: Clinical & Laboratory Standards Institute; 2016. https://clsi.org/standards/products/clinical-chemistry-and-toxicology/documents/c24/. Accessed 11 Sept 2024.
6. CLSI C. C62Ed2 | Liquid chromatography-mass spectrometry methods, 2nd Edition. In: Clinical & Laboratory Standards Institute; 2024a. https://clsi.org/standards/products/clinical-chemistry-and-toxicology/documents/c62/. Accessed 11 Sept 2024.
7. CLSI C-A. C50-A: mass spectrometry in the clinical laboratory. In: Clinical & Laboratory Standards Institute; 2007. https://clsi.org/standards/products/clinical-chemistry-and-toxicology/documents/c50/. Accessed 11 Sept 2024.
8. CLSI E. EP10 Ed4 | Preliminary evaluation of quantitative medical laboratory measurement procedures, 4th ed. In: Clinical & Laboratory Standards Institute; 2024b. https://clsi.org/standards/products/method-evaluation/documents/ep10/. Accessed 11 Sept 2024.
9. CLSI EA. EP05 A3: evaluating quantitative measurement precision. In: Clinical & Laboratory Standards Institute; 2014. https://clsi.org/standards/products/method-evaluation/documents/ep05/. Accessed 11 Sept 2024.
10. Crews BO, Drees JC, Greene DN. Data-driven quality assurance to prevent erroneous test results. Crit Rev Clin Lab Sci. 2019;57:146–60. https://doi.org/10.1080/10408363.2019.1678567.
11. Dolan J. Troubleshooting basics, part IV: Peak shape problems. 2012;30:564–9.
12. Grant R, Rappold B. Development and validation of small molecule analytes by LC–tandem mass spectrometry. In: Tietz textbook of clinical chemistry and molecular diagnostics. 6th ed. St. Louis: Elsevier Inc.; 2018. p. 326.
13. Hage D. Chromatography. In: Tietz textbook of clinical chemistry and molecular diagnostics. 6th ed. Elsevier Inc.; 2018. p. 266–94.

14. Haymond S. System performance monitoring in clinical liquid chromatography-tandem mass spectrometry (LC–MS/MS). In: Garg U, editor. Clinical applications of mass spectrometry in biomolecular analysis: methods and protocols. New York: Springer US; 2022. p. 13–25.
15. Henderson CM, Shulman NJ, MacLean B, et al. Skyline performs as well as vendor software in the quantitative analysis of serum 25-hydroxy vitamin D and vitamin D binding globulin. Clin Chem. 2018;64:408–10. https://doi.org/10.1373/clinchem.2017.282293.
16. Kushnir MM, Rockwood AL, Nelson GJ, et al. Assessing analytical specificity in quantitative analysis using tandem mass spectrometry. Clin Biochem. 2005;38:319–27. https://doi.org/10.1016/j.clinbiochem.2004.12.003.
17. Mineva EM, Schleicher RL, Chaudhary-Webb M, et al. A candidate reference measurement procedure for quantifying serum concentrations of 25-Hydroxyvitamin D3 and 25-Hydroxyvitamin D2 using isotope-dilution liquid chromatography-tandem mass spectrometry. Anal Bioanal Chem. 2015;407:5615–24. https://doi.org/10.1007/s00216-015-8733-z.
18. R Core Team R: A Language and Environment for Statistical Computing.
19. Rappold BA. Review of the use of liquid chromatography-tandem mass spectrometry in clinical laboratories: part II-operations. Ann Lab Med. 2022;42:531–57. https://doi.org/10.3343/alm.2022.42.5.531.
20. Rappold BA. Best practices for routine operation of clinical mass spectrometry assays. In: Mass Spectrometry for the Clinical Laboratory, Elsevier Inc.; 2017. p. 77–106.
21. Richards K, Rijntjes E, Rathmann D, Köhrle J. Avoiding the pitfalls when quantifying thyroid hormones and their metabolites using mass spectrometric methods: the role of quality assurance. Mol Cell Endocrinol. 2017;458:44–56. https://doi.org/10.1016/j.mce.2017.01.032.
22. Sempos CT, Vesper HW, Phinney KW, et al. Vitamin D status as an international issue: national surveys and the problem of standardization. Scand J Clin Lab Invest Suppl. 2012;243:32–40. https://doi.org/10.3109/00365513.2012.681935.
23. Toghi Eshghi S, Auger P, Mathews WR. Quality assessment and interference detection in targeted mass spectrometry data using machine learning. Clin Proteomics. 2018;15:33. https://doi.org/10.1186/s12014-018-9209-x.
24. United States Pharmacopeia (USP). The harmonised general chapter chromatography. 2021.
25. Vesper HW, Miller WG, Myers GL. Reference materials and commutability. Clin Biochem Rev. 2007;28:139–47.
26. Vicente FB, Lin DC, Haymond S. Automation of chromatographic peak review and order to result data transfer in a clinical mass spectrometry laboratory. Clin Chim Acta. 2019;498:84–9. https://doi.org/10.1016/j.cca.2019.08.004.
27. Victoria Zhang Y, Garg U. Mass spectrometry in clinical laboratory: applications in therapeutic drug monitoring and toxicology. Methods Mol Biol. 2024;2737:1–13. https://doi.org/10.1007/978-1-0716-3541-4_1.
28. Vitamin D Standardization-Certification Program. https://www.cdc.gov/clinical-standardization-programs/php/vitamin-d/index.html
29. Vogeser M, Seger C. Quality management in clinical application of mass spectrometry measurement systems. Clin Biochem. 2016;49:947–54. https://doi.org/10.1016/j.clinbiochem.2016.07.005.
30. Wahab MF, Armstrong D, Patel DC. Peak shapes and their measurements: The need and the concept behind total peak shape analysis. LC-GC North America. 2017;35:846–53.
31. Winters BD, Cvach MM, Bonafide CP, et al. Technological distractions (part 2): a summary of approaches to manage clinical alarms with intent to reduce alarm fatigue. Crit Care Med. 2018;46:130–7. https://doi.org/10.1097/CCM.0000000000002803.
32. Zeng W, Bateman KP. Quantitative LC-MS/MS. 1. Impact of points across a peak on the accuracy and precision of peak area measurements. J Am Soc Mass Spectrom. 2023;34:1136–44. https://doi.org/10.1021/jasms.3c00077.

Regulatory Considerations for LC-MS/MS-Based Clinical Assays

11

Rebecca Ann Flugrad, Kyla Marie Jorgenson, Patricia Jones, and Y. Victoria Zhang

Introduction

Mass spectrometry (MS)-based assays have become critical tools in clinical diagnostics, offering unique tests with unparalleled sensitivity, specificity, and flexibility. However, the regulatory landscape governing these tests is complex and evolving.

Most MS-based assays are examples of laboratory-developed tests (LDTs). LDTs are tests developed within a single laboratory, in general, intended to be utilized for that laboratory's patient population. In many cases, the LDTs are developed as there is no FDA-approved test available that meets the patient needs. LDTs have been regulated under the Clinical Laboratory Improvement Amendments (CLIA) of 1988, administered by the Centers for Medicare & Medicaid Services (CMS). CLIA regulations ensure laboratory quality, focusing on personnel qualifications, assay validation, and quality control measures. The analytical utility and quality of the LDT are well covered by CLIA; however, clinical utility is not part of CLIA and is one of the aspects that have prompted the FDA to pursue regulation of these assays. Thus, recent discussions at the federal level regarding LDT regulations may be changing the landscape of MS assays, including such variables as which

R. A. Flugrad · K. M. Jorgenson
Department of Pathology and Laboratory Medicine, University of Rochester Medical Center, Rochester, NY, USA

P. Jones (✉)
Children's Medical Center, Dallas, TX, USA
e-mail: Patricia.Jones@UTSouthwestern.edu

Y. V. Zhang (✉)
Department of Pathology and Laboratory Medicine, University of Rochester Medical Center, Rochester, NY, USA
e-mail: Victoria_Zhang@urmc.rochester.edu

Y. V. Zhang, U. Garg (eds.), *Practical Guide to Implementing Liquid Chromatography Mass Spectrometry in Clinical Laboratories*,
https://doi.org/10.1007/978-3-032-03852-4_11

laboratories offer testing, the variety of analytes assessed, and which manufacturers continue production of instrumentation.

In this chapter, we will examine the current regulatory requirements for mass spectrometry-based LDTs under CMS and CLIA, introduce the history of federal regulations of clinical laboratory testing, and share the development and discussions on the FDA's 2024 final rule on LDTs. We hope that by understanding this regulatory environment, laboratories can navigate compliance challenges while continuing to innovate in personalized medicine and advanced diagnostics, and continue to advance the practice of laboratory medicine.

Early Stages of FDA and Its Regulations of Laboratory Services

The regulations of clinical laboratory services have a long and evolving history (Fig. 11.1). The 1938 Federal Food, Drug, and Cosmetic Act (FD&C Act), signed into law by President Franklin D. Roosevelt, established the Food and Drug Administration as the Federal agency with the authority to oversee and regulate standards for the production, marketing, sale, and distribution of food, drugs, and cosmetics. The FDA is thus responsible for ensuring the safety and effectiveness of these items, the creation and enforcement of quality standards, inspection of manufacturing facilities, regulation of prescription drug and device advertising, as well as product labeling and health claims on food and dietary supplements. Additionally, the FDA has the authority to recall or seize unsafe products and is responsible for approving new entities [1, 2].

Also signed by President Franklin D. Roosevelt, the 1944 Public Health Service Act consolidated existing public health laws into a single framework, thereby centralizing and expanding the federal government's role in protecting public health. It authorized the US Public Health Service (PHS) to cooperate with state and local health departments on a broader scale and to offer technical and financial assistance

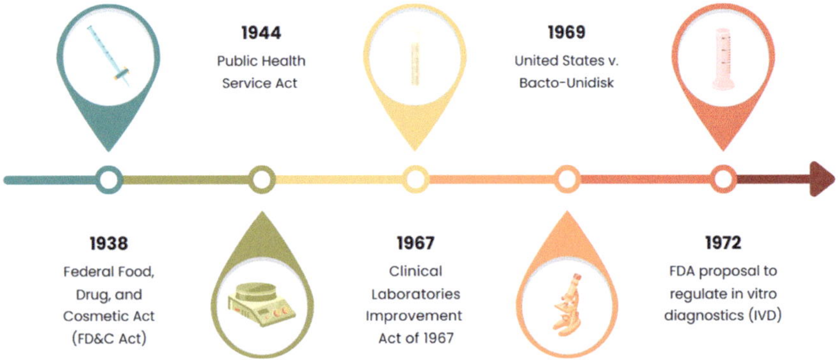

Fig. 11.1 Early stages of regulations of clinical laboratories

to support local public health programs [3–5]. This broad mandate to protect public health can be seen as the foundation for many later health programs and policies, including laboratory oversight, as the act provided a structure for the federal government to standardize medical and health services.

The "Partnership for Health Amendments of 1967" (Public Law 90–174) was enacted by Congress, with the intent to "improve the performance of clinical laboratories", among other goals. The law regulated hospital-based labs and labs engaged in interstate commerce. Laboratory licensure was required in order to accept or request specimens; however, licensure procedures were not well-established by the law, although some guidance was provided [6–8]. Licensure requirements included the maintenance of a quality control program, records, equipment, and facilities for proper operation, a qualified director and other personnel, and participation in proficiency testing. The law also established grounds for licensure revocation [6].

In 1962, the government seized an interstate shipment of antibiotic sensitivity discs, claiming that they were "drugs" and not "devices", as defined by the Federal Food, Drug, and Cosmetic Act. Because of the presence of antibiotics in the discs, they needed to meet the requirements of the FDA's pre-market process. In 1969, United States v. Bacto-Unidisk, 394 U.S. 784, the United States District Court for the Eastern District of Michigan determined that the discs did not meet the definition of a drug, and this decision was upheld by the Court of Appeals for the Sixth Circuit. The Supreme Court, however, reversed both decisions and ruled that the discs must meet the FDA's regulations for pre-market approval [9].

Rapid advancement of in vitro diagnostic (IVD) products along with increasingly widespread use prompted the FDA to reconsider their safety and efficacy, and a proposal was developed in 1972 to further regulate these products. Drugs and devices used for diagnosis, prevention or treatment of disease, including those used for pregnancy detection, blood typing, or presence of antibodies were included in the category of IVDs. In vitro diagnostics were defined as "those reagents, instruments and kits which perform no anatomical, physiological, or therapeutic function, which are not injected into humans, and which are used solely to provide information on specimens taken from the human body." Because IVDs were considered devices and/or drugs, the FDA would have jurisdiction over them. Required labeling information was also discussed in the proposal, including the scientific basis of the product, its intended use, and technical details regarding performance characteristics, such as specificity and sensitivity [10].

FDA Regulations of In Vitro Diagnostics and CLIA'88

Congress amended the Federal Food, Drug and Cosmetic Act with the Medical Device Amendments of 1976 (MDA) (Fig. 11.2). This allowed the FDA to regulate medical devices intended for use in humans, including in vitro diagnostics, and devices that entered interstate commerce or were distributed between state borders [8, 11]. The amendments established a risk-based classification system for medical

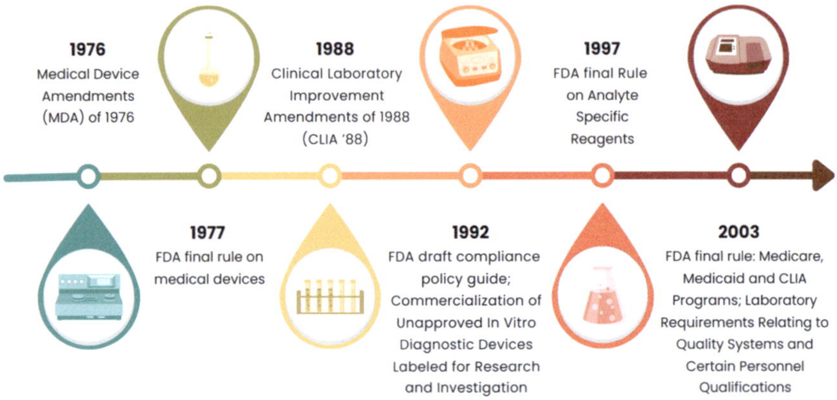

Fig. 11.2 Major events for FDA regulations of in vitro diagnostics

devices and created a process for premarket approval (PMA) and premarket notification (510(k)). Post-market requirements were also enacted, including listing devices with the FDA, good manufacturing practices, and adverse event reporting [11, 12].

The FDA was given authority to regulate LDTs under the MDA because laboratory-developed tests were considered a medical device, and more specifically, an in vitro diagnostic. However, as of the time when we write this chapter, there are two lawsuits against FDA's decision, which claim that LDTs are not "devices" but are services within the practice of medicine, and the FDA cannot regulate the practice of medicine. From FDA's perspective, at the time, enforcement discretion was observed for LDTs because of their particular characteristics; home brew tests were generated in small volumes, used for rare diseases or for local patient populations, were created and used in a single laboratory associated with the treating facility, utilized manual techniques and used reagents that were already FDA compliant [13].

In the final rule on medical devices published in 1977, the FDA described exemptions from institution registration. Because clinical laboratories provided a benefit to the consumer through the use of medical devices, they were not required to register with the FDA [8].

Between 1967 and 1988, technological advancements allowed for laboratory tests that were much simpler to perform. In addition, laboratory instrument footprints were smaller, making their installation more common in non-CLIA certified laboratories, such as at physician office laboratories and small clinics. These sites often did not adhere to clinical laboratory standards, and untrained individuals were performing testing. At the time, there was public concern about adverse patient outcomes caused by improperly performed Papanicolaou smears. The response by Congress was to establish CLIA '88, or Public Law 100–578 [14, 15].

Although the Partnership for Health Amendments of 1967 established regulations for laboratories involved in interstate commerce, CLIA '88 established quality standards for all laboratories. Congress sought to improve the accuracy, reliability, and timeliness of patient test results, regardless of where testing was performed. The regulations were applicable to labs engaging in interstate commerce and those participating in Medicare and Medicaid programs [7].

In the 1992 FDA document "Commercialization of Unapproved In Vitro Diagnostic Devices Labeled for Research and Investigation," the FDA stated that laboratories have been manufacturing "home brew" products for diagnostic purposes, and that these products are to be regulated in the same way as any other unapproved medical device [16]. Draft policy guidelines to regulate LDTs as medical devices were published by the FDA at this time. Laboratory professionals argued that home brew assays were already regulated under CLIA, and that the FDA did not have the legal authority to further regulate this category of testing. The FDA stated that its institution had the appropriate authority; however, it withdrew its proposal [17].

In 1997, the FDA enacted the Final Rule on Analyte Specific Reagents, a policy to regulate analyte-specific reagents (ASRs), but refrained from enacting regulation on in vitro diagnostics in which the ASRs were used. ASRs were defined as any analyte that had specific binding or a chemical reaction with substances in a specimen. Many reagents fell under this classification, including antibodies, cancer markers, oligonucleotides, or microbiological nucleic acids [17]. ASRs were classified as restricted devices under the FD&C Act, creating restrictions on sale, distribution, and use. The rule did not apply to reagents sold in non-clinical settings, or to those used as components in an FDA-approved test [18]. Additionally, the FDA recognized the importance of homebrew tests, and stated that their further regulation would have a negative effect on public health [17]. However, laboratories producing LDTs were to be considered manufacturers of medical devices, and are thus under the FDA's jurisdiction [8].

The 2003 final rule, "Medicare, Medicaid, and CLIA Programs; Laboratory Requirements Relating to Quality Systems and Certain Personnel Qualifications", Pub. L. 100–578, designated requirements for quality control (QC), personnel performing testing, quality assurance, and changed how proficiency testing (PT) was graded, lowering the passing score from 90% to the current 80% [19]. Under the final rule, laboratories that use LDTs were to establish performance characteristics for their home-brew tests, including accuracy, precision, analytical sensitivity and specificity, reportable range, and reference intervals [8, 20].

In summary, the regulatory landscape for in vitro diagnostics and laboratory-developed tests (LDTs) has evolved significantly over the decades, shaped by advances in technology, clinical needs, and public health concerns. Beginning with the Medical Device Amendments of 1976, the FDA classified LDTs as medical devices but exercised enforcement discretion due to their limited scope and use in specialized settings. LDTs were regulated under CLIA'88, which established universal quality standards for all laboratories, regardless of their participation in interstate commerce or federal programs. While FDA started to try to introduce additional layers of regulation, enforcement remained selective. These initial attempts signaled the FDA's intention to further their oversight of LDTs.

FDA Regulations of Laboratory Developed Tests

Since the early 2000s, the FDA has increasingly expressed concerns regarding laboratory-developed tests (LDTs) and has more frequently signaled its intent to implement regulatory oversight of these tests (Fig. 11.3).

In June 2010, the FDA announced that a public meeting would occur on July 19th and 20th to discuss increased oversight of LDTs. The notice states that in 1976, homebrew tests were considered relatively simple, well-characterized, and low-risk,

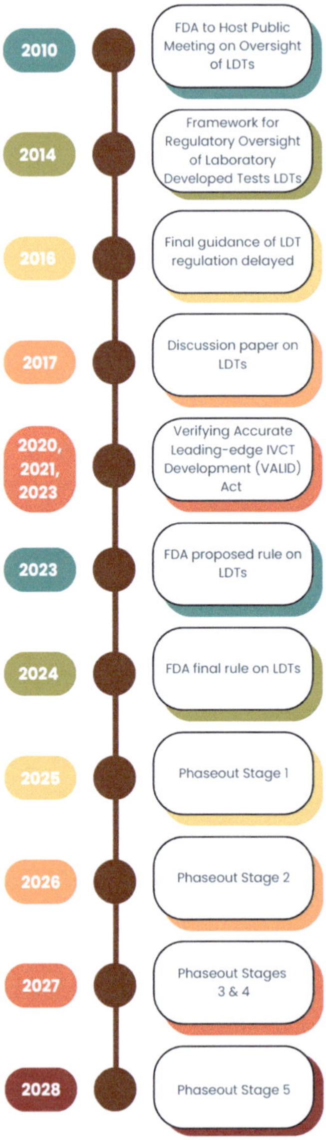

Fig. 11.3 Recent FDA regulations of laboratory developed tests

and were performed within a single healthcare entity in which the patient was being treated. Since that time, however, technological leaps have allowed commercial laboratories to have greater geographic reach, and LDTs became more accessible to patients. In addition, many providers and patients were relying more heavily on LDTs for information on which to base critical clinical decision-making. At the public meeting, the FDA discussed enforcement discretion, stating that the law for regulating LDTs was already in effect; however, there was no active enforcement [8, 21].

The FDA issued a document outlining how regulation would be enforced for LDTs in 2014 (Framework for Regulatory Oversight of Laboratory Developed Tests, LDTs), which would halt enforcement discretion [8]. The change in the FDA's interest in regulating home-brew tests was due to another leap in technological advances that led to increasingly complex testing, faster transportation of specimens, and a less centralized model of test reporting. Many commercial labs, unaffiliated with a hospital, were now offering tests to patients regardless of where they lived in relation to the laboratory [21]. At this time, tests that were "intended for clinical use and designed, manufactured, and used within a single laboratory" were defined as LDTs [22].

The FDA intended to use risk-based assessment to determine the level of oversight for individual LDTs [22]. LDTs with particular characteristics would still be under enforcement discretion, such as those created and used within a single lab operating within an associated healthcare facility, for patients being treated in said facility. Also excluded from enforcement were assays that used components or instruments that were FDA approved and that were interpreted by laboratory professionals without automated instrumentation or software [22]. In addition, the draft guidance laid out the FDA notification process and requirements for notification, reporting, and a possible approach to quality system regulation. A second document, titled *FDA Notification and Medical Device Reporting for Laboratory Developed Tests (LDTs),* detailed FDA notification of LDTs and adverse event reporting requirements [8].

After the election results, on November 18, 2016 the FDA halted efforts to finalize guidance of regulations of LDTs, stating that they would wait for the new administration [23, 24]. However, in 2017, since the FDA had not yet issued formal regulatory guidance for LDTs, the agency published a document with the intent to encourage continued discussion on the topic, which summarized stakeholder and public feedback elicited after the 2014 draft guidance [25].

The Verifying Accurate Leading-edge IVCT Development (VALID) Act was first introduced in 2020 by the House Energy and Commerce committee as H.R.6102 [26] and by the Senate Health, Education, Labor, and Pensions (HELP) committee as S.3404 [27]. It was reintroduced in 2021 by the same committees as H.R.4128 [28], and S.2209 [29], respectively. This bill is intended to amend the FD&C Act to include, in addition to drugs and devices, a new category termed 'in vitro clinical tests' (IVCT).

An IVCT was defined as a test intended by its developer to be used in the collection, preparation, analysis, or in vitro clinical examination of specimens taken or derived from the human body for the purpose of (i) identifying or diagnosing a disease or condition; (ii) providing information for diagnosing, screening, measuring, detecting, predicting, prognosing, analyzing, or monitoring a disease or condition, including by making a determination of an individual's state of health; or (iii) selecting, monitoring, or informing therapy or treatment for a disease or condition; and may include (i) a test protocol or laboratory test protocol; (ii) an instrument; (iii) a specimen receptacle; (iv) software; and is not part of an exclusion [27–29]. This new category thus would encompass both IVDs and LDTs.

IVCTs are further subdivided into low- and high-risk categories. Low-risk tests are exempt from premarket review, while high-risk ICVTs would require preapproval review. A low-risk test is one where an undetected inaccurate result would cause minimal or no harm, or minimal or no disability, or immediately reversible harm, or would lead to only a remote risk of adverse patient impact or adverse public health impact, or has a high risk but there are mitigating measures established to prevent, detect, or otherwise mitigate the risk of inaccurate results. A high-risk test is one where an undetected inaccurate result would present unreasonable risk for serious or irreversible harm or death to a patient or patients, or would otherwise cause serious harm to the public health, or is potentially likely to result in the absence, significant delay, or discontinuation of life-supporting or life-sustaining medical treatment [27–29].

As the bill was not passed in 2021, it was again reintroduced by the House Energy and Commerce committee, this time in conjunction with the House Ways and Means committee, as H.R.2369 in 2023; however, this too did not pass, and did not have a related Senate bill [30].

On October 3, 2023, the FDA proposed to amend its definition of "in vitro diagnostic products" to confirm that all IVDs, including those manufactured by laboratories, are considered devices under the FD&C Act (FDA proposed rule on LDTs) [31]. Further, the FDA's amendment aimed to clarify the regulatory landscape and align LDTs with other IVDs by phasing out the FDA's historical policy of general enforcement discretion for LDTs and subjecting them to the same regulatory requirements as other IVDs.

On May 6, 2024, the FDA published its final rule, essentially finalizing its 2023 proposed rule, that effective July 5, 2024, (i) IVDs are devices under FD&C Act, including when the manufacturer of the IVD is a laboratory; and (ii) the general enforcement discretion approach for LDTs would be phased out so that IVDs manufactured by a laboratory will generally fall under the same enforcement approach as other IVDs. However, targeted enforcement discretion policies will exist for several categories of IVDs manufactured by a laboratory in certain circumstances. Categories where some or all of the applicable requirements will generally not be enforced include: Public Health Surveillance tests, 1976-type LDTs, HLA tests for transplantation, forensic tests, LDTs manufactured and performed within the Department of Defense and Veterans Health Administration, LDTs for unmet needs manufactured and performed by labs integrated in the healthcare system treating the patient, currently marketed IVDs offered as LDTs first marketed prior to rule publication date and not modified beyond scope described in preamble, non-molecular antisera LDTs for rare red blood cell antigens, LDTs approved by New York State Clinical Laboratory Evaluation Program, and modified version of another manufacturer's 510(k) cleared or De Novo authorized test [32].

The phaseout period is set to occur over a four-year period and will include five stages. Stage 1 will call for compliance with medical device reporting requirements, correction and removal reporting requirements, and quality system requirements regarding complaint files. Stage 2 will cover requirements not included in other stages, such as registration, labeling, and investigational use requirements. Stage 3 will expect compliance with quality system requirements other than the complaint files covered by Stage 1. In Stage 4, unless a premarket submission has been received, premarket review is expected for high-risk IVDs, and Stage 5 will expand this to include moderate- and low-risk IVDs [32].

The New York State Regulations on LDTs

In the FDA's final rule, assays that were approved by the New York State (NYS) Clinical Laboratory Evaluation Program (CLEP) were considered as a separate category. This section provides an overview of the LDTs approval process for NYS CLEP [32].

The CLEP is a regulatory framework overseen by the New York State Department of Health (NYSDOH) to ensure the quality and accuracy of clinical laboratory testing, including LDTs. CLEP requires laboratories to obtain permits from the NYSDOH and to be compliant with both CLIA standard and additional state-specific rigorous requirements before performing clinical testing on specimens from New York residents [33].

New York State requires laboratories to submit detailed validation data for all LDTs and to undergo a rigorous approval process before implementation. Those validation data include analytical performance (accuracy, precision, linearity, sensitivity, and specificity, and reference ranges), clinical validity and utility, and quality assurance documentation. Tests are reviewed to ensure they meet the required analytical and clinical performance criteria. Laboratories may not offer an LDT until it is officially approved. CLEP conducts ongoing inspections to monitor laboratories' adherence to regulations. Approved LDTs are subject to periodic review to ensure ongoing compliance [33, 34].

Both CLEP and FDA categorize testing using a risk-based assessment. For CLEP, a Risk Attestation form is completed, and the organization then undergoes a review process to place the assay into high, moderate, or low risk. Testing may not be offered clinically until the review process has determined an assay's level of risk [32–34].

Conditional approval can be given to some testing, however high risk LDTs are not eligible, and full approval must be achieved before the assay is offered to patients. In the case of a moderate risk test, conditional approval is given when the laboratory holds a permit in the relevant testing category. CLEP also outlines requirements for adverse reporting, documentation, and proficiency testing, among other considerations (e.g., facility design, human resources) [34, 35].

In summary, the CLEP program establishes one of the most stringent oversight systems for LDTs in the United States. By mandating pre-approval, validation, and ongoing monitoring, New York State ensures that laboratory-developed tests meet high standards of quality and reliability, safeguarding patient care and outcomes.

Impact of the FDA Final Rules on LDTs

At the current time, the impact of the FDA final rule on LDTs is mostly conjecture; however, having witnessed the amount of additional work, personnel, and cost required when labs moved to meet CLIA requirements in the 1990s, it is not hard to see where this new regulation could make significant impacts. Additionally, the final rule will result in labs performing LDTs being subject to duplicative regulation by two federal agencies. This section will attempt to outline the possible impacts of the FDA final rule on the laboratories performing LDTs, on the patients who benefit from LDTs, and on the healthcare systems and providers who rely on LDTs.

Impact on the Lab

Currently, there is little to no information available from the FDA on how exactly labs need to go about meeting the requirements of each phase, even though stage 1 is due in May 2025, less than 4 months at the time of writing this chapter. For example, stage 1 calls for compliance with medical device reporting requirements, correction and removal reporting requirements, and quality system requirements regarding complaint files. No doubt, documentation and forms will need to be submitted to the FDA for each LDT performed in order to accomplish this stage; however, there has been no information forthcoming yet on how to do that, where to find the forms, exactly what forms are required, etc. Most clinical labs, especially hospital labs, have no experience with the FDA or with FDA's processes for submitting a test or test information to the FDA. Thus, labs will most likely need to hire people with this experience if they wish to continue performing LDTs. Resources of time, money, and personnel may need to be added and will be tied up with this effort, especially if the lab is performing many LDTs.

Stage 2 covers registration, labeling, and investigational use requirements, and although it is generally understood that the FDA will charge fees for registration of LDTs, there has been no information on what those fees will be, or even if they will be per LDT or per institution. The cost to a lab that performs many LDTs may be high enough that institutions may not support it, and labs may decide not to continue or not to start performing LDTs. Certainly, even more thought and planning than usually happens before developing a test will be necessary if the development includes FDA processes, costs, and timelines.

Thus, it is likely that becoming compliant with the FDA final rule will be both costly and resource expensive for labs that currently perform many LDTs. Even tests which are currently exempt from some requirements, like unmet need tests, will cost money and take time to be registered and meet the requirements they will still need to meet. Currently, exempt tests still need to meet the requirements of stages 1, 2, and part of 3.

Impact on Patients

Many patients are currently benefitting from the results of LDTs. An example of this is current testing for inborn errors of metabolism (IEM), most of which is performed using mass spectrometry. These tests currently fall into the "unmet need" category and are critically important because normal development and a normal life for an infant with an IEM depend almost entirely on how fast the diagnosis is made and treatment is begun. If labs can no longer afford to develop and run these LDTs, fewer and fewer labs will have this testing available. Infants and families may be required to travel long distances to find a lab still performing the tests, or their samples may take extra time to reach a lab performing them. The delay can make a difference between a normal life and a compromised one for the infant, and in the case of some IEM, between life or death.

IEM testing is an extreme example; however, less extreme examples are equally impactful to the patients who rely on these tests. Currently, antifungal drug testing is almost entirely performed by mass spectrometry LDTs. If labs are unable to continue providing this testing, and the patient samples must be sent out to a distant reference lab, the potential exists for the patient to spend extra days in the hospital while awaiting the results of his antifungal test so that dosing can be adjusted or have to make multiple trips to the healthcare facility for dosing adjustments. Adjusting a dose, waiting 3 days for a new drug level, then adjusting the dose again, and again waiting 3 days, is not good healthcare.

A third example of the impact of FDA regulation of LDTs on patients is toxicology testing, and especially emergency toxicology testing. While most chemistry analyzers have a panel of drugs that can be tested in urine samples by immunoassay, many of those drugs are reported as a class of drugs, i.e., positive for benzodiazepines. Additionally, immunoassays are highly susceptible to interferences via cross-reacting compounds, leading to false positives or false negatives, and cannot be adapted to changing drugs being seen in the community. Mass spectrometry-based LDTs are the only good way of detecting and reporting specific drugs accurately at the lower limits and across a broad dynamic range. These tests are also the only ones adaptable enough to attempt to keep up with changing patterns of synthetic and non-synthetic drugs out on the streets. If laboratories stop offering these tests due to FDA regulation, the patient impact could be as severe as death from unknown substance overdoses. Even without that extreme, treatment of patients without the testing available to determine what drugs are onboard may be empiric and ineffective.

These are only three of many examples of the direct impact the FDA's final rule will have on patients.

Impact on Healthcare

One of the primary reasons that LDTs exist is that there is not an FDA-approved test that meets the needs of the patient population being served. Currently, developing and completely validating an LDT may cost a lab several thousand dollars and take roughly a year. IVD companies can spend up to several million dollars and over 5 years to develop and bring a new test to market through the FDA process. In an era when technology is advancing so rapidly, FDA's process is almost ludicrous.

In 1977, the FDA described exemptions from its oversight because clinical laboratories provided a benefit to the consumer through the use of medical devices. The benefit to patients and to the entire healthcare field is more pronounced today than ever before. In the same way that IVD manufacturers currently hesitate to improve their assays if it means resubmitting them through the FDA, currently exempt LDTs may not be improved upon, and new ones will not be developed under FDA regulation. LDTs can currently be produced and provide the necessary and timely benefits to patient care. That ability to make timely healthcare possible will be lost under the FDA's final rule. Hospital labs do not have the resources, time, or money to take a test through the FDA and will not continue to develop LDTs. Thus, innovative new test solutions for immediate patient care will likely become a thing of the past.

Future of the Regulatory Landscape of MS-Based Assays

The future of the regulatory landscape is hard to predict at this time. The FDA's final rule is being challenged in court by two court cases, maintaining that the FDA has no authority to regulate LDTs because they are not "devices." LDTs are services performed within the practice of medicine by medical professionals, and the FDA CANNOT regulate the practice of medicine. Whether the final rule will be enacted or not is unknown, as there are pending court challenges at this moment. Other things that may happen first include: The US Department of Health and Human Services (HHS) could revoke the final rule; Congress could act to legislate the regulation of LDTs in place of the final rule, giving LDT regulation back to CLIA and CMS; the plaintiffs could win the lawsuit and the final rule be struck down, or lose it and the final rule would go into effect or be challenged by additional lawsuits.

In this day of rapidly advancing technology, the FDA's regulation of the entire IVD landscape needs to be overhauled, a topic that is beyond the scope of this chapter. In the meantime, mass spectrometry-based testing will continue to be developed as it is often the only way or the best way to measure necessary analytes and meet the healthcare needs of the patients. If the FDA indeed regulates LDTs, labs will find a way to meet the regulatory requirements and continue to provide the needed testing.

At the final stage of reviewing this chapter, a significant legal development occurred. On March 31, 2025, US District Court Judge Sean D. Jordan struck down the FDA's final rule asserting regulatory authority over laboratory-developed tests (LDTs), ruling that the agency lacked statutory authority to regulate them. This decision marks a pivotal moment in the ongoing debate over LDT oversight and reinforces longstanding arguments made by the laboratory community. Rather than revising earlier discussions in this chapter, we have opted to preserve them in their original form so that readers can fully appreciate the process that led to this ruling. The progression of perspectives, advocacy efforts, and regulatory debates outlined throughout this chapter provides important context for understanding the implications of this decision.

Conclusion

Mass spectrometry-based assays have been an integral part of clinical diagnostics to support critical patient needs. The superior, adaptable characteristics of these assays are essential to ensure the highest quality possible results are provided for patients. Mass spectrometry assays have always been regulated under the CLIA regulations. Although regulation of clinical laboratories and medical devices has been ongoing since 1938, there has been recent focus on LDTs, or home-brew tests, by the Food and Drug Administration (FDA). The FDA has broadcast its concerns and intention to regulate LDTs as any other laboratory test, beginning in 2010, with a public meeting. A framework for regulation and several iterations of the VALID Act attempted to more fully regulate laboratory-developed tests, however, all iterations were defeated, and nothing changed. With technological advances, more widespread use of clinical laboratory testing, and safety concerns, the federal government has repeatedly asserted its authority to ensure that laboratories are accountable for the safety and efficacy of their test menus. As more contemporary technology, transportation methods, and de-centralized laboratory testing have gained momentum, FDA intends to fully regulate all laboratory testing, including those developed and used within a single laboratory. As of May 2024, the FDA published its new rule to regulate LDTs, and a four-year-long phaseout process has begun, which will ensure that all testing is compliant with the FDA's regulations. Whether this final rule will stand up in court to lawsuits claiming the FDA has no authority to regulate LDTs and be enacted is as yet unknown. Whatever the outcome, mass spectrometry-based testing will continue to be developed to meet patients' healthcare needs.

References

1. Part II. Food, drug, cosmetic act. U.S. Food & Drug Administration; 1938. 29/2024. https://www.fda.gov/about-fda/changes-science-law-and-regulatory-authorities/part-ii-1938-food-drug-cosmetic-act

2. Lam C, Patel P. Food, drug, and cosmetic act. StatPearls Publishing. Updated 2023 Jul 31. https://www.ncbi.nlm.nih.gov/books/NBK585046/.
3. Public Health Service Act. Public Health Rep. 1944;59(28):468.
4. Snyder L. Passage and significance of the 1944 Public Health Service Act. Public Health Rep. 1994;109(6):721–4.
5. Wilcox A. The Public Health Service Act, 1944. Soc Secur Bull. 1944;August:15–7.
6. Partnership for Health Amendments of 1967. (PL 90–174, December 5, 1967) United States Statutes at Large, 81 (1967) pp. 533–42.
7. Rivers PA, Dobalian A, Germinario FA. A review and analysis of the clinical laboratory improvement amendment of 1988: compliance plans and enforcement policy. Health Care Manag Rev. 2005;30(2):93–102. https://doi.org/10.1097/00004010-200504000-00003.
8. Genzen JR, Mohlman JS, Lynch JL, Squires MW, Weiss RL. Laboratory-developed tests: a legislative and regulatory review. Clin Chem. 2017;63(10):1575–84. https://doi.org/10.1373/clinchem.2017.275164.
9. United States v. Bacto-Unidisk, 394 U.S. 784 (1969).
10. 37 Fed. Reg. 160 (August 17, 1972) pp. 16613–7.
11. Medical Device Amendments of 1976. (PL94–295, May 28, 1976) United States Statutes at Large, 90 (1976) pp. 539–83.
12. Center for Devices and Radiological Health. A history of medical device regulation and oversight in the US. U.S. Food and Drug Administration, FDA; 2023. www.fda.gov/medical-devices/overview-device-regulation/history-medical-device-regulation-oversight-united-states.
13. Congress, Medical Device Amendments to the FD&C Act. Library of Congress (1976), pp. 94–295.
14. Public Law 100–578, Section 353 Public Health Service Act (42 USC 263a) October 31, 1988.
15. Brophy MA. The clinical laboratory improvement program: not your ordinary regulatory program. Mil Med. 2000;165(7 Suppl 2):48–51.
16. FDA. Draft compliance policy guide: commercialization of unapproved in vitro diagnostic devices labeled for research and investigation; 1992.
17. Shapiro JK, Prebula RJ. FDA's regulation of analyte-specific reagents; 2003, p. 25.
18. 62 Fed. Reg. 225 (November 21, 1997) pp. 62243–60.
19. 68 Fed. Reg. 16 (January 24, 2003) pp. 3641–714.
20. 68 Fed. Reg. 16 (January 24, 2003) p. 3707.
21. FDA News Release. June 16, 2010. https://wayback.archive-it.org/7993/20161023122106/http:/www.fda.gov/NewsEvents/Newsroom/PressAnnouncements/2010/ucm215766.htm (Accessed November 14, 2024).
22. 79 Fed. Reg. 192 (October 3, 2014) p. 59776–79.
23. Brennan Z. FDA delays finalization of lab-developed test draft guidance. RAPS.Org, Regulatory Affairs Professionals Society; 2016. www.raps.org/News-and-Articles/News-Articles/2016/11/FDA-Delays-Finalization-of-Lab-Developed-Test-Draf.
24. Gibbs JN. LDTs: the Saga continues. Update Magazine, Food and Drug Law Institute; 2017.
25. Discussion paper on laboratory developed tests. Food and Drug Administration; 2017. https://www.fda.gov/downloads/MedicalDevices/ProductsandMedicalProcedures/InVitroDiagnostics/LaboratoryDevelopedTests/UCM536965.pdf (Accessed November 2024).
26. H.R.6102 - 116th Congress (2019–2020): VALID Act of 2020. (2020, March 5). https://www.congress.gov/bill/116th-congress/house-bill/6102/text
27. S.3404 - 116th Congress (2019–2020): VALID Act of 2020. (2020, March 5). https://www.congress.gov/bill/116th-congress/senate-bill/3404/text
28. H.R.4128 - 117th Congress (2021–2022): VALID Act of 2021. (2021, June 25). https://www.congress.gov/bill/117th-congress/house-bill/4128/text
29. S.2209 - 117th Congress (2021–2022): VALID Act of 2021. (2021, June 24). https://www.congress.gov/bill/117th-congress/senate-bill/2209/text
30. H.R.2369 - 118th Congress (2023–2024): VALID Act of 2023. (2023, April 7). https://www.congress.gov/bill/118th-congress/house-bill/2369/text

31. 88 Fed. Reg. 190 (October 3, 2023), p. 68006–68031, https://www.govinfo.gov/content/pkg/FR-2023-10-03/pdf/2023-21662.pdf
32. 89 Fed. Reg. 88 (May 6, 2024) p. 37286–37445.
33. Tiered evaluation of laboratory developed tests policy. Wadsworth Center, New York State Department of Health; 2023. www.wadsworth.org/sites/default/files/WebDoc/Tiered_LDT_Review_Policy_Jan2020.pdf.
34. General systems standards. Wadsworth Center, New York State Department of Health; 2021. https://www.wadsworth.org/sites/default/files/WebDoc/EFFECTIVE_GeneralSystems_May2021_FINAL.pdf
35. Califf RM. AHA letter to the FDA on laboratory developed tests (LDTs) proposed rule. American Hospital Association; 2023. www.aha.org/lettercomment/2023-12-01-aha-letter-fda-laboratory-developed-tests-ldts-proposed-rule.

Bringing It All Together: Integrated Evaluation of Core Concepts of LC-MS/MS Applications in Clinical Laboratories

12

Y. Victoria Zhang and Uttam Garg

Chapter 1: Introduction

1. **Who is credited with introducing adsorption chromatography, marking the beginning of LC?**

   A. John Fenn
   B. Csaba Horváth
   C. Mikhail Tswett
   D. F.W. Aston

2. **What was one of the earliest clinical applications of mass spectrometry?**

   A. Vitamin D quantification
   B. Newborn screening for metabolic disorders
   C. Drug of abuse confirmation
   D. Thyroid hormone analysis

3. **Which ionization technique, developed by John Fenn, was instrumental for analyzing large biomolecules?**

   A. MALDI
   B. Electron ionization

Y. V. Zhang (✉)
Department of Pathology and Laboratory Medicine, University of Rochester Medical Center, Rochester, NY, USA
e-mail: Victoria_Zhang@urmc.rochester.edu

U. Garg
Pathology and Laboratory Medicine, Children's Mercy Hospital and University of Missouri-Kansas City School of Medicine, Kansas City, MO, USA

Y. V. Zhang, U. Garg (eds.), *Practical Guide to Implementing Liquid Chromatography Mass Spectrometry in Clinical Laboratories*,
https://doi.org/10.1007/978-3-032-03852-4_12

C. Electrospray ionization (ESI)
D. TOF-MS

4. **Why is LC-MS/MS considered the gold standard for drug of abuse testing?**

   A. Low operational cost
   B. Rapid analysis time
   C. High sensitivity and specificity
   D. Use of radioactive tracers

5. **Which assay was pivotal in demonstrating the limitations of immunoassays in low concentration measurement?**

   A. Vitamin D
   B. Testosterone
   C. Thyroglobulin
   D. Cortisol

6. **Which of the following is a limitation of mass spectrometry in peptide analysis?**

   A. Low resolution
   B. High reagent cost
   C. Missed detection of unknown variants
   D. Inability to measure steroids

7. **What type of mass spectrometer has dominated clinical applications so far?**

   A. Orbitrap
   B. Ion trap
   C. Triple quadrupole
   D. Time-of-flight

8. **Which clinical application relies heavily on LC-MS/MS for accurate dosing?**

   A. Toxicology screening
   B. Therapeutic drug monitoring
   C. Lipid profiling
   D. CBC analysis

9. **What major concern is raised when a peptide variant is biologically active but undetected by MS?**

   A. Increased false positives
   B. Extended run times
   C. Misdiagnosis due to inaccurate concentration
   D. Unnecessary retesting

10. **What is one advantage of MS over traditional immunoassays?**

    A. Lower maintenance needs
    B. Shorter instrument lifespan

C. Improved specificity for structurally similar analytes
D. Broader cross-reactivity

11. **Which is a key challenge in implementing LC-MS/MS in clinical labs?**

A. Low throughput
B. Automated vendor service contracts
C. Incompatibility with analyzers
D. Lack of reproducibility

12. **Which mass spectrometry imaging method offers analyte-specific visualization similar to histopathology?**

A. NMR
B. PET-CT
C. MS imaging
D. Western blot

Answer Key

1. C. Mikhail Tswett
2. B. Newborn screening for metabolic disorders
3. C. Electrospray ionization (ESI)
4. C. High sensitivity and specificity
5. B. Testosterone
6. C. Missed detection of unknown variants
7. C. Triple quadrupole
8. B. Therapeutic drug monitoring
9. C. Misdiagnosis due to inaccurate concentration
10. C. Improved specificity for structurally similar analytes
11. A. Low throughput
12. C. MS imaging

Chapter 2: Fundamentals of Mass Spectrometry

1. **Which ionization technique is best suited for analyzing large biomolecules like proteins and peptides with minimal fragmentation?**

A. Electron Ionization (EI)
B. Electrospray Ionization (ESI)
C. Chemical Ionization (CI)
D. Atmospheric Pressure Chemical Ionization (APCI)

2. **What was a major limitation of early GC–MS applications in clinical laboratories?**

A. Inability to analyze small molecules
B. Requirement for chemical derivatization of non-volatile compounds

C. Low sensitivity
D. Excessive fragmentation of biomolecules

3. **Which Nobel Prize-winning technique enables the analysis of solid-phase samples like crystallized specimens?**

A. Matrix-assisted laser desorption/ionization (MALDI)
B. Electrospray ionization (ESI)
C. Chemical ionization (CI)
D. Atmospheric pressure chemical ionization (APCI)

4. **What advantage does LC-MS/MS offer over immunoassays in clinical diagnostics?**

A. Lower cost
B. Faster turnaround time
C. Higher specificity and reduced cross-reactivity
D. Elimination of the need for sample preparation

5. **Which component of a mass spectrometer is responsible for converting neutral molecules into charged ions?**

A. Mass analyzer
B. Detector
C. Ion source
D. Collision cell

6. **In ESI, what phenomenon occurs when droplets reach the Rayleigh limit?**

A. Solvent evaporation stops
B. Droplets undergo fission or emit ions
C. Analyte degradation occurs
D. Ion suppression increases

7. **Which ionization technique is most suitable for nonpolar compounds like lipids and polycyclic aromatic hydrocarbons?**

A. ESI
B. APCI
C. APPI
D. MALDI

8. **What is the primary function of the matrix in MALDI?**

A. To separate ions by m/z
B. To absorb laser energy and assist in desorption/ionization
C. To fragment large molecules
D. To stabilize the sample in the gas phase

9. **Which mass analyzer is known for its high resolution and use of Fourier transform to generate mass spectra?**

A. Quadrupole
B. Ion trap
C. Orbitrap
D. TOF

10. **What is the main advantage of a triple quadrupole (QQQ) mass spectrometer?**

A. High resolution for untargeted analysis
B. High sensitivity and specificity for targeted quantification
C. Ability to analyze large proteins
D. Structural elucidation of unknown compounds without standards

11. **Which scan mode in QQQ-MS monitors specific precursor-product ion transitions for known compounds?**

A. Full scan
B. Product ion scan
C. Neutral loss scan
D. Selected reaction monitoring (SRM)

12. **What is the key difference between data-dependent acquisition (DDA) and data-independent acquisition (DIA)?**

A. DDA fragments all ions, while DIA selects ions based on abundance.
B. DDA selects abundant ions for MS/MS, while DIA fragments predefined m/z windows.
C. DDA is used only with MALDI, while DIA is for ESI.
D. DDA requires higher resolution than DIA.

13. **Which technology enables real-time molecular analysis during surgery by thermally ablating tissue?**

A. MasSpec Pen
B. iKnife (REIMS)
C. DESI
D. DART

14. **What is the primary challenge hindering widespread adoption of MS in clinical laboratories?**

A. Lack of specificity
B. Lack of sensitivity
C. Complexity, high cost, and need for expertise
D. Inability to analyze small molecules

15. **Which of the following is NOT a soft ionization technique?**

A. ESI
B. APCI
C. EI

D. MALDI

16. **What role does collision-induced dissociation (CID) play in tandem MS?**

    A. Ionizes neutral molecules
    B. Fragments precursor ions to generate product ions
    C. Separates ions by m/z
    D. It accelerates ions toward the detector to improve sensitivity

17. **Which mass analyzer is best suited for rapid, high-throughput microbial identification?**

    A. Quadrupole
    B. Ion Trap
    C. TOF
    D. Orbitrap

18. **What emerging technology could replace liquid chromatography (LC) by separating ions in the gas phase based on size, shape, and charge?**

    A. AI-driven spectral analysis
    B. Ion mobility spectrometry (IMS)
    C. Ambient ionization MS
    D. Fourier transform MS

Answer Key

1. B. Electrospray ionization (ESI)
2. B. Requirement for chemical derivatization of non-volatile compounds
3. A. Matrix-assisted laser desorption/ionization (MALDI)
4. C. Higher specificity and reduced cross-reactivity
5. C. Ion source
6. B. Droplets undergo fission or emit ions
7. C. APPI
8. B. To absorb laser energy and assist in desorption/ionization
9. C. Orbitrap
10. B. High sensitivity and specificity for targeted quantification
11. D. Selected reaction monitoring (SRM)
12. B. DDA selects abundant ions for MS/MS, while DIA fragments predefined *m/z* windows
13. B. iKnife (REIMS)
14. C. Complexity, high cost, and need for expertise
15. C. EI
16. B. Fragments precursor ions to generate product ions
17. C. TOF
18. B. Ion mobility spectrometry (IMS)

Chapter 3: Fundamentals of Liquid Chromatography

1. **The main difference between liquid chromatography (LC) and gas chromatography (GC) is:**

   A. LC uses a solid stationary phase, while GC uses a liquid stationary phase
   B. Sample injection method
   C. Nature of mobile phase
   D. Required temperature for separation of analytes

2. **What is the retention factor (k) used to describe in liquid chromatography (LC)?**

   A. Column length
   B. The maximum pressure a column can withstand
   C. Compound retention relative to void time
   D. Particle size

3. **Which liquid chromatography (LC) technique uses a non-polar stationary phase and a polar mobile phase?**

   A. Ion-exchange chromatography
   B. Reversed-phase LC (RPLC)
   C. Hydrophilic interaction LC (HILIC)
   D. Normal-phase LC

4. **A separation factor (α) greater than 1 indicates:**

   A. Complete peak overlap
   B. No retention
   C. Baseline separation
   D. Some degree of separation between peaks

5. **Increasing the flow-rate in LC will generally:**

   A. Sharpen all the peaks
   B. Reduces back-pressure
   C. Increase peak broadening and decrease resolution
   D. Always improve resolution

6. **Size-exclusion chromatography separates compounds primarily based on:**

   A. Charge
   B. Hydrophobicity
   C. Polarity
   D. Molecular size

7. **Which stationary phase is commonly used in hydrophilic interaction LC (HILIC)?**

   A. C18

B. Ion-exchange
C. Polar surface with water layer
D. Polystyrene resin

8. **A peak asymmetry factor (A/B) less than 1 indicates:**

A. Peak tailing
B. Peak fronting
C. Poor resolution between peaks
D. Broad baseline

9. **An advantage of HILIC over RPLC is:**

A. Faster analysis time
B. Better separation of non-polar compounds
C. Better separation of polar or charged compounds
D. No need for gradient elution

10. **In ion-exchange chromatography (IEC), increasing ionic strength of the mobile phase will:**

A. Increase retention time
B. Decrease retention time
C. Cause peak fronting
D. Improve peak shape

11. **What is a typical feature of UPLC compared to HPLC?**

A. Lower pressure than HPLC
B. Smaller particle sizes for faster separations
C. Slower run times
D. Lower resolution

12. **Gradient elution is most beneficial for:**

A. Single compound analysis
B. Separating compounds with similar polarities
C. Complex mixtures with variable retention
D. Volatile analytes

13. **Affinity chromatography differs from other LC types by:**

A. Using charge interactions
B. Using molecular size for separation
C. Using specific interaction with an immobilized-ligand
D. Requiring organic solvents

14. **Ion-pair chromatography is used for:**

A. Retaining neutral molecules
B. Using counter ions to retain ionic compounds on non-polar columns
C. Separating compounds based on their polarity in a hydrophobic environment

D. Size-based separation

Answer Key

1. C. Nature of mobile phase
2. C. Compound retention relative to void time
3. B. Reversed-phase LC (RPLC)
4. D. Some degree of separation between peaks
5. C. Increase peak broadening and decrease resolution
6. D. Molecular size
7. C. Polar surface with water layer
8. B. Peak fronting
9. C. Better separation of polar or charged compounds
10. B. Decrease retention time
11. B. Smaller particle sizes for faster separations
12. C. Complex mixtures with variable retention
13. C. Using specific interaction with an immobilized-ligand
14. B. Using counter ions to retain ionic compounds on non-polar columns

Chapter 4: Sample Preparation for LC-MS/MS Analysis

1. **What is the primary purpose of sample preparation in LC-MS/MS analysis?**

   A. To increase the speed of analysis
   B. To reduce the cost of the analysis
   C. To eliminate the need for internal standards
   D. To separate the analyte(s) of interest from the biological matrix

2. **Which ionization source typically exhibits more matrix effects in LC-MS/MS?**

   A. Atmospheric pressure chemical ionization (APCI)
   B. Electrospray ionization (ESI)
   C. Matrix-assisted laser desorption/ionization (MALDI)
   D. Fast atom bombardment (FAB)

3. **What is a major disadvantage of protein precipitation (PPT)?**

   A. It requires very large sample volumes
   B. It cannot be automated
   C. It introduces significant matrix effects due to residual phospholipids
   D. It is too expensive for routine use

4. **Which technique combines principles of LLE with a solid support material to improve efficiency?**

A. SPE
B. Ion mobility
C. Immunoprecipitation (IP)
D. Supported liquid extraction (SLE)

5. **What is the primary advantage of supported liquid extraction (SLE) over traditional LLE?**

A. Lower cost
B. No need for organic solvents
C. Faster extraction time
D. Reduced risk of emulsion formation and better automation compatibility

6. **Which sample preparation method is most selective for weakly acidic or basic analytes?**

A. Mixed-mode SPE
B. Reversed-phase SPE
C. Hydrophilic interaction liquid chromatography (HILIC)
D. Phospholipid depletion (PLD)

7. **What is a key limitation of dilute and shoot (D&S)?**

A. It cannot be used for urine samples
B. It requires derivatization
C. It introduces all matrix components into the LC-MS/MS system
D. It is only suitable for high-concentration analytes

8. **What is the primary use of derivatization in LC-MS/MS?**

A. To reduce sample volume
B. To enhance detection sensitivity for certain analytes (e.g., hormones)
C. To increase the volatility of analytes for easier ionization
D. To speed up chromatography

9. **What is a major challenge in dried blood spot (DBS) analysis?**

A. High sample volume requirements
B. Inability to use internal standards
C. Hematocrit effect causing variability in analyte recovery
D. DBS samples are unstable at room temperature

10. **Which technique is commonly used for protein/peptide analysis in bottom-up proteomics?**

A. Dilute and shoot
B. Protein precipitation
C. Trypsin digestion followed by SPE or IP
D. QuEChERS

11. **Which of the following is an advantage of online SPE?**

A. No need for evaporation steps
B. Lower instrument cost
C. Simpler method development
D. No matrix effects

12. **What is a common issue with manual liquid–liquid extraction (LLE)?**

A. Inability to concentrate analytes
B. Risk of incomplete phase separation and emulsion formation
C. High cost of organic solvents
D. LLE requires derivatization

13. **Which technique is best suited for concentrating analytes from large sample volumes?**

A. D&S
B. PPT
C. SPE
D. PLD

14. **What is the primary benefit of using 96-well plates in sample preparation?**

A. Reduced sample volume
B. Lower matrix effects
C. No need for internal standards
D. Higher throughput and automation compatibility

15. **What is the main purpose of tracking system suitability test (SST) parameters in LC-MS/MS?**

A. To reduce sample preparation time
B. To eliminate the need for internal standards
C. To automate data analysis
D. To monitor instrument performance and detect degradation over time

Answer Key

1. D. To separate the analyte(s) of interest from the biological matrix
2. B. Electrospray ionization (ESI)
3. C. It introduces significant matrix effects due to residual phospholipids
4. D. Supported liquid extraction (SLE)
5. D. Reduced risk of emulsion formation and better automation compatibility
6. A. Mixed-mode SPE
7. C. It introduces all matrix components into the LC-MS/MS system
8. B. To enhance detection sensitivity for certain analytes (e.g., hormones)
9. C. Hematocrit effect causing variability in analyte recovery
10. C. Trypsin digestion followed by SPE or IP
11. A. No need for evaporation steps

12. B. Risk of incomplete phase separation and emulsion formation
13. C. SPE
14. D. Higher throughput and automation compatibility
15. D. To monitor instrument performance and detect degradation over time

Chapter 5: Specific Lab Techniques for LC-MS/MS Analysis

1. **What is the first step in implementing LC-MS/MS in a clinical laboratory?**

   A. Vendor qualification
   B. Defining the clinical need and site preparation
   C. Reagent selection
   D. Hiring staff

2. **What is the minimum resistivity required for type I water used in LC-MS/MS?**

   A. 10 MΩ-cm
   B. 18 MΩ-cm
   C. 5 MΩ-cm
   D. 1 MΩ-cm

3. **Why are isotopically labeled internal standards preferred in LC-MS/MS?**

   A. They mimic the behavior of the analyte and reduce variability
   B. They eliminate the need for sample preparation
   C. They require no method validation
   D. They improve chromatographic separation between analytes

4. **What is the purpose of a system suitability test (SST) in LC-MS/MS?**

   A. To qualify vendors
   B. To calibrate the MS
   C. To verify chromatographic and MS performance before analysis
   D. To prepare mobile phases

5. **What is the recommended technique for handling viscous liquids with an air displacement pipette?**

   A. Forward mode
   B. No pre-wetting
   C. Using a syringe
   D. Reverse mode with wide-bore tips

6. **Why should guard columns be used in LC-MS/MS systems?**

   A. To increase flow rate
   B. To protect the analytical column from contaminants
   C. To reduce the need for mobile phases

D. To enhance the sensitivity of the mass spectrometer

7. **Which mobile phase modifier is recommended to avoid salt buildup in the MS source?**

   A. Ammonium formate
   B. Sodium phosphate
   C. Potassium chloride
   D. Sulfuric acid

8. **What is the minimum recommended air changes per hour (ACH) for occupied laboratories using chemicals?**

   A. 4 ACH
   B. 8 ACH
   C. 12 ACH
   D. 2 ACH

9. **Which of the following is NOT a recommended step for column conditioning?**

   A. Using non-volatile buffers for equilibration
   B. Flushing with 10 column volumes of storage solvent
   C. Transitioning to the desired mobile phase gradually
   D. Avoiding bacterial growth by purging with organic solvent

10. **What is the primary advantage of using positive displacement pipettes for volatile liquids?**

    A. Lower cost
    B. Faster dispensing
    C. Reduced impact of environmental conditions on measurement accuracy
    D. Compatibility with all tip types

11. **What is the primary risk of leaving aqueous solutions in an idle LC-MS/MS system?**

    A. Decreased backpressure
    B. Improved column longevity
    C. Bacterial growth and clogging
    D. Enhanced detector performance

12. **What is the purpose of pre-wetting pipette tips in forward mode pipetting?**

    A. To reduce tip cost
    B. To condition the air inside the tip and improve accuracy
    C. To increase dispensing speed
    D. To avoid touching the container wall

13. **Which of the following is a recommended practice for mobile phase preparation?**

    A. Using non-volatile salts
    B. Preparing large batches to save time
    C. Mix solvents directly in the LC reservoir
    D. Storing mobile phases in airtight containers to prevent contamination

Answer Key

1. B. Defining the clinical need and site preparation
2. B. 18 MΩ-cm
3. A. They mimic the behavior of the analyte and reduce variability
4. C. To verify chromatographic and MS performance before analysis
5. D. Reverse mode with wide-bore tips
6. B. To protect the analytical column from contaminants
7. A. Ammonium formate
8. B. 8 ACH
9. A. Using non-volatile buffers for equilibration
10. C. Reduced impact of environmental conditions on measurement accuracy
11. C. Bacterial growth and clogging
12. B. To condition the air inside the tip and improve accuracy
13. D. Storing mobile phases in airtight containers to prevent contamination

Chapter 6: Method Development and Validation for LC-MS/MS Analysis

1. **What is the FIRST step in developing an LC-MS/MS method for clinical use?**

   A. Optimizing collision energy
   B. Defining the intended clinical application
   C. Selecting a mass spectrometer vendor
   D. Preparing calibrators

2. **Which of the following is a key advantage of using MRM mode in triple quadrupole MS?**

   A. Ability to analyze large biomolecules without fragmentation
   B. High specificity via selective precursor/fragment ion monitoring
   C. Lower cost compared to single-stage MS
   D. No need for chromatographic separation

3. **What is the primary purpose of a calibration curve in quantitative LC-MS/MS?**

A. To reduce matrix effects
B. To shorten analysis time
C. To diagnose instrument malfunctions
D. To establish the relationship between analyte concentration and detector response

4. **Which parameter is critical for assessing method precision?**

A. Relative standard deviation (RSD) of replicate measurements
B. Limit of detection (LOD)
C. Retention time
D. Column temperature

5. **What does "selectivity"refer to in method validation?**

A. The speed of chromatographic separation
B. The sensitivity of the mass spectrometer
C. The method's ability to distinguish the analyte from interferents
D. The purity of the mobile phase

6. **A common cause of ion suppression in LC-MS/MS is:**

A. Co-eluting matrix components (e.g., phospholipids)
B. High flow rate
C. Low column temperature
D. Use of a long LC column

7. **Why is dwell time optimization important in MRM methods?**

A. To reduce instrument cost
B. To eliminate the need for internal standards
C. To ensure sufficient data points per chromatographic peak (12–20 points)
D. To shorten method development time

8. **Which ionization source is preferred for polar molecules in LC-MS/MS?**

A. APCI
B. Electron impact (EI)
C. Electrospray ionization (ESI)
D. MALDI

9. **What is the purpose of a "matrix factor" assessment?**

A. To quantify ion suppression/enhancement caused by sample matrix
B. To calculate column lifetime
C. To determine optimal LC flow rate
D. To validate software integration

10. **Why are stable isotope-labeled internal standards (SIL-IS) preferred in LC-MS/MS?**

A. They are cheaper than chemical analogs

B. They eliminate the need for chromatographic separation
C. They reduce data file size
D. They closely mimic analyte behavior during extraction/ionization

11. **Which of the following is a key metric for assessing chromatographic performance?**

A. Retention factor (k) between 2 and 10
B. Dwell time <1 ms
C. Mobile phase pH >7
D. Column length >150 mm

12. **What is the primary goal of sample preparation in LC-MS/MS?**

A. To increase analyte volatility
B. To isolate the analyte from matrix interferents
C. To reduce MS resolution requirements
D. To eliminate the need for calibration

13. **Which sample preparation technique is most effective for removing phospholipids?**

A. Protein precipitation
B. Solid-phase extraction (SPE) with phospholipid removal plates
C. Derivatization
D. Dilute-and-shoot

14. **What is the purpose of "parallelism" experiments during method development?**

A. To optimize collision energy
B. To validate software algorithms
C. To compare LC columns from different vendors
D. To evaluate commutability between calibration matrix and patient samples

15. **Which of the following is a critical component of system suitability testing (SST)?**

A. Monitoring RT reproducibility and peak shape in replicate injections
B. Assessing laboratory staff training records
C. Validating LIMS integration
D. Calculating patient reference intervals

16. **Why is method robustness tested during pre-validation?**

A. To reduce the number of calibrators
B. To eliminate the need for QC samples
C. To shorten chromatographic run times
D. To ensure consistent performance across reagent lots/instruments

17. **What is the typical acceptance criterion for accuracy at the LLMI during validation?**

    A. ±5%
    B. ±20%
    C. ±50%
    D. No criteria required

18. **Which statistical method is used to evaluate method comparison data?**

    A. Student's *t*-test
    B. ANOVA
    C. Chi-square test
    D. Passing-Bablok regression

19. **How many samples are typically required to establish reference intervals?**

    A. 20
    B. 120
    C. 500
    D. 1000

20. **What is the primary goal of method validation?**

    A. To reduce instrument maintenance
    B. To eliminate matrix effects
    C. To automate data analysis
    D. To confirm reliability and accuracy for clinical use

Answer Key

1. B. Clinical application defines performance requirements.
2. B. MRM provides specificity via selective ion transitions.
3. D. Calibration curves quantify concentration-response relationships.
4. A. Precision is measured via RSD.
5. C. Selectivity ensures no interferents skew results.
6. A. Matrix components suppress ionization.
7. C. Dwell time ensures adequate peak sampling.
8. C. ESI is ideal for polar molecules.
9. A. Matrix factor quantifies ion suppression/enhancement.
10. D. SIL-IS tracks analyte behavior.
11. A. Retention factor balances resolution and peak broadening.
12. B. Sample prep removes interferents.
13. B. Phospholipid removal plates reduce matrix effects.
14. D. Parallelism ensures matrix commutability.
15. A. Monitoring RT reproducibility and peak shape in replicate injections
16. D. To ensure consistent performance across reagent lots/instruments

17. B. ±20% is common for LLMI accuracy.
18. D. Passing-Bablok evaluates method agreement.
19. B. 120 samples ensure statistical significance.
20. D. Validation confirms clinical reliability.

Chapter 7: Instrument and Assay Maintenance for LC-MS/MS Analysis

1. **What is the primary goal of a comprehensive LC-MS/MS maintenance program?**
   A. To reduce the cost of reagents and the need for trained personnel
   B. To eliminate the need for service contracts
   C. To shorten method validation time
   D. To ensure continuous high-quality results and trouble-free instrument operation
2. **Which of the following is NOT typically included in an LC-MS/MS maintenance SOP?**
   A. Autosampler needle replacement frequency
   B. Mass spectrometer source cleaning procedures
   C. Experimental methods for developing new assays
   D. Mobile phase preparation guidelines
3. **Why should PEEK tubing be cut at a perfect right angle?**
   A. To reduce solvent consumption
   B. To prevent dead volume and peak broadening
   C. To make the tubing easier to bend during installation
   D. To increase flow rate
4. **What is the primary indicator of column degradation?**
   A. Increased autosampler speed
   B. Retention time shifts or peak shape distortion
   C. Higher gas generator pressure
   D. Decrease in mobile phase pressure
5. **What is the most common cause of decreased MS sensitivity?**
   A. Contamination of the ion source or capillary electrode
   B. Use of shorter LC columns
   C. High pump pressure
   D. Using a low flow rate during LC separation
6. **How often should mass accuracy calibration is typically performed?**
   A. Daily

B. Monthly
C. Biannually or annually
D. Every 5 years

7. **What is the purpose of a diverter valve in LC-MS/MS systems?**

A. To increase sample throughput
B. To divert HPLC outflow to waste outside acquisition windows
C. To reduce solvent consumption
D. To automate column switching

8. **What is the recommended frequency for full system backups?**

A. Non needed if the instrument is running well
B. Regularly or after significant software updates
C. Only during annual maintenance
D. When storage is full

9. **Why is brand fidelity critical for assay reagents and calibrators?**

A. To reduce paperwork
B. It simplifies purchasing
C. CAP requires single-brand use
D. Minor differences between manufacturers can impact method performance

10. **How should new lots of calibrators be verified?**

A. By visual inspection
B. By checking the expiration date and assuming accuracy if within range
C. Using patient comparisons, linearity assessment, or proficiency samples
D. Skipping verification if calibrators are certified

11. **What is the primary purpose of SST samples?**

A. To replace calibrators
B. To reduce mobile phase consumption
C. To automate column cleaning
D. To verify LC-MS/MS system performance before batch analysis

12. **Which parameters are commonly monitored in SST?**

A. Retention time, peak area, signal-to-noise ratio
B. Sample volume and injector pressure
C. Laboratory temperature
D. Gas generator pressure

13. **What is a common standard used for mass spectrometer performance verification during routine system testing (RST)?**

A. Solvent blank
B. Unfiltered serum
C. Sample matrix from previous runs

D. Polypropylene glycol (PPG) or certified reference materials

Answer Key

1. D. To ensure continuous high-quality results and trouble-free instrument operation
2. C. Experimental methods for developing new assays
3. B. To prevent dead volume and peak broadening
4. B. Retention time shifts or peak shape distortion
5. A. Contamination of the ion source or capillary electrode
6. C. Biannually or annually
7. B. To divert HPLC outflow to waste outside acquisition windows
8. B. Regularly or after significant software updates
9. D. Minor differences between manufacturers can impact method performance
10. C. Using patient comparisons, linearity assessment, or proficiency samples
11. D. To verify LC-MS/MS system performance before batch analysis
12. A. Retention time, peak area, signal-to-noise ratio
13. D. Polypropylene glycol (PPG) or certified reference materials

Chapter 8: Troubleshooting for LC-MS/MS

1. **System suitability testing is primarily used to:**

   A. Adjust the mass spectrometer's tuning parameters
   B. Replace calibration curves
   C. Clean the mass spectrometer
   D. Confirm that the analytical system is performing adequately before analyzing patient or study samples

2. **If a mass spectrometer passes vendor calibration but still exhibits application-specific issues, what should be done?**

   A. Ignore the problem since vendor calibration is sufficient
   B. Assume the instrument is fully functional
   C. Clean the MS or contact the vendor
   D. Reduce the mobile phase flow rate

3. **What is the most likely cause of *no chromatographic peaks* with normal baseline noise?**

   A. Mass spectrometer hardware failure
   B. Extraction error or autosampler misinjection
   C. High mobile phase viscosity
   D. Excessive dwell time

4. **A gradual decrease in signal intensity is often caused by:**

A. Sudden mobile phase contamination
B. Dirty ion optics or column degradation
C. Incorrect autosampler wash solvent
D. High gas supply pressure

5. **High background/noise in LC-MS/MS is typically due to:**

A. Mobile phase contamination or gas supply issues
B. Insufficient vacuum pressure in the mass analyze
C. Low flow rate
D. Low column temperature

6. **Peak fronting is often caused by:**

A. Column overloading or incorrect mobile phase pH
B. Weak injection solvent strength
C. Dead volume in tubing
D. Incorrect detector settings

7. **Choppy peaks are most likely due to:**

A. Poorly cut PEEK tubing
B. Detector noise
C. Excessive mobile phase degassing
D. Suboptimal electrospray ionization or insufficient dwell time

8. **Peak splitting may result from:**

A. Detector saturation
B. Excessive mobile phase flow rate
C. High signal-to-noise ratio
D. Dead volume or incorrect elution strength of the injected solution

9. **Low pressure in an LC system may indicate:**

A. Column blockage
B. Leak or air in the system
C. High mobile phase viscosity
D. Pump malfunction causing high backpressure

10. **High pressure is most often caused by:**

A. Incorrect mobile phase
B. Low mobile phase flow rate
C. Protein buildup on the column head
D. Air bubbles in the detector

11. **Carryover in LC-MS/MS is often caused by:**

A. Low mobile phase flow rate
B. Low signal intensity
C. Autosampler wash issues or column retention

D. High dwell time

12. **A downward trend in internal standard (IS) signal across a batch indicates:**

    A. Contamination of the mass spectrometer
    B. Gradual sample degradation
    C. Mobile phase evaporation
    D. High column efficiency

13. **If a system suitability test passes but patient samples fail, the issue likely lies in:**

    A. Mass spectrometer calibration
    B. LC hardware
    C. High pump pressure
    D. Extraction or sample-specific matrix effects

14. **Improperly cut PEEK tubing can lead to:**

    A. Improved peak symmetry
    B. Reduced mobile phase viscosity
    C. Dead volume and peak tailing
    D. Lower system backpressure

Answer Key

1. D. Confirm that the analytical system is performing adequately before analyzing patient or study samples
2. C. Clean the MS or contact the vendor
3. B. Extraction error or autosampler misinjection
4. B. Dirty ion optics or column degradation
5. A. Mobile phase contamination or gas supply issues
6. A. Column overloading or incorrect mobile phase pH
7. D. Suboptimal electrospray ionization or insufficient dwell time
8. D. Dead volume or incorrect elution strength of the injected solution
9. B. Leak or air in the system
10. C. Protein buildup on the column head
11. C. Autosampler wash issues or column retention
12. A. Contamination of the mass spectrometer
13. D. Extraction or sample-specific matrix effects
14. C. Dead volume and peak tailing

Chapter 9: Data Analytics for LC-MS/MS Platform

1. **Which parameter is most commonly used to define the width of a chromatographic peak?**

A. Baseline width
B. Full Width at Half Maximum (FWHM)
C. Total peak area
D. Peak apex duration

2. **What does Savitzky-Golay (S-G) filtering accomplish in peak detection?**

A. Eliminates all baseline drift
B. Transforms time domain to frequency domain
C. Smooths data while preserving peak shape and height
D. Matches peak shapes using convolution

3. **Which method uses the second derivative of a Gaussian function for peak detection?**

A. Savitzky–Golay filter
B. Continuous wavelet transform
C. Trapezoidal rule
D. Fourier transform

4. **What is the primary advantage of weighted regression in calibration?**

A. Eliminates the need for internal standards
B. Ensures all data points are equally important
C. Reduces bias at low concentration levels
D. Corrects measurement errors in the calibration standards

5. **Why is smoothing important before derivative-based peak detection?**

A. To reduce the retention time
B. To amplify the noise
C. To stabilize baseline variation
D. To reduce noise and improve derivative calculation

6. **What metric is most useful for identifying systematic error in a calibration curve?**

A. R^2 value
B. Percent difference
C. Total ion count
D. First derivative

7. **Which rule detects large random errors in Levey–Jennings plots?**

A. 2–2 s rule
B. R-4 s rule
C. 1–3 s rule
D. 3–1 s rule

8. **What does heteroscedasticity refer to in mass spectrometry calibration?**

A. Constant variance across concentrations

B. Variance increasing with concentration
C. Lack of baseline correction
D. Use of external calibration only

9. **Why is Simpson's Rule preferred over the trapezoidal method in LC-MS quantification?**

A. It better matches the curved shapes of chromatographic peaks
B. It does not require peak boundaries
C. It eliminates the need for baseline correction
D. It uses fewer data points

10. **The $1/x^2$ weighting scheme is most appropriate when:**

A. Variance is constant
B. Signal decreases with concentration
C. Variance increases proportionally with concentration
D. Baseline noise is negligible

11. **Which XML-based format is considered the most robust for MS data exchange?**

A. mzXML
B. ANDI-MS
C. JCAMP-DX
D. mzML

12. **In Levey-Jennings plots, what does clustering of QC values within ±1 SD typically indicate?**

A. Systematic bias
B. Increased imprecision
C. Normal assay performance
D. Random outliers

13. **What does total allowable error (TEa) combine?**

A. Precision and calibration drift
B. Bias and imprecision
C. Baseline and noise
D. Resolution and accuracy

14. **Why is internal standard normalization critical in quantitative LC-MS studies?**

E. To reduce background noise
F. To replace external calibration
G. To account for variability in ionization and recovery
H. To simplify integration

Answer Key

1. B. Full width at half maximum (FWHM)
2. C. Smooths data while preserving peak shape and height
3. D. Fourier transform
4. C. Reduces bias at low concentration levels
5. D. To reduce noise and improve derivative calculation
6. B. Percent difference
7. C. 1–3 s rule
8. B. Variance increasing with concentration
9. A. It better matches the curved shapes of chromatographic peaks
10. C. Variance increases proportionally with concentration
11. D. mzML
12. C. Normal assay performance
13. B. Bias and imprecision
14. C. To account for variability in ionization and recovery

Chapter 10: Quality Assurance Programs for LC-MS/MS Platform

1. **Which of the following quality assurance (QA) metrics is primarily used to assess chromatographic separation between analyte and nearby peaks?**

   A. Peak area
   B. Peak symmetry
   C. Retention time
   D. Resolution

2. **What is the recommended minimum signal-to-noise ratio (S/N) for samples at the lower limit of quantification according to CLSI C62?**

   E. 5:1
   F. 10:1
   G. 15:1
   H. 20:1

3. **What does a peak symmetry factor significantly less than 1.0 typically indicate?**

   A. Tailing
   B. Gaussian shape
   C. Fronting
   D. Baseline noise

4. **What is one main advantage of using internal standards in LC-MS/MS?**

A. Enhance resolution
B. Normalize for ion suppression
C. Decrease run time
D. Increase signal noise

5. **What is a common cause of peak tailing?**

A. Low sample volume
B. Column overload
C. Worn stationary phase
D. Low ion ratio

6. **The SST sample should ideally contain analytes at:**

A. Only the lowest LLOQ
B. Zero concentration
C. Middle of AMR or near medical decision points
D. Twice the highest calibrator concentration

7. **Baseline chromatographic resolution is generally considered adequate when R is at least:**

A. 1.00
B. 1.25
C. 1.50
D. 2.00

8. **What does a high false alert rate in QA metrics lead to?**

A. Improved sensitivity
B. Reduced maintenance
C. Alert fatigue
D. More accurate calibrations

9. **Ion ratio failures are more common at:**

A. High analyte concentrations
B. Mid-analyte concentrations
C. Low analyte concentrations
D. Stable internal standard levels

10. **Which metric is used to detect co-eluting peaks and verify analyte identity?**

A. Signal-to-noise
B. Ion ratio
C. Peak area
D. Internal standard recovery

11. **If peak shape, ion ratio, and resolution fail but relative RT passes, the issue is likely due to:**

A. Correct peak integration

B. Poor LC/MS maintenance
C. Mis-integration
D. Interfering peak

12. **What is the best strategy to minimize false alerts during QA metric development?**

A. Use only vendor defaults
B. Employ wide acceptance ranges
C. Use a data-driven approach
D. Ignore low-level interferences

Answer Key

1. D. Resolution
2. D. 20:1
3. C. Fronting
4. B. Normalize for ion suppression
5. C. Worn stationary phase
6. C. Middle of AMR or near medical decision points
7. B. 1.25
8. C. Alert fatigue
9. C. Low analyte concentrations
10. B. Ion ratio
11. D. Interfering peak
12. C. Use a data-driven approach

Chapter 11: Regulations and LDT of LC-MS/MS Assays

1. **What is the primary purpose of CLIA '88?**

A. To regulate the manufacturing of laboratory equipment
B. To ensure quality laboratory testing for patient care
C. To replace FDA regulations
D. To eliminate the need for proficiency testing

2. **Which organization provides accreditation for clinical laboratories beyond CLIA requirements?**

A. FDA
B. College of American Pathologists (CAP)
C. CDC
D. OSHA

3. **What does ISO 15189 accreditation emphasize?**

A. Competence and quality management in medical laboratories
B. Instrument calibration only
C. Research-use-only (RUO) assays
D. FDA compliance for LDTs

4. **Under CLIA, what is the minimum frequency for proficiency testing (PT) for non-waived tests?**

A. Monthly
B. Quarterly
C. Annually
D. Biannually

5. **Which regulation requires laboratories to document personnel qualifications (e.g., technical supervisors)?**

A. CLIA '88 (42 CFR Part 493)
B. FDA 21 CFR Part 11
C. ISO 13485
D. USP <1058>

6. **Which CLIA category applies to laboratory developed tests like LC-MS/MS?**

A. Waived
B. Moderate complexity
C. High complexity
D. Exempt

7. **Which document provides guidelines for LC-MS/MS method validation in clinical labs?**

A. CLSI C62
B. FDA Food Safety Modernization Act
C. HIPAA Security Rule
D. USP <1225>

8. **What is required for a laboratory to perform LDTs under CLIA?**

A. CLIA certification and validation data
B. FDA premarket approval (PMA)
C. ISO 9001 certification
D. CAP accreditation only

9. **What is the purpose of the CAP Checklist for mass spectrometry?**

A. To assess compliance with CLIA and additional quality standards
B. To replace FDA inspections
C. To eliminate proficiency testing
D. To evaluate the efficiency of mass spectrometer detectors

10. **Which FDA phase requires premarket review for high-risk IVDs under the 2024 final rule?**
    A. Stage 1
    B. Stage 3
    C. Stage 4
    D. Stage 5
11. **What is the primary critique of FDA's 2024 LDT final rule by laboratories?**
    A. Duplicative regulation (FDA + CLIA) and high compliance costs
    B. Lack of focus on mass spectrometry
    C. Elimination of proficiency testing
    D. Overemphasis on ISO 15189
12. **Which category of LDTs is exempt from FDA's 2024 final rule?**
    A. Public health surveillance tests
    B. High-risk molecular assays
    C. Tests using RUO reagents
    D. All LDTs in CAP-accredited labs
13. **What was the outcome of the March 2025 court ruling on FDA's LDT final rule?**
    A. FDA's authority to regulate LDTs was struck down
    B. The rule was expanded to include RUO tests
    C. CLIA '88 was repealed
    D. The VALID Act was enacted

Answer Key

1. B. CLIA '88 ensures quality testing for patient care.
2. B. CAP provides accreditation beyond CLIA.
3. A. ISO 15189 emphasizes lab competence/quality management.
4. D. PT is required three times a year and minimum twice a year for non-waived tests.
5. A. CLIA '88 mandates personnel qualification documentation.
6. C. LC-MS/MS is high-complexity under CLIA.
7. A. CLSI C62 guides LC-MS/MS validation.
8. A. CLIA certification + validation are required for LDTs.
9. A. CAP Checklist ensures CLIA+/additional standards compliance.
10. C. Stage 4 requires premarket review for high-risk IVDs.
11. A. Labs critique duplicative regulation and costs.
12. A. Public health surveillance tests are exempt.
13. A. March 2025 ruling struck down FDA's LDT authority.

Index

Y. V. Zhang, U. Garg (eds.), *Practical Guide to Implementing Liquid Chromatography Mass Spectrometry in Clinical Laboratories*,
https://doi.org/10.1007/978-3-032-03852-4